Andrea Pieroni, PhD
Lisa Leimar Price, PhD
Editors

Eating and Healing
Traditional Food As Medicine

Pre-publication
REVIEWS,
COMMENTARIES,
EVALUATIONS . . .

"Eating and Healing explores the contemporary significance of the primordial recognition by humans that food and medicine represent a continuum rather than the artificial categories typically imposed in Western science. By bringing together the experiences of researchers working with traditional populations around the world, it demonstrates both the universality and the continued relevance of this relationship. In drawing on current research and methodologies at the interface between the biological and social sciences, the authors offer exciting new insights into an underexplored theme in the ethnobotanical literature and provide a timely focus of theoretical and practical importance linking human health with the conservation and use of biodiversity.

Several chapters specifically address issues tied to global change. Rural subsistence and urban populations together face health problems related to the simplification of diets and erosion of biocultural diversity. The consequences can be understood increasingly from insights into functional health benefits offered by food and dietary supplements beyond basic nutrition, including hypoglycemic, antioxidant, immunostimulant, and antibiotic activities. Understanding of traditional practices provides health-relevant information for populations adapting to rapid change in developing countries as well as for people in industrial countries. Here the multidisciplinary approaches and focus of the authors on both biological and cultural components of foods as medicines offer a valuable basis for promoting positive behaviors through food culture. That traditional systems once lost are hard to re-create underlines the imperative for the kind of documentation, compilation, and dissemination of eroding knowledge of biocultural diversity represented by this volume."

Timothy Johns, PhD
Professor of Human Nutrition,
McGill University

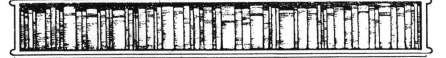

Food Products Press®
An Imprint of The Haworth Press, Inc.
New York • London • Oxford

Eating and Healing
Traditional Food As Medicine

FOOD PRODUCTS PRESS®
Crop Science
Amarjit S. Basra, PhD
Editor in Chief

The Lowland Maya Area: Three Millennia at the Human-Wildland Interface edited by A. Gómez-Pompa, M. F. Allen, S. Fedick, and J. J. Jiménez-Osornio

Biodiversity and Pest Management in Agroecosystems, Second Edition by Miguel A. Altieri and Clara I. Nicholls

Plant-Derived Antimycotics: Current Trends and Future Prospects edited by Mahendra Rai and Donatella Mares

Concise Encyclopedia of Temperate Tree Fruit edited by Tara Auxt Baugher and Suman Singha

Landscape Agroecology by Paul A. Wojtkowski

Concise Encyclopedia of Plant Pathology by P. Vidhyasekaran

Molecular Genetics and Breeding of Forest Trees edited by Sandeep Kumar and Matthias Fladung

Testing of Genetically Modified Organisms in Foods edited by Farid E. Ahmed

Fungal Disease Resistance in Plants: Biochemistry, Molecular Biology, and Genetic Engineering edited by Zamir K. Punja

Plant Functional Genomics edited by Dario Leister

Immunology in Plant Health and Its Impact on Food Safety by P. Narayanasamy

Abiotic Stresses: Plant Resistance Through Breeding and Molecular Approaches edited by M. Ashraf and P. J. C. Harris

Teaching in the Sciences: Learner-Centered Approaches edited by Catherine McLoughlin and Acram Taji

Handbook of Industrial Crops edited by V. L. Chopra and K. V. Peter

Durum Wheat Breeding: Current Approaches and Future Strategies edited by Conxita Royo, Miloudi M. Nachit, Natale Di Fonzo, José Luis Araus, Wolfgang H. Pfeiffer, and Gustavo A. Slafer

Handbook of Statistics for Teaching and Research in Plant and Crop Science by Usha Rani Palaniswamy and Kodiveri Muniyappa Palaniswamy

Handbook of Microbial Fertilizers edited by M. K. Rai

Eating and Healing: Traditional Food As Medicine edited by Andrea Pieroni and Lisa Leimar Price

Physiology of Crop Production by N. K. Fageria, V. C. Baligar, and R. B. Clark

Plant Conservation Genetics edited by Robert J. Henry

Introduction to Fruit Crops by Mark Rieger

Sourcebook for Intergenerational Therapeutic Horticulture: Bringing Elders and Children Together by Jean M. Larson and Mary Hockenberry Meyer

Agriculture Sustainability: Principles, Processes, and Prospects by Saroja Raman

Introduction to Agroecology: Principles and Practice by Paul A. Wojtkowski

Handbook of Molecular Technologies in Crop Disease Management by P. Vidhyasekaran

Handbook of Precision Agriculture: Principles and Applications edited by Ancha Srinivasan

Dictionary of Plant Tissue Culture by Alan C. Cassells and Peter B. Gahan

Handbook of Potato Production, Improvement, and Postharvest Management edited by Jai Gopal and S. M. Paul Khurana

Eating and Healing
Traditional Food As Medicine

Andrea Pieroni, PhD
Lisa Leimar Price, PhD
Editors

Food Products Press®
An Imprint of The Haworth Press, Inc.
New York • London • Oxford

For more information on this book or to order, visit
http://www.haworthpress.com/store/product.asp?sku=5254

or call 1-800-HAWORTH (800-429-6784) in the United States and Canada
or (607) 722-5857 outside the United States and Canada

or contact orders@HaworthPress.com

Published by

Food Products Press®, an imprint of The Haworth Press, Inc., 10 Alice Street, Binghamton, NY 13904-1580.

PUBLISHER'S NOTE
The development, preparation, and publication of this work has been undertaken with great care. However, the Publisher, employees, editors, and agents of The Haworth Press are not responsible for any errors contained herein or for consequences that may ensue from use of materials or information contained in this work. The Haworth Press is committed to the dissemination of ideas and information according to the highest standards of intellectual freedom and the free exchange of ideas. Statements made and opinions expressed in this publication do not necessarily reflect the views of the Publisher, Directors, management, or staff of The Haworth Press, Inc., or an endorsement by them.

This book has been published solely for educational purposes and is not intended to substitute for the medical advice of a treating physician. Medicine is an ever-changing science. As new research and clinical experience broaden our knowledge, changes in treatment may be required. While many potential treatment options are made herein, some or all of the options may not be applicable to a particular individual. Therefore, the author, editor, and publisher do not accept responsibility in the event of negative consequences incurred as a result of the information presented in this book. We do not claim that this information is necessarily accurate by the rigid scientific and regulatory standards applied for medical treatment. **No warranty, expressed or implied, is furnished with respect to the material contained in this book. The reader is urged to consult with his/her personal physician with respect to the treatment of any medical condition.**

Copyright acknowledgments can be found on page xviii.

Cover photographs courtesy of Andrea Pieroni.

Cover design by Jennifer M. Gaska.

Library of Congress Cataloging-in-Publication Data

Eating and healing : traditional food as medicine / Andrea Pieroni, Lisa Leimar Price, editors.
    p. ; cm.
   Includes bibliographical references and index.
   ISBN-13: 978-1-56022-982-7 (hc. : alk. paper)
   ISBN-10: 1-56022-982-9 (hc. : alk. paper)
   ISBN-13: 978-1-56022-983-4 (pbk. : alk. paper)
   ISBN-10: 1-56022-983-7 (pbk. : alk. paper)
   1. Medicinal plants. 2. Diet therapy. 3. Ethnobotany. 4. Traditional medicine. 5. Wild plants, Edible—Therapeutic use.
   [DNLM: 1. Diet Therapy. 2. Medicine, Traditional. 3. Plants, Edible. 4. Plants, Medicinal. WB 400 E14 2005] I. Pieroni, Andrea. II. Price, Lisa Leimar.
RS164.E26 2005
615'.321—dc22
                                                              2005009084

CONTENTS

ABOUT THE EDITORS

Andrea Pieroni, PhD, is an ethnobotanist/pharmacognosist and Lecturer in Pharmacognosy at the School of Pharmacy of the University of Bradford, United Kingdom. He is also part-time associate professor in the Department of Social Sciences at the Wageningen University in the Netherlands. Currently he is the scientific coordinator of a European Union–funded research project dealing with a circum-Mediterranean ethnobotanical study on wild and neglected plants for food and medicine. He is a member of the Board of the International Society for Ethnopharmacology and of the International Society of Ethnobiology, and has authored numerous scientific articles and books in this field. Dr. Pieroni's present research focuses on traditionally gathered wild food and medicinal plants in the Mediterranean.

Lisa Leimar Price, PhD, is an anthropologist and associate professor in the Department of Social Sciences, Wageningen University, the Netherlands. She has been a Rockefeller Fellow for Social Scientists in Agriculture, a Ford Foundation Fellow, and a Fulbright Fellow. Prior to joining Wageningen University, she was a senior scientist at the International Rice Research Institute in the Philippines. She has undertaken strategic farm level research throughout Asia and has served as a consultant on gender in research for the World Bank, the Netherlands Ministry of Foreign Affairs, and the International Rice Research Institute. She is the author of numerous publications on wild plant foods and ethnoscience. Dr. Price specializes in gender studies, agrobiodiversity, natural resource management, and ethnoscience.

CONTRIBUTORS

Jens Aagaard-Hansen has a double background as anthropologist and medical doctor. In addition to his 13 years of clinical work and specialization as a general practitioner, he has been involved with applied medical anthropology, cross-disciplinary research management, and research capacity strengthening in Africa and Asia for the past 11 years. He has wide experience in research, consultant work, and teaching.

Jeff Adelmann (The Herb Man) is a medicinal herb grower/producer operating out of Farmington, Minnesota. He has significant botanical expertise and experience in plants used by diverse cultures. He coordinates plant propagation and species documentation for the Medicinal Herb Network and is a member of the Organic Herb Producers Cooperative.

Alpina Begossi is a researcher in human ecology, fisheries ecology, and ethnobiology, and lectures in human ecology at the Graduate Group in Ecology, UNICAMP, Campinas, S. P. Brazil. She has been doing research for about 20 years on the Atlantic Forest coast and in the Brazilian Amazon.

Helen Clifton is an elder of the Gitga'at Nation of Hartley Bay, British Columbia. Her late husband, Chief Johnny Clifton (Wahmoodmx), was born at the seaweed camp at Princess Royal Island, and Helen has been harvesting seaweed there since she was a young woman, learning about the old ways of seaweed harvesting from her mother-in-law, Lucille Clifton, and other elders of previous generations. A fluent speaker of Sm'algyax (Tsimshian language), she has participated in and witnessed the changes in plant resource harvesting and processing for over five decades.

Mohamed Eddouks is a phytopharmacologist/physiologist and professor at Moulay Ismail University, Faculty of Sciences and Techniques, Errachidia. He is also the research director of UFR Physiology of the Nutrition and Endocrine Pharmacology. His research focuses on phytopharmacology and pathophysiology of diabetes mellitus and medicinal plants in Morocco.

Daimy Godínez has a degree in biological sciences from the University of Santiago de Cuba and a master's degree in plant taxonomy from the University of La Habana. She holds a research position in the Biodiversity Division of the CIMAC (Centro de Investigaciones de Medio Ambiente de Camagüey), a research center of the Cuban Academy of Sciences. She specializes in management and conservation of Cuban biodiversity and related ethnobotanical themes.

Louis E. Grivetti is a geographer trained in nutrition science. He is professor of nutrition at the University of California, Davis. He and his students have conducted research on edible wild plants in Africa (Sahel states and eastern Botswana), Asia (northern Thailand), and the Americas (Southeast Asian immigrant urban gardens).

Christopher A. Hafner has over 20 years experience as a fully licensed and accredited practitioner of Traditional Chinese Medicine. He now practices at Crocus Hill Oriental Medicine in St. Paul, Minnesota. He is adjunct faculty with the University of Minnesota, an expert herbalist wild-crafter, and leads the network initiative investigating medicinal herb quality.

Natalia Hanazaki is an ecologist and professor in the Department of Ecology and Zoology at the Universidade Federal de Santa Catarina, Brazil. She is also an associate researcher at the Centre of Environmental Studies (NEPAM) of the Universidade de Campinas, Brazil. Her research is focused on human ecology and ethnobiology, especially the use of natural resources, and ethnobotany.

Craig A. Hassel is an associate professor and extension specialist in food and nutrition in the Department of Food Science and Nutrition at the University of Minnesota, St. Paul. He received his PhD in nutritional science at the University of Arizona. His current research interests include cross-cultural understandings of food as medicine and health/nutrition.

Thomas W. Kuyper is a fungal ecologist at Wageningen University. His main interest is the role of fungi in ecosystem functioning in temperate and tropical forests and agro-ecosystems.

Ana H. Ladio is an ethnobotanist and ecologist. She is a researcher in the Ecology Department of the Universidad Nacional del Comahue,

Argentina. Her research focuses on wild edible and medicinal plant use in northwest Patagonia from an ecological perspective.

Ramón Morales is a botanist/ethnobotanist and researcher at Real Jardín Botánico de Madrid, CSIC (Spain). His research focuses on the Labiatae family and ethnobotany in Spain, especially food and medicinal plants.

Charles Ogoye-Ndegwa has a background in medical and nutritional anthropology. He previously focused on breast-feeding and childhood and pregnancy food taboos. With over ten years of progressive involvement in research, he now focuses on the social modeling of trade-offs between gender, disease, and development. He works at the Kenyan Agricultural Research Institute (KARI).

Patrick L. Owen is a PhD candidate at the School of Dietetics and Human Nutrition and the Centre for Indigenous Peoples' Nutrition and Environment at McGill University, Montreal, Canada. His research interests are ethnonutrition and ethnobotany in relation to metabolic diseases.

Manuel Pardo de Santayana is a botanist/ethnobotanist and researcher at Real Jardín Botánico de Madrid, CSIC (Spain). He researches Spanish ethnopharmacology and ethnotaxonomy and is also working on the Labiatae family in the Flora Iberica Project.

Nivaldo Peroni is an agronomist with a master's degree in genetics and doctoral degree in plant biology. He is associate researcher at the Centre of Environmental Studies (NEPAM) of the Universidade de Campinas (UNICAMP), Brazil. His research focuses on ethnobotany and plant domestication, especially the use, conservation, and amplification of genetic resources.

Cassandra L. Quave is a doctoral candidate in the Department of Biology, Center for Ethnobiology and Natural Products at Florida International University. Her research focuses on the bioactivity of medicinal plants used in traditional healing practices in the Mediterranean.

Marsha B. Quinlan is a medical anthropologist in the Department of Anthropology at Washington State University. Her research focuses on ethnomedicine, health behavior in families, and ethnobotany.

Robert J. Quinlan is a biocultural anthropologist and assistant professor in the Department of Anthropology at Ball State University in

Muncie, Indiana. His research is in the areas of human evolutionary ecology and health.

Rossano M. Ramos graduated with a degree in biological sciences from the Universidade de Campinas, Brazil, and is a graduate student in the Environmental Sciences Program at Universidade de São Paulo, Brazil. His research is focused on game and foraging strategies in the Amazon, at the Reserva Extrativista do Alto Juruá.

Elia San Miguel is an ethnobotanist and researcher at Real Jardín Botánico de Madrid, CSIC (Spain). She is researching the ethnobotany of the Asturias region of Spain.

Sabino Sanca is the president of the semiformal traditional healers' association AMETRAC (Associación de Médicos Tradicionales) from the Andean community Apillapampa, Cochabamba Department, Bolivia. He was initiated into traditional medicine more than 25 years ago and has traveled to other Latin American countries for workshops on medicinal plants.

Renne Soberg has been growing medicinal herbs organically for over ten years in Lakeville, Minnesota. He founded the Organic Herb Producers Cooperative and leads the Medicinal Herb Network initiatives on field trials and feasibility studies of medicinal herb production, as well as postharvest processing and essential oil production.

Nancy J. Turner is located at the School of Environmental Studies, University of Victoria, Victoria, British Columbia. She is a professor of ethnoecology.

Ina Vandebroek is a biologist with PhD in medical sciences. She has carried out two years of postdoctoral fieldwork in the Bolivian Andes and the Amazon to study the use of medicinal plants for community health care and knowledge variability among traditional healers. She is currently a researcher at the New York Botanical Garden.

Gabriele Volpato is an ethnobotanist and biologist who has been working in Cuba for the past four years, first as a student of the Department of Biology at the University of Padua and currently in the Department of Social Sciences at Wageningen University, the Netherlands. His research focuses on ethnobiological and ecological issues in the use of Cuban traditional food and medicinal plants.

Acknowledgments

We would like to express our deepest gratitude to our colleague Professor Anke Niehof for her encouragement and generous support during the preparation of this manuscript. We also thank Michael G. Price and Joy Burroughs for their patience in assisting in the difficult task of the scientific copy editing.

COPYRIGHT ACKNOWLEDGMENTS

Introduction

Andrea Pieroni
Lisa Leimar Price

We both have childhood memories of the way women in our lives would arrange the cuisine so that it served as both food and medicine. Pieroni recalls chestnut-meal polenta boiled in the new red wine: that was one of the most common cough remedies used by grandmothers in Pieroni's home region in the mountains of northern Tuscany during the cold winter months. Price recalls her childhood in the United States and the chicken soup served to ease the discomfort of and speed recovery from a common cold, as well as the inevitable prune juice to relieve childhood constipation.

Since the days of our childhoods, these foods have become recognized as "functional foods." However, the link to culture and tradition is barely visible in scientific undertakings. In fact, what we both learned in our respective formal educations in pharmacy and anthropology was that food and medicine were two different arenas. Only recently are we learning the importance of the food-medicine linkages.

Plants may be used both as medicine and food, and it is difficult to draw a line between these two areas: food may be medicine, and vice versa. Plant resources in traditional societies, especially wild greens, are often used multicontextually as food and medicine. The gathering or cultivation, preparation, and consumption of these species are rooted in the emic perceptions of the natural environments coupled with available resources, local cuisine and medical practices, taste appreciation, and cultural heritage (Johns, 1990, 1999; Etkin, 1994, 1996; Price, 1997; Heinrich, 1998; Pieroni, 2000; Pieroni et al., 2002).

Much is still to be discovered about the fascinating links between food and medicine among different cultures, even more than 20 years after the superb work of Nina Etkin and Paul Ross (1982) on the medicinal plant uses among the Hausa in Nigeria, where out of 235 noncultivated medicinal plants, 63 taxa were also used as food. A number of studies on the potential health benefit aspects of traditional foods show that such plants have specific pharmacological effects. For example, Timothy Johns and co-workers (Johns and Kokwaro, 1991; Uiso and Johns, 1995; Johns, Mhoro, and Sanaya, 1996; Johns, Mhoro, and Uiso, 1996; Johns et al., 1999; Owen and Johns, 2002) have demonstrated how the overlap of food and medicine are related to the ingestion of phytochemicals that can explain very diverse cultural food behaviours and health outcomes. For example, in the case of the Maasai paradox, the Maasai obtain 66 percent of calories from fat, yet they do not suffer from illnesses typical of high-fat diets found in Western cultures. This has been attributed to the high level of saphins (which bind cholesterol) in the 25 or so different plants they combine into a soup along with their high-fat foods. Although we have had few but very important contributions in the area of plant foods as medicines, much less is known about traditional consumption of animal food-medicines such as fish (Begossi, 1998).

This book explores this gray area between food and medicine and the diverse ways in which these two cosmos overlap and penetrate each other in traditional and indigenous cultures.

We have placed Louis Grivetti's contribution as the first chapter in this book. Grivetti (along with Britta Ogle) made an important and lasting early contribution to understanding traditional food and medicine through his investigations into wild-food plant gathering and consumption (for example, Ogle and Grivetti, 1985a, b, c, d). The contemporary contributions of Grivetti and his collaborators and students continue this tradition of providing exciting and challenging insights (Grivetti and Ogle, 2000; Johnson and Grivetti, 2002a, b; Ogle et al., 2003). Thus, it is a great pleasure for us that Louis Grivetti agreed to place his contribution in the introductory position of the book, starting the volume off with his reflections on 30 years of research in the field of edible wild plants as food and medicine.

The main research themes in Grivetti's group have been the cultural and nutritional aspects of the use of edible wild plants; studies of cultural diversity in geographical regions of environmental similarity (culture variable/environment constant); or studies of cultures that occupy different ecological niches (environmental variable/culture constant). Three efforts have characterized Grivetti's work: (1) procurement and dietary uses of wild plants during periods of drought or social unrest; (2) maintenance of the ability to recognize edible wild species; and (3) nutrient analysis of key species. The chapter by Grivetti summarizes this amazing work and concludes with selected topics for further investigation.

The contributions in the book look at many of the aspects descried by Grivetti, analyzing diverse case studies from around the globe through the lens of cultural, environmental, and/or biopharmacological aspects of the traditional consumption of biological resources.

The chapters that come after Grivetti's are arranged according to geographic regions of the world: two contributions for Asia, two for Europe, two for North America, two for the Caribbean, four for South America, and three for Africa. While this division represents different geographic areas, the reader will find that certain topics and themes within each chapter are common in multiple regions.

ASIA

Patrick Owen's contribution on Tibetan foods and medicines examines antioxidants in the Tibetan diet as potential mediators of high-altitude nutritional physiology. He reviews biotic and abiotic influences on high-altitude nutritional physiology. Tibetan highlanders have a low incidence of heart disease despite a diet rich in saturated fat. His work shows that an interplay of factors and protective elements are involved in the low incidence of cardiovascular disease and proposes that the highlander Tibetans have incorporated foods that contain prophylactic elements.

Lisa Price's chapter has a double function. She provides a background to wild/semidomesticated plant foods gathered in agricultural environments that provides a framework for a deeper understanding of these plants at the interface of foods and food-medicines. This framework is married to her own field research in Northeast Thailand and the role of wild plant foods in rural life. She goes on to discuss her findings on the overlap of gathered food plants with medicines and as functional foods and explores the multiple-use value of these plants in farmer's deciding to establish gathering restrictions for selected species they perceive as rare. Throughout the chapter, the roles of women in general, and in Northeast Thailand in particular, are discussed.

EUROPE

Andrea Pieroni and Cassandra Quave provide a comparative study on the consumption of wild plants among ethnic Albanians and Italians living in southern Italy. They distinguish between wild plants used in separate contexts as food or medicine, as functional foods, or as food-medicines. The research populations do not perceive functional foods to have specific medical properties, but just consider them to be "healthy," while medicinal foods (food-medicines) have clear folk medical prescriptions.

Pieroni and Quave's research on the medicinal or nutraceutical value of many of these plants has demonstrated high antioxidant activity and potential as therapeutic agents for the management and prevention of chronic diseases such as diabetes, stroke, and coronary heart disease. Their high levels of antioxidants may be especially important in the prevention and management of age-related diseases (ARDs). The authors suggest that recording and conserving traditional knowledge regarding the use of plants is of utmost importance, not only for the biocultural conservation of the communities/environments studied but also for future medical advancements in the prevention and management of chronic diseases. Given the current socioeconomic and cultural shifts in rural southern Italy, conservation and restoration of the plants and plant knowledge must be undertaken soon.

Manuel Pardo de Santayana, Elia San Miguel, and Ramón Morales analyze the digestive beverages used as medicinal food in a cattle-breeding community in northern Spain (Campoo, Cantabria). They note a tremendous erosion of traditional knowledge about wild plants and their uses. For example, they note that only 20 percent of the wild food species previously consumed are still eaten today. A few exceptions were represented by infusions. These infusions are frequently ingested for both the tasty flavor and medicinal digestive properties. One example is the homemade digestive spirits, such as *pacharán*, prepared with blackthorn fruits *(Prunus spinosa)*. Their chapter illustrates the considerable interest in southern Europe to examine changes in lifeways and habits among traditional rural societies and the potential use of traditional knowledge for the development and marketing of new "old" nutraceuticals. In order to economically diversify and revitalize rural areas such as Campoo we should look back and rediscover valuable traditional practices and knowledge, maintain active ones, and adopt strategies for exchanging information and experiences with other, similar cultures and regions.

NORTH AMERICA

For the region of North America, Nancy Turner and Helen Clifton collaborated to study the harvesting and consumption of seaweed among the Gitga'at, a Sm'algyax- (Tsimshian-) speaking people of Hartley Bay in British Columbia, Canada. Their work illustrates how the harvesting and consumption of seaweed reflects a complex, traditional ecological knowledge system that links the land and the sea, people and other life-forms, and culture to nature. Their study is about eating rather than the healing aspects of seaweed consumption, but it still provides an important contribution to this book because of the links made between nutritional, cultural, and environmental knowledge on an underresearched, traditional wild food resource. Helen Clifton, as a member of the Gita'at Nation of Hartley Bay, brings particular cultural richness to this chapter.

In the modern metropolitan U.S. context, Craig Hassel, Christopher Hafner, Renne Soberg, and Jeff Adelmann analyze how traditional Chinese medicine (TCM) practitioners use descriptive sensory analysis procedures to assess the quality of medical herbs, and how that challenge inspired a joint network of herb growers and Chinese practitioners to improve the quality of TCM drugs. They provide information about foods used as medicine in the CM tradition and the dilemmas faced by CM practitioners in the United States when the Chinese medicinal epistomology is not accounted for in the Western biomedical paradigm.

THE CARIBBEAN

In the Caribbean, Marsha and Robert Quinlan report on the "bush medicine" (home health care) practiced in Dominica (Lesser Antilles) and show how the system is based on a version of New World hot/cold humoral theory. All body tissues and fluids, especially blood and mucus, are assumed to react to heat and cold. Cold illnesses are associated with respiratory problems or are stress induced and require hot remedies, ingested as seasonings and herbal "teas," to thin secretions and to help sufferers relax. Hot illnesses have to do with increased body heat, redness, and swelling and are usually thought to stem from dirt or feces in the body. These illnesses are treated with cold foods and "teas" that often have laxative properties. Moreover, a food or herb's humoral quality is determined by how it affects illnesses and the body.

Gabriele Volpato and Daimy Godínez studied the medicinal foods of Cuban households and demonstrate how economic factors, ethnicity, and historic antecedents play a role in the dynamic strategies that people adopt to heal minor troubles by using food preparations.

SOUTH AMERICA

For South America, Alpina Begossi, Natalia Hanazaki, and Rossano Ramos offer a unique contribution on animal-derived food medicines. They examine the various fish species that are recommended in the diets of invalids, as well as the medicinal fish used among the Caiçaras of the Brazilian Atlantic forest coast and the Caboclos of the Brazilian Amazon. By using interviews based on questionnaires and direct observations during long fieldwork periods on the islands of Búzios, Gipóia, and Vitória, and in the coastal communities of Juréia and Ubatuba on the Atlantic Forest coast, they discover that fish recommended for invalids tend to have a diet based on vegetal matter, detritus, or invertebrates. They propose that the use of nonpiscivorous prey (i.e., fish that do not feed on other fish) in the diet of invalids may be associated with the reduced risk of accumulating toxins from fish from lower trophic levels compared with fish from high trophic levels.

Natalia Hanazaki, Nivaldo Peroni, and Alpina Begossi address the comparative uses of edible and healing plants of native inhabitants of the Amazon and Atlantic Forest areas of Brazil. They collected data through interviews with 433 native residents whose livelihood is based mainly on fisheries and small-scale agriculture. They found that about 20 percent of the plants mentioned in the Amazon area were used for both food and medicine, while the proportion in the Atlantic Forest area consisted of approximately half of the documented species.

In their contribution, Ina Vandebroek and Sabino Sanca analyze the use of food medicines in the Bolivian Andes. They discovered that 50 percent of the 43 species they document as overlapping as food and medicine are wild species. Eleven of these are "weeds" growing around agricultural fields. Aerial parts and fruits are used most frequently for food as well as for medicine.

Ana Ladio investigated the gathering activity of wild plant foods with medicinal use in a Mapuche Community of Northwest Patagonia in Argentina. She shows how the selection of edible and medicinal plants in the Cayulef community is influenced by botanical, ecological, and sociocultural aspects that lead to distinct patterns of species use. Cayulef people know and use a variety of wild edible plants, some of which are also utilized as medicine—representing a substantial overlap of edible and medicinal species (63 percent). These medicinal foods enlarge the opportunities to cure illness and improve the well-being of families at the same time. Moreover, wild food species with medicinal and nonmedicinal uses belong to diverse botanical families that are distinct from the botanical families of the exclusively edible species. Ladio proposes that chemotaxonomical differences between the plants utilized as food-medicine can explain the existence of a systematic and evolutionary pattern in wild plant use.

AFRICA

Charles Ogoye-Ndegwa and Jens Aagaard-Hansen's chapter explores the dietary and medicinal use of traditional herbs among the Luo of Western Kenya. They studied the cultural aspects (perceptions, attitudes, and practices) of traditional herbs with regard to dietary and medicinal use over a period of four years. They identified 72 different edible plants, most of which grow wild. Out of these 72, 65 were perceived to have medicinal value as well as being used for food. The authors emphasize how these herbs are an underutilized resource and how they could represent a precious potential for dealing with both food insecurity and the need for preventive health care in vulnerable communities.

In the context of southern Cameroon, Thomas Kuyper analyzes how different populations (Bantu, Bagyeli) differ in patterns of mushroom consumption for dietary and medicinal purposes. He shows how these differences depend on the mushroom species that occur in the various ecosystems, their phenology, and the habitats in which local populations collect and cultivate their food sources. Extensive mushroom knowledge does not automatically imply a high social valuation of mushrooms and hence a high consumption. Kuyper points out the importance of understanding social and cultural factors that affect mushroom consumption when proposing interventions such as mushroom cultivation as a source for improving food security.

Mohamed Eddouks reports on the overlap between food and medicine and ethnopharmacology in Morocco. Eddouks demonstrates how food medicines represent an integral part of the health care system in Morocco and how many pathologies have been traditionally treated using foods. He provides cultural insights as well as a list of foods used as medicine in Morocco and examines phytotherapy in different regions of the country. He also notes that women frequently use more medicinal plants than men. He concludes that phytotherapy should not be used by only the poor but be a real tool of medicine for all people.

REFERENCES

Begossi, A. (1998). Food taboos: A scientific reason? In Prendergast, H.D.V., N.L. Etkin, D.R. Harris, and P.J. Houghton (Eds.), *Plants for food and medicine*. Kew, UK: The Royal Botanical Gardens.

Etkin, N.L. (1994). The cull of the wild. In Etkin, N.L. (Ed.), *Eating on the wild side*. Tucson: University of Arizona Press.

Etkin, N.L. (1996). Medicinal cuisines: Diet and ethnopharmacology. *International Journal of Pharmacognosy* 34: 313-326.

Etkin, N.L. and P.J. Ross (1982). Food as medicine and medicine as food: An adaptive framework for the interpretation of plant utilisation among the Hausa of northern Nigeria. *Social Science and Medicine* 16: 1559-1573.

Grivetti, L.E. and B.M. Ogle (2000). Value of traditional foods in meeting macro- and micronutrients needs: The wild plant connection. *Nutrition Research Review* 13: 31-46.

Heinrich, M. (1998). Plants as antidiarrhoeals in medicine and diet. In Prendergast, H.D.V., N.L. Etkin, D.R. Harris, and P.J. Houghton (Eds.), *Plants for food and medicine*. Kew, UK: The Royal Botanical Gardens.

Johns, T. (1990). *With bitter herbs they shall eat it*. Tucson: University of Arizona Press.

Johns, T. (1999). Plant constituents and the nutrition and health of indigenous peoples. In Nazarea, V.D. (Ed.), *Ethnoecology—Situated knowledge, located lives*. Tucson: University of Arizona Press.

Johns, T. and J.O. Kokwaro (1991). Food plants of the Luo of Siaya District, Kenya. *Economic Botany* 45: 103-113.

Johns, T., R.L.A. Mahunnah, P. Sanaya, L. Chapman, and T. Ticktin (1999). Saponins and phenolic content in plant dietary additives of a traditional subsistence community, the Bateni of Ngorongoro District, Tanzania. *Journal of Ethnopharmacology* 66: 1-10.

Johns, T., E.B. Mhoro, and P. Sanaya (1996). Food plants and masticants of the Batemi of Ngorongoro District, Tanzania. *Economic Botany* 50: 115-121.

Johns, T., E.B. Mhoro, and F.C. Uiso (1996). Edible plants of Mara Region, Tanzania. *Ecology of Food and Nutrition* 35: 71-80.

Johnson, N. and L.E. Grivetti (2002a). Environmental change in Northern Thailand: Impact on wild edible plant availability. *Ecology of Food and Nutrition* 41: 373-399.

Johnson, N. and L.E. Grivetti (2002b). Gathering practices of Karen women: Questionable contribution to beta-carotene intake. *International Journal of Food Sciences and Nutrition* 53: 489-501.

Ogle, B.M. and L.E. Grivetti (1985a). Legacy of the chameleon: Edible wild plants in the kingdom of Swaziland, southern Africa. A cultural, ecological, nutritional study. Part I—Introduction, objectives, methods, Swazi culture, landscape and diet. *Ecology of Food and Nutrition* 16: 193-208.

Ogle, B.M. and L.E. Grivetti (1985b). Legacy of the chameleon: Edible wild plants in the kingdom of Swaziland, southern Africa. A cultural, ecological, nutritional study. Part II—Demographics, species, availability and dietary use, analysis by ecological zone. *Ecology of Food and Nutrition* 17: 1-30.

Ogle, B.M. and L.E. Grivetti (1985c). Legacy of the chameleon: Edible wild plants in the kingdom of Swaziland, southern Africa. A cultural, ecological, nutritional study. Part III—Cultural and ecological analysis. *Ecology of Food and Nutrition* 17: 31-40.

Ogle, B.M. and L.E. Grivetti (1985d). Legacy of the chameleon: Edible wild plants in the kingdom of Swaziland, southern Africa. A cultural, ecological, nutritional study. Part IV—Nutritional values and conclusions. *Ecology of Food and Nutrition* 17: 41-64.

Ogle, B.M., H.T. Tuyet, H.N. Duyet, and N.N.X. Dung (2003). Food, feed or medicine: The multiple functions of edible wild plants in Vietnam. *Economic Botany* 57: 103-117.

Owen, P.L. and T. Johns (2002). Antioxidant in medicines and spices as cardioprotective agents in Tibetan highlanders. *Pharmaceutical Biology* 40: 346-357.

Pieroni, A. (2000). Medicinal plants and food medicines in the folk traditions of the upper Lucca Province, Italy. *Journal of Ethnopharmacology* 70: 235-273.

Pieroni, A., S. Nebel, C. Quave, H. Münz, and M. Heinrich (2002). Ethnopharmacology of *liakra:* Traditional weedy vegetables of the Arbëreshë of the Vulture area in southern Italy. *Journal of Ethnopharmacology* 81: 165-185.

Price, L. (1997). Wild plant food in agricultural environments: A study of occurrence, management, and gathering rights in Northeast Thailand. *Human Organization* 56: 209-221.

Uiso, F. and T. Johns (1995). Risk assessment of the consumption of a pyrrolizidine alkaloid containing indigenous vegetable *Crotalaria brevidens* (Mitoo). *Ecology of Food and Nutrition* 35: 111-119.

Chapter 1

Edible Wild Plants As Food and As Medicine: Reflections on Thirty Years of Fieldwork

Louis E. Grivetti

INTRODUCTION

Ethnobotanical themes have characterized the efforts of my research group for nearly three decades. The first portion of this chapter reviews the genesis that led to my professional interest in ethnobotany, includes an overview of my initial research conducted nearly three decades ago in the eastern Kalahari Desert of southern Africa, and presents unpublished fieldwork data related to the theme of the present volume. The second portion of this chapter summarizes the research of our team since 1976. The concluding section of this chapter identifies promising research themes.

GENESIS

I am not a trained botanist: I took no formal botanical course work during my undergraduate or graduate training. In fact, I expressed little interest in the plant kingdom until the middle years of my life. That ethnobotany has been one of the major themes in my geographical and nutritional research during the past three decades, therefore, needs a brief explanation. As an undergraduate and graduate student at the University of California, Berkeley (1956-1962), I majored in paleontology with complementary interests in anthropology, geology, and zoology. Ethnobotany was an acquired interest, initially peripheral, but it then became central to my doctoral training in geography at the University of California, Davis (1970-1976).

My dissertation supervisor was Professor Frederick Simoons. He guided me in cultural food practices and encouraged me to explore the nutritional consequences of food-related behavior. Simoons was a geographer, and through his training I was exposed to the general theories of plant and animal domestication, especially the works of Edgar Anderson and Carl Sauer. I was intrigued by Anderson's nonconformist view that the rationale for plant domestication was not food, but aesthetics, beauty, and color. I also admired Anderson's creative idea of "the garbage dump," whereby ancient hunter-gatherers ultimately came to recognize the potential value of having supplies of plant foods adjacent to human encampments (Anderson, 1952). As a graduate student I listened intently when Carl Sauer lectured and related his thesis that maize had been exchanged across the Pacific and/or Atlantic Oceans well before 1492 (Sauer, 1969). I also was intrigued with Sauer's view that "sophisticated fisher-folks" living at midelevations in mountainous terrain adjacent to lakes may have been the first humans to domesticate plants and that future excavations at highland regions within the tropics would confirm his thesis (Sauer, 1952).

I selected a dissertation problem in the Republic of Botswana: Why had the Tswana peoples of the eastern Kalahari thrived during eight years of drought between 1965-1973, when a drought of similar intensity and timing in the West African Sahel had caused the untimely deaths of more than 2 million people? The enigma was obvious: two similar agro-economic systems in similar environmental niches—but the Kalahari cultures thrived while the Sahel cultures experienced social disruption and death.

In order to secure funding for my fieldwork, I was employed as the Administrative Officer for the Meharry/Botswana Maternal and Child Health Project and seconded to the Botswana Ministry of Health. My wife and I arrived in Gaborone, the national capital, in April 1973. My dissertation topic was submitted to and reviewed by the Botswana Office of the President, and I was approved to work among the baTlokwa ba Moshaweng, a Tswana society whose tribal capital, Tlokweng, lay a short distance east of Gaborone. My project-related responsibilities kept me at the Ministry during the day, where I backstopped a team of professionals and public health educators who provided nursing in-service training. During evenings and on weekends and holidays I worked at Tlokweng and the bushlands adjacent to the baTlokwa settlement and collected data for my dissertation.

I had prepared extensively for fieldwork prior to arrival in Botswana and had summarized the cultural monographs and geographical works on the pre- and postcolonial era in southern Africa; I had read and outlined scores of historical works and articles that described the movements, settlement, and cultural organization of Tswana peoples in the eastern Kalahari. Especially enlightening were eighteenth- and nineteenth-century accounts by explorers, missionaries, and traders that described the food base of Tswana societies, one characterized by hunting, gathering, agriculture, horticulture, animal husbandry, as well as barter and cash exchanges. These documents mentioned the role of edible wild plants as components of the Tswana diet, but I was unprepared to find that such "lesser foods"—often deprecated by nineteenth-century authors and twentieth-century agricultural developers—were critical to Tswana survival in their eastern Kalahari thirst-land.

I was welcomed by baTlokwa elders and introduced to tribal members, and I hired field assistants and held focus-group interviews with elderly women and men. Villagers at Tlokweng had not suffered during the recent eight-year drought (1965-1973) that preceded my arrival. I looked for evidence of malnutrition but saw none: no evidence of kwashiorkor, marasmus, avitaminosis, or mineral defiencies. Primary medical problems included alcoholism, upper respiratory diseases, and tuberculosis. Why had the baTlokwa survived eight years of drought when so many hundreds of thousands of their cultural counterparts had died in the environmentally similar Sahel of western Africa? What had sustained the baTlokwa, nutritionally, during the difficult drought years when their livestock died and their field and garden crops had withered?

One key to baTlokwa nutritional success was their sustained ability to identify and use edible wild plants during years of good rainfall or drought. Tribal elders provided me with the names of more than 200 edible wild plants and identified an additional 100-plus species used in nonfood contexts (i.e., household and stockade construction, decoration, dye, fiber, magic, medicine, thatch, toys and leisure pursuits, and even as props to teach moral lessons). I learned that many species were critical components of diet after domesticated cultivars had vanished. It was obvious early in my fieldwork that elderly baTlokwa held the key to plant identifications and uses in this arid thirst-land, whereas younger children, especially teenagers, did not recognize the broad spectrum of edible plants available within tribal territory. This dichotomy presented another enigma: if the information on how to recognize and use edible wild plants was not being passed to future generations of baTlokwa youth, there would come a time when a drought of severe magnitude would hammer the people and many would starve in the midst of food plenty.

The timing was fortuitous. I arrived in the eastern Kalahari when knowledge of the environment and edible wild species was still maintained by village elders and could be passed to younger generations. The baTlokwa children and young adults I interviewed expressed little interest in plant lore and were eager to adopt "Western" cultural icons of behavior, dress, and fast-food. Further, their school training ignored traditional cultural practices that had sustained health and nutrition during drought years. Most evenings and weekends elderly men and women greeted me with conversations that began something like this: "Welcome to Tlokweng, I have so much to tell you about the plants. My grandchildren do not care. They do not know the most basic ones. Please write this down."

I immersed myself in collecting cultural, historical, and botanical data and probed for information and insights from baTlokwa elders. Two elderly men recommended by the tribal council were assigned to teach me the "local botany." By this time I had trained myself how to key and identify species and had access to the most important published Kalahari floras. The first working day out in the bush my teachers identified seven local species of *Acacia (A. eurubescens, A. fleckii, A. grandicornuta, A. karroo, A. mellifera, A. robusta,* and *A. tortilis).* I dutifully recorded their comments in my field notebook; recorded the local seTswana names; and referenced the distinctive barks, spine and leaf configurations, canopy development (or lack thereof) and pod/seed shapes. The second day when we resumed our work my teachers quizzed me. To my amazement they told me I had failed! I presumed that my teachers were just pulling my leg, but they were serious and informed me: "You are a very slow learner. Even the youngest of our children would not make such mistakes. You should know better."

But I *had* keyed the species correctly: I *had* matched the seTswana terms provided by my teachers with the correct Latin names. In the days and weeks that passed, my teachers regularly shook their heads in amused frustration as they attempted to teach me the eastern Kalahari flora. On such walks they taught me other things as well: how to make fire (with both drill and flint/steel methods); how to identify wild animal spoor; how not to get lost; how to identify medicinal plants; and terms for plant assemblages that otherwise would have escaped me.

During this "initiation" period I prepared a master list of seTswana names of wild plants, wrote down their culinary, medicinal, or other uses, and prepared my first botanical checklist. There came a time when I administered the expanded checklist to a stratified sample of 200 baTlokwa households to seek information on which species, if any, had been consumed during the recent drought. After three or four interviews I determined that something was wrong. But what? Ultimately, the realization came that I had made a classical error: traditional baTlokwa plant taxonomy bore no relationship to classical Linnaean genus/species designations. Each woody species could be called by one of four distinct names, depending on whether or not the representative specimen was "tall" versus "short" or "in fruiting season" versus "out of fruiting season." In some instances these differences were relatively minor, as with *mosu* (*Acacia tortilis:* mature form) and *mosuane* (*Acacia tortilis:* immature form). In other instances, however, differences were profound, as with *mothatha* (*Pappea capensis:* not in fruiting season) and *mopennengwe* (*Pappea capensis:* mature tree with fruit). This revelation required me to winnow my floral checklist and was my first introduction to folk taxonomies.

For more than 100 years the baTlokwa of the eastern Kalahari Desert of Botswana had not experienced famine or social disruption during drought. Nutritional success in this land was due to a balance between environmental offerings and cultural decisions. The eastern Kalahari offered a great diversity of edible wild plants and the baTlokwa regularly utilized these available resources. The primary message that emerged after two years of fieldwork was drought did *not* cause famine, and one explanation for the Sahel disaster was cultural inability to recognize and use available wild food resources—foods that once were sustaining during drought. I argued in my dissertation and in subsequent publications that "semi-arid environments continue to offer potential opportunities to societies able to recognize and utilize them" and urged further work on the so-called "lesser plants of agriculture," or what members of my research team ultimately would call the "edible weeds of agriculture" (Grivetti, 1976 and 1979).

Magic, Medicine, and Morality

The baTlokwa attached magical considerations to several local Kalahari plants. Perhaps the most interesting was *ntige* (collected; identity uncertain). This low shrub with tiny, paired leaves and sturdy crown root was associated ecologically with stands of *mogonono (Terminalia sericea)* and was present only in the eastern portion of the study area near the border with South Africa. Slices of *ntige* root produced an unusual sensation when chewed for the first time; the tongue became numb. Thereafter, the sensation was not repeated (confirmed by personal test). *Ntige* had a pleasing, sweet, cinnamon-like flavor but produced no other physiological effect. The baTlokwa elders stated that chewing several pieces of *ntige* at once was wasteful, since there was no accumulative effect as with alcoholic beverages. In past times, baTlokwa warriors chewed *ntige* before battle in the belief that they would become invincible and a rapid decisive victory would be assured. Elders also reported that if a snip of *ntige* root was worn on the body, that person would be protected against false representation and, if accused wrongly of assault, robbery, or other offense, a small piece of *ntige* root placed in one's pocket or shoe would assure acquittal (Grivetti, 1976).

Another Kalahari species combined magical and medical properties. If a menstruating woman purposefully or accidentally visited a woman recently delivered, the new mother was considered unclean and polluted *(go gata)*. A repurification ceremony then was conducted: the leaves of *thola e tona (Solanum incanum)* were ground and mixed with sorghum porridge and milk. After eating this mixture, the new mother was considered ritually clean (Grivetti, 1976).

Roots of *mosokalatsebeng (Sansevieria aethiopica)* were cooked, ground, and prepared as a paste. A quantity of paste was given to young children to stimulate appetite *(go pallwa ke dijo)*. *Mogwong-wolo* roots (identity uncertain; not collected) were ground and added to boiling water. The fluid was blended with porridge and eaten by patients to relieve diarrhea, stomach cramps, or other common intestinal problems *(mala a iteirisa)*. *Mmaketiketi* roots (identity uncertain; not collected) were gathered and sections cut from the fleshy portions. After cleaning, these roots were chewed, a well-masticated piece spit into the hand, and the mass sniffed to relieve headache *(tlhogo e a opa)*. *Kgomo ya buru* roots *(Bulbine tortilifolia)* were ground and boiled, whereupon the resulting fluid was drunk by elderly men to relieve kidney pain *(tlhogo jwa diphilo)*. Barks stripped from the east side of *moomane* trees *(Maeura schinzii)* were ground, boiled, and infusions drunk by women who suffered prolonged labor *(go tlhoka go balaga)*. The barks were said to relieve pain and relax muscles, to facilitate rapid and easy delivery. *Mosunyana* leaves *(Acacia tortilis:* immature form) were boiled and the liquid drunk to settle the stomach and severe vomiting. *Kgopane* leaves *(Aloe zebrine)* were dried, ground on a stone mortar, and the powder mixed with water and drunk to alleviate *sehuba,* or cough (Grivetti, 1976).

Considerations of magic required that timber cut for household and stockade construction or for thatching needs had to be stored off of the ground on special drying racks. Such trees and grasses identified included *Acacia robusta, A. eurbescens, A. mellifera, Combretum imberbe, Comniphora* spp., *Dichrostachys cinera, Spirostachys africana,* and *Terminalia sericea,* as well as *Cymbopogon plurinoidis, Eragraosis pallens, Heteropogon contortus,* and *Panicum maximum.* The baTlokwa held that if timber and thatch grasses remained on the ground, unseasonable hail and crop destruction would result. Further, should stored thatch be insufficient for construction needs, additional grass could be cut, but only with a hoe, never a metal sickle, otherwise hailstorms would result. This focus on regulation of hailstorms also influenced decisions not to cut certain bushes or trees during the agricultural season lest hailstorms result. Such plants included *Burkea africana, Peltophorum africanum, Sclerocarya caffra, Terminalia sericea, Vangueria* spp., and *Ziziphus mucronata.* Other plants, specifically *Vangueria* spp. and *Ximenia* spp., were not burned during the planting season lest the decision also cause hailstorms (Grivetti, 1981b).

Stout branches cut from Kalahari bushes or trees served as threshing sticks *(meotlwana).* The most suitable branches were from *Acacia caffra, Croton gratissimus,* and *Ziziphus mucronata.* Branches from *Croton gratissimus* were especially sought because of a magical association between the tree name, *moologa,* and the verb *go loga* (to increase). Respondents stated that if grain was threshed using sticks from *moologa,* the quantity of grain that resulted would be greater than if threshing sticks from other species were used. To protect the family's harvested grain from theft, the baTlokwa collected six roots of *Uriginea sanguinea* and used them to make a protective design on the threshing floor before the first surface coat of mud was applied to the threshing floor. Four roots were planted at each corner of the rectangular threshing area, and the fifth planted in the center. After the mud coat had dried, the sixth root was smeared over the completed floor, completing the design of an "X" that connected the four corners through the centrally planted root (Grivetti, 1981b).

Resin from *moretlwa (Grewia flava)* was used by the baTlokwa to teach a moral lesson. Appearance of this resin was said to be a rare event and once located it was to be handled with great care because if dropped it became difficult to find because of its high clarity index. A young child was given a piece of *moretlwa* resin as a gift and instructed to hold the present tightly and not to drop or set it down (instructions, of course, that never could be followed). The resin always was lost and the child taught the lesson that something valuable should be protected, otherwise, it would disappear and never return (Grivetti, 1976).

Famine Foods

A number of species were consumed by the baTlokwa during drought, plants that ordinarily would not be eaten. Such foods, commonly called "famine foods" in the ethnobotanical literature, are items having potential dietary use, but not regularly eaten during normal rainfall years. Famine foods used by the baTlokwa included fruits and seeds of *magabala (Cucumis metuliferous);* fruits and seeds of *mokapana (Cucumis myriocarpus);* leaves of *moologa (Croton gratissimus);* and roots of *motlopi (Boscia albitrunca).* Leaves of *moologa* commonly served as agricultural charms to protect crops, but during drought they were cooked and served as an onion substitute. Roots of *motlopi* were ground and prepared as a porridge substitute when sorghum crops failed. Under conditions of normal rainfall, *magabala* and *mokapana* generally were cattle or goat fodder and eaten by humans only as drought intensified (Grivetti, 1976).

THREE DECADES OF ETHNOBOTANICAL RESEARCH

Upon completion of my dissertation in 1976, I joined the Departments of Geography and Nutrition at the University of California, Davis. My Kalahari work ultimately came to the attention of USAID, and I was invited to lecture at in-service training programs. My presentations focused on two topics: the importance of edible wild plants in maintaining sound nutrition during drought and periods of social unrest, and the paradox of agricultural development, whereby heavy reliance upon herbicides, paradoxically, reduced food security in many regions of the globe because the "edible weeds of agriculture" were being eliminated.

After these presentations my research team was awarded a USAID contract to prepare three position papers summarizing current knowledge about edible plants and their roles in traditional societies in Africa, Central and South America, and South and East Asia and the Pacific Basin. The purpose of these reports was to provide information to decision makers at embassy/consulate levels regarding the potential role of edible wild plants in local food traditions. We identified the relative dietary-nutritional importance of selected species and examined the research potential for such species within the context of agricultural development. The basic questions posed and answered included the following:

1. Are edible wild species central or peripheral to maintaining dietary quality?
2. Is their use seasonal, or are species utilized throughout the agricultural/calendar year?
3. Do wild species complement or duplicate energy and nutrients obtained from domesticated field crops? and
4. What role do wild species play in maintaining nutritional quality of diet during drought and periods of social unrest?

Our team used the term *edible weeds of agriculture* and cautioned that agricultural development should not be at the expense of these species, many of which critical if the quality of local diets was to be maintained (Grivetti, 1980a, b, 1981a).

We expanded our work and next focused on Africa. Evidence suggested that dietary use of edible wild plants remained an integral component of the diets of many sub-Saharan societies. All traditional societies surveyed used edible wild species throughout the calendar year, and many species were especially important during the periods just before harvest, the "hungry months." Our findings emphasized the need for caution when planners and economists embarked upon agricultural development, since expansion of agricultural fields into bush lands merely to produce more acres/hectares of domesticated cultivars—at the expense of edible wild plant habitats—was a short-sighted policy. We did not know whether or not edible wild species duplicated or complemented nutrients provided by domesticated species, since so few had been analyzed for nutrient content. However, we documented the important role of edible wild plants used to maintain the dietary status of individuals, families, and social groups during periods of drought and social unrest, and the importance of "famine foods" that individuals/families consumed during periods of drought or civil disturbances. Although thousands of accounts had been published in Africa and elsewhere, publications that identified edible wild plants in a global context, we reported that no region of the world had been investigated systematically. In essence, thousands of wild species continued to be used by traditional peoples in Africa, the Americas, Asia and the Pacific region, and even rural Europe, and we noted that most had not been analyzed for their nutritional content (Grivetti et al., 1987).

Work by my student Lawrence Pauling in the Cayagan Valley of northern Luzon in the Philippines confirmed that local farmers utilized a broad range of wild plants growing in their rice paddies—species that served as fodder for livestock and for human consumption. In order to achieve higher rice yields, extension specialists recommended use of herbicides to eliminate these so-called "weeds of agriculture." Pauling reported that many of these so-called weeds served critical, dual purposes: food for humans and fodder for livestock. He identified 31 useful species growing in rice paddies: local farmers ate 14 while 5 were important medicinal plants. Further, 19 of these species served as fodder resources for water buffalo, horses, and pigs. Pauling recommended that herbicides not be employed until a better understanding of the cultural ecology and food production system of the Cayagan Valley had been achieved (Pauling and Grivetti, 1984).

Linda Gilliland and I met with representatives of the Kashaya Pomo Nation of north-central California. The Kashaya Pomo were concerned that elderly members of the tribe had been denied the right to eat traditional foods while hospitalized, since registered dietitians and physicians were uncertain of the energy and nutritional content of such foods. When the elders refused to eat standard hospital food—thought too bland by the patients—the term *hospital anorexia* was coined. The Kashaya Pomo requested that we conduct proximate and mineral analyses of a suite of traditional plant and animal foods. We compared nutrient values of traditional foods against representative commercial items: fresh and cooked acorn preparations from *Quercus agrifolia, Q. douglassii, Q. dumosa,* and *Q. wislizenii* were compared to enriched white bread; seeds and nuts from *Avena fatua, Juglans hindsii, Salvia columbariae,* and *S. leucophylla* were evaluated against sunflower kernels; berries and fruits from *Hereromeles arbutifolia, Rubus procerus,* and *Sambucus mexicana* were compared to raw apple; leafy vegetables from *Brassica campestris, Chlorogalum pomeridianum,* and *Claytonia perfoliata* were evaluated against uncooked spinach; stalks and stems of *Typha angustifolia* against fresh, uncooked asparagus stalks; and bulbs and corms of *Brodiaea laxa, B. pulchella, C. hlorogalum pomeridianyum* against white potatoes (Gilliland, 1985).

The acorn data from our study were enlightening. During the second decade of the twentieth century, C. Hart Merriam reported the first nutrient values for California acorns, and his paper (Merriam, 1918) had been regularly cited to support the contention that acorns were excellent sources of protein. Our analysis of fresh acorns provided by the Kashaya Pomo revealed protein content to be low and variable, between 6.7 and 2.4 percent protein per 100 g edible portion. Acorns that Merriam had analyzed had been stored for ten years and were extremely dry; fresh acorns we analyzed were approximately 46 percent water (hence the lower protein values). Ground, dried acorn powder consumed by the Kashaya Pomo contained a mean of 5.6 percent protein by weight; leached acorns had even lower values at 2.1 percent; and traditional acorn bread was similar at 2.2 percent protein. Traditional seed foods used by the Kashaya Pomo, however, were good sources of protein and energy, and they exhibited higher mineral values than commercial sunflower seeds. Traditional fruits were low in sodium, with elevated values of calcium, iron, magnesium, and potassium when compared to raw apple. Leaves of *Claytonia perfoliata* and various bulbs also exhibited high values for calcium and iron. Overall, we recommended that these traditional foods could be used in hospital dietetic exchange lists (Gilliland, 1985).

Two Research Paridigms

As a cultural geographer trained in nutrition science, I have trained my students to take a cultural-ecological approach when investigating cultural patterns of food and diet. Environments offer opportunities to social groups and our research objective has been to dissect and separate environmental from cultural determinants of diet. In conducting such work, two research paradigms have been used through the years. The first is to investigate how different cultures interact within the same environmental setting. One characteristic approach, therefore, has been to study two to four cultures that occupy a flat-plain landscape where soils and vegetation, climate and weather, and geological structure and relief are variables that present specific problems for the different cultures to solve (environment constant : culture variable). The alternative approach has been to study a single culture within a highly diversified landscape of mountains, valleys, and lowlands to investigate how this culture adapts or modifies their food procurement practices up and down slope (culture constant : environment variable).

Research of the first type was represented by my early experiences in the Republic of Botswana, where I investigated baTlokwa and other Tswana societies and how they hunted-gathered, produced, and distributed food in the flatlands of the eastern Kalahari Desert. The flatland, cultural variable approach taken in Botswana revealed how the majority baTlokwa and minority communities secured adequate, nutritious food resources even during the peak of drought. These different Tswana societies maintained sound food-related practices and were able to utilize a vast array of edible wild plants and animals during drought, when food sources from domesticated cultivars and livestock declined or were lost. In this geographical setting the environment presented similar "offerings" to members of these Tswana societies, and the Kalahari thirst-land might even be called an edible wild plant "supermarket" with a wide diversity of species available during both rainy and dry seasons (Grivetti, 1976, 1978, 1979).

Britta Ogle used the second approach, where culture was the constant and environment the variable, in the kingdom of Swaziland. It was logical that Ogle return to Swaziland for her field investigation, since she had lived there several years previously, spoke rudimentary setSwasi, and already had established a friendship network of home economists and extension specialists to draw upon for fieldwork assistance. She identified the different arrays of edible wild plants in each primary niche (high-veld; middle-veld; low-veld; lubombo). Ogle's data were enlightening: nearly 40 percent of respondents indicated that wild plants contributed more to their annual diet than domesticated cultivars. Many species were utilized locally and were unfamiliar to Swazi living in different niches. She also documented that more than 40 percent of respondents cultivated edible wild plants in household gardens. One unusual finding was that local school children exhibited more extensive knowledge of edible wild species than many elders (the opposite of my Kalahari data), explained, in part, because of the geographical location of schools at boundary lines between two distinctive ecological niches. Given such school settings, children collected different arrays of plants as they walked to and from school—going up and down slope—and experienced a greater exposure to edible wild species than their parents or grandparents, who lived exclusively within a specific niche. Ogle recommended that schools continue to be constructed at these critical ecological boundaries to maintain this important knowledge (Ogle and Grivetti, 1985a, b, c, d).

Research Opportunities and Minimal Budgets

Two factors have characterized our ethnobotanical research themes: previous experience overseas (opportunism) and low cost. Students in my research group have been regularly invited to return to Africa for investigations on edible wild plants because of previous affiliations with the American Peace Corps or with nongovernmental or private volunteer organizations (NGOs and PVOs). We have funded our ethnobotanical studies primarily on minigrants in the range of $4,000 to $8,000 per student for a research period between three and six months.

Carol Humphry wanted to study edible wild plants, and she returned to Niger where previously she had served as a Peace Corps volunteer. Humphry compared plant use in two Hausa villages located in different ecological niches and collected data on foraging strategies. She identified 84 common edible wild plants, and nearly 50 percent of these were regularly consumed by the majority of Hausa interviewed. Half of the villagers could identify more than 60 wild species, while 10 percent of respondents reported other edible plants had disappeared as a result of recent droughts (Humphry et al., 1993).

The so-called "edible weeds of agriculture" played prominent roles in Hausa agricultural and dietary traditions. Humphry reported that nearly all villagers (93 percent) protected such plants and did not remove them by hoeing. She reported that drought always had been a companion of the Hausa, and that villagers had grown more and more dependent upon the cultivation of non-drought-adapted domesticated cultivars—activities that placed the villagers at risk. Humphry also noted that only 10 percent of those interviewed recognized or consumed "famine foods," identified as leaves of *Balanites aegyptia, Boscia salicifolia, Cassia occidentalis, Commiphora africana, Ficus thonningii, Gynandropsis gynandra, Hibiscus canabinus, Jacquemontia tamnifolia, Maerua angolensis* and *M. crassifolia, Melochia corchonifolia, Tribulus terrestris,* and *Sclerocarya birrea;* seeds of *Cenchrus biflorus;* and fruits of *Lagenaria siceraria* and *Parkia biglobosa* (Humphry et al., 1993).

Garrett Smith, a former Peace Corps volunteer with previous experience in West Africa, conducted his edible wild plant fieldwork in Burkina Faso, exploring dietary use of selected species during drought and nutritional roles of species in regard to potential vitamin-A blindness. He reported that 36 percent of the vegetables consumed in villages were edible wild plants, and such species accounted for approximately 20 percent of all regional dietary products. The most commonly consumed wild species included: *Adansonia digitata, Sclerocarya birrea,* and *Tamarandus indica.* Smith noted that wild plants were gathered primarily by women and girls (81 percent) who collected for family use, whereas men and boys gathered mainly for personal consumption. Gathering required considerable energy expenditure since primary collection sites were eight to ten kilometers distant. He reported that knowledge and use of traditional famine foods had declined in recent years because government and international relief agencies had supplied food to drought-affected areas. This decline in knowledge—partially caused by governmental and international "good deeds"—was viewed by Smith as ominous, since food relief ultimately could result in cultural inability to identify life-sustaining foods growing near villages. He reported that many species were outstanding dietary sources of the trace minerals copper, iron, manganese, magnesium, and zinc and reasonable sources for beta-carotene (Smith et al., 1995, 1996).

Cassius Lockett conducted his fieldwork on edible wild plants in eastern Nigeria and worked among rural Fulani at two settlements. Lockett examined dietary patterns of children under five, pregnant and lactating women, and the elderly; identified food procurement strategies for edible wild plants; and determined whether or not these strategies changed during periods of drought compared to times of normal rainfall. Focus-group discussions among Fulani elderly revealed the names of 36 species gathered during the dry season; among these were fruits, leaves, and seeds of *Adansonia digitata* and *Balanites aegyptiaca;* fruits and seeds of *Dererium microcarpum* and *Tamarindus indica;* and fruits of *Ziziphus mauritiana.* Important species available and eaten during the wet season included *Aden microcephala, Lannea schiniperi,* and *Ximenia americana* (Lockett and Grivetti, 2000; Lockett et al., 2000).

Lockett reported that many local species were not eaten universally by Fulani but were associated by age, gender, or physiological status. Wild foods considered beneficial to neonates and infants included bark of *Adansonia digitata* (in the belief that consumption enabled infants to gain weight); fruits of *Ficus sycomorus* and roots of *Cissus cornifolia* (eaten to alleviate stomach ache); fruits of *Bridelia ferruginea* (to treat diarrhea); and leaves of *Veronia colorate* (to protect the stomach of infants and reduce the incidence of vomiting and diarrhea). A minority of respondents stated that fruits of *Bridelia ferruginea* were used to treat children with malaria, while fruits of *Dererium microcarpum* were consumed especially by children during drought to alleviate hunger (Lockett and Grivetti, 2000).

Wild plants commonly associated with pregnancy and lactation included *Annona senegalensis, Balanites aegyptiaca, Bridelia ferru-

ginea, Dererium microcarpum, Gardenia aqualla, Grewia mollis, Lannea schiniperi, Parkia biglobosa, Prosopos africana, Tamarindus indica, and *Ximenia americana.* Fulani women ate fruits of *Ficus thonningii* during the last weeks of pregnancy to reduce labor time and to ease pain. No edible wild plants were identified as harmful to pregnant women, although bitter foods in general, as well as mango, potato, and commercial granulated sugar, were avoided in the belief that consumption caused spontaneous abortion, stillbirth, or fetal abnormalities. During postpartum, several preparations of edible wild plants were consumed in the belief that breast-milk production would be increased; among these were porridge mixed with fruits of *Tamarindus indica* or *Ximenia americana.* Further, leaves of *Veronia colorate* were pounded and the extracted fluid drunk to increase breast-milk production. A minority of Hausa respondents stated that *Pseudoedrela kotshyi* commonly was eaten by elderly men in order to maintain vigor and strength (Lockett and Grivetti, 2000).

Lockett also noted many edible wild plants used by the Hausa served both as food and as medicine, and many health practitioners regularly used wild plants in their pharmacopia. Bark of *Adansonia digitata* was ground and given to Hausa children to make them gain weight, leaves of *Veronia colorate* were eaten to expel intestinal parasites, and seeds of *Parkia biglobosa* were eaten to alleviate headache (Lockett et al., 2000).

At the request of the editors of *Nutrition Research Reviews,* Britta Ogle and I prepared a review on the value of traditional foods in meeting macro- and micronutrient needs. We reviewed the basic themes and problems associated with wild plant research: historical studies; salvage ethnobotany and famine foods; the hidden harvest or "edible weeds of agriculture"; problems of incomplete nutrient databases; difficulties when scholars and professionals in different fields fail to communicate; and problems of inconsistent project design, diversified methods, and variables in laboratory analysis of micronutrients (Grivetti and Ogle, 2000).

We called for further studies on how, when, and why edible wild plants were used to feed infants and young children or adult women during pregnancy and lactation. We argued that edible wild plants were part of global agricultural systems, and that "agricultural development should not be at the expense of nutritional quality of human diet where edible wild species play critical roles." We also echoed the perceptive comments of Joyce Doughty, issued more than 25 years earlier, that "nutritional quality of diet may decline with agricultural development unless edible wild species that provide essential micronutrients to the diet are considered part of the total food system" (Doughty, 1979a, b). We lamented the fact that many agricultural specialists and planners stressed production of domesticated field crops and commonly ignored or dismissed the so-called lesser species. We presented information that many individuals—and some societies— starve in the midst of food plenty because they have lost the ability to identify and utilize the edible wild plant base available in the surrounding bushlands, and that it would be "tragic if in the rush to become modern, humans lost the ability to identify and use species available to them" (Grivetti and Ogle, 2000).

Noelle Johnson previously served in the Peace Corps in West Africa. During her work in Burkina Faso, Johnson prepared a training manual on how to identify edible wild plants: an educational module that stressed the importance of such species in maintaining the quality of traditional diets (personal communication). She elected to implement her edible wild plant study in a different geographical region of the world and chose to work among Karen women in northern Thailand. Johnson's objectives were to identify the most important edible wild species; determine seasonality, food preparation techniques, and dietary uses by age and gender; and to identify why certain wild species were removed from bushlands and incorporated into Karen home gardens. She identified nearly 50 important edible wild species regularly used as part of Karen traditional diet and reported that 31 had declined significantly during the past ten years and an additional seven local species already had disappeared. The majority of women interviewed (69 percent) reported they cultivated edible wild species in household gardens; 17 of these plants were observed and collected. When Johnson asked why certain wild species were cultivated and not others, the women replied that they already had experimented with some varieties: some simply had not flourished as expected, some needed more shade or water than was available, and others would have taken too long to reach maturity. Her most important conclusion, however, was a redefinition of the term extinction:

> Certain edible wild plants could be ecologically stable and present throughout a given geographical area—but in actuality be *nutritionally extinct*—because such plants no longer are recog-

nized by family members and no longer contribute to household food intake. (Johnson and Grivetti, 2002a)

Johnson also reported the beta-carotene content of the most important local edible wild species. She concluded that although the Karen diet was rich in edible wild greens and provided modest to good sources of energy and minerals, the presence and bioavailability of beta-carotene was marginal. Traditional food preservation and preparation techniques, specifically storage under conditions of high temperature and humidity and boiling for long time periods, reduced the dietary content of this provitamin. Further, most edible greens with reasonable quantities of beta-carotene were not consumed at the same meal with a fat source (Johnson and Grivetti, 2002b).

Mary Dalsin returned to former Soviet Asia and worked in Kazakstan as part of a binational team of American and Kazak scholars to evaluate dietary patterns in livestock-owning households before and after economic reforms. Dalsin considered hunting and gathering in Kazak society as one part of her work and sought data on the importance of these activities in maintaining quality of diet during "hard times." She reported that 25 percent of households regularly gathered edible wild plants, with most efforts focused on securing berries, bulbs (especially wild garlic and onion), fruits, medicinal herbs, and mushrooms. Dalsin identified an underlying fear related by some Kazaks that edible wild plants might not be safe, with presumed danger related to possible residual radiation from atmospheric testing conducted during the peak of the Cold War during the 1950s. Other Kazaks, however, dismissed such dangers and blamed the decline in dietary use of edible wild plants upon lack of petrol supplies for their personal inability to travel to former plant-collection areas (Dalsin et al., 2002).

Jan Corlett, another of my students with extensive international service in both Africa and Asia, elected to work among Hmong immigrants to Sacramento, California. Corlett's objectives were to identify the most common Hmong culinary herbs grown in urban gardens and examine whether or not such species posed potential health risks to consumers from possible heavy-metal contamination (arsenic, cadmium, chromium, or lead). She identified 25 exotic species: items imported surreptitiously to the United States, purchased within California through brokers, or exchanged through friendship networks. The most commonly grown included *Acorus gramineus, Dendran-*

thema indicum, Eupatorium lindleyana, Polygonum odoratum, and *Sedum* cf. *spectabile.* Several of these exotic species commonly served as both food and medicine: *Acorus gramineus*—cooked with chicken and prescribed by traditional healers to women during postpartum periods; *Basella alba*—cooked with chicken and prescribed to alleviate arthritis and back pain; and *Dendranthema indicum*—cooked with chicken and prescribed as a general tonic to relieve cough, but also applied externally to reduce bruising. *Polygonum* cf. *cymosum* was identified as a famine food in Laos, but in urban Sacramento, California, leaves of this plant were applied externally on the stomach to lessen stomachache. Although the Hmong women cultivated their gardens on an abandoned site in urban Sacramento, a location with an unknown history, none of the samples analyzed had detectable levels of heavy metals (Corlett et al., 2001; Corlett et al., 2003).

REFLECTIONS AND POTENTIAL RESEARCH AREAS

Historical Texts and Use of Edible Wild Plants in Human Diet

During the past three decades my historical work has included efforts to search broadly for references to edible wild plant use in both ancient and contemporary societies. Even a cursory inspection of ancient texts reveals the important, prominent role of such species throughout history, whether in ancient Egypt, Greece, and Rome; India and China; or even in Aztec and Mayan cultures. One such text will suffice, and presented here are two selected passages from *The Deipnosophists* (philosophers at dinner) by Athenaeus of Naucratis, that date to c. 200 CE:

> And Socrates was many a time found walking up and down in front of his house in the late afternoon, and to those who asked, "What are you doing at this hour?" he would reply, "Gathering a relish for my dinner. . . ." (Athenaeus, V:157:E-F)
>
> Shoots of marjoram, set deep in a pot, may be forced [transplanted and forced to grow] by manure, so too young sprouts of the frankincense tree and all other plants that our gardens provide to make wreaths for toiling men. Yes, there are slender

ferns and oak resembling white poplar, and the crocus closing in spring-time, henna, too, and mint with pungent smell and all the beauties which a meadow rears without cultivation in hollow watered places. (Athenaeus, XV:684:A-C)

Despite the richness and wide availability of these ancient works, too numerous to mention, no scholar has searched such texts systematically to identify and catalog uses of edible wild species by ancient cultures.

Use of Edible Wild Plants During Military Conflict

The importance of edible wild plants during periods of social unrest and war is also well documented but has not been searched systematically. The example cited here dates to the American Revolutionary War era, and the author—well-known for his military and political careers—is not a name that most ethnobotanists would cite:

As there is a plenty of common and French sorrel; lamb's quarters, and water cresses, growing about camp; and as these vegetables are very conducive to health, and tend to prevent the scurvy and all putrid disorders . . . the General recommends to the soldiers the constant use of them, as they make an agreeable salad, and have the most salutary effect. The regimental officer of the day [is] to send to gather them every morning, and have them distributed among the men. (Washington, 1777)

One rewarding avenue of ethnobotanical research would be to continue the pursuit of edible wild plant use during civil unrest and to interview soldiers and survivors of recent military campaigns who maintained reasonable caloric intakes and overall nutritional status by use of edible wild plants. Such geographical areas, globally, might include: Algeria, Angola, Bosnia, Cambodia, Iran, Iraq, Laos, Lebanon, Northern Ireland, Palestine/West Bank, Rwanda, Serbia, Vietnam, and Zimbabwe.

Antonia Leda-Matalas, my colleague at Harokopio University, Athens, Greece, has encouraged her students to interview elderly Greeks at senior centers in Athens, asking them to recall the different types of edible wild plants consumed during the Athens famine of World War II. These reports currently are being summarized for publication (Leda-Matalas, personal communication). Britta Ogle, working recently in Vietnam, produced a wonderful monograph titled *Wild Vegetables and Micronutrient Nutrition: Studies on the Significance of Wild Vegetables in Women's Diets in Vietnam* (Ogle, 2001). Ogle's work also clarified how edible wild plants sustained civilians during the American-Vietnamese War, and she drew attention to the important efforts by Nguyen Tien Ban and Bui Minh Duc, who earlier in their careers had prepared a military manual on edible wild plants for use during that tragic period (Nguyen and Bui, 1994).

Safety and Toxic Analogues

It has been known for many decades that the plant kingdom is not a smorgasbord of safe foods on which to dine. By some estimates, 90 percent of plants in any ecological niche may be toxic to humans (Leopold and Ardrey, 1972). One subtheme in the search for safe edible species is to investigate "toxic analogues," defined as species that are poisonous in one environmental setting but safe in another, or two plants closely affiliated on the basis of external morphology, one being safe and the other toxic. An extension of this theme applies directly to the health of persons who emigrate from one geographical area to another. Those who gather wild plants must first solve what is safe to eat, and this is done quickly—so long as individuals remain and inhabit the same environmental niche. When societies/individuals move geographically from one niche to another, as from Cambodia, Laos, or Vietnam to northern California during recent decades, poisonings have been caused by incautious selection and eating of plants presumed to have been safe (but in fact misidentifications or toxic analogues). Recent immigrants from Southeast Asia who forage incautiously among stands of wild plants growing in Golden Gate Park, San Francisco, for example, sometimes have found themselves as patients in hospital emergency rooms when plants thought to be safe have turned out to be poisonous.

Archaeology and Plant Dispersals

Anthropologists, geographers, and ethnobotanists argue over the implications of how and when certain plants were dispersed globally. All evidence, for example, suggests that maize and chili peppers were domesticated in central Mexico. The prevailing scholarly opinion holds that both foods did not disperse globally until after arrival of the Spanish in 1519 CE. It is interesting, therefore, that images of what appear to be maize are carved on the walls of Hindu temples in southern India—sites that predate the thirteenth century CE (Johannessen and Parker, 1989). Such art-related evidence suggests pre-Columbian trade across the Pacific Ocean, but pollen evidence is lacking.

Ethnobotanists, especially those with interests in the subfield of palynology, could do much to clarify and document the presence of maize and chili peppers, and whether or not these crops were transferred from Mesoamerica to Asia prior to 1492. The techniques are simple: core representative samples of mud bricks that can be dated to specific pre-Columbian periods and search for maize/chili pollen. Such efforts would not be expensive, probably less than $20,000 for a well-designed survey period in which trained palynologists work hand in hand with agronomists and social scientists.

Another fruitful avenue of ethnobotanical enquiry would be to examine further the cultural and medicinal uses of cacao (Dillinger et al., 2000). The phylogenetic origins of cacao remain unclear: was *Theobroma cacao* domesticated initially in the western Amazon and independently in Mexico/northern Guatemala, or did the genus spread from north to south (alternatively south to north)? Given the relatively short germination time for cacao beans, were the early dispersals of *Theobroma* via seeds or seedlings? Following such questions, how and when did the early explorers/traders along the east and west coasts of Central America and the western and northern coasts of South America initiate global trade and exchange in cacao beans/ trees?

Nutrition and Nutrient Databases

Much work is needed, globally, on improving and expanding the nutrient databases of the major and minor edible wild species within the Sahel and other arid or semiarid zones and within the high, cold deserts of southern Asia north of the Himalayas. Hundreds of plant collectors, ethnobotanists, anthropologists, geographers, and others have worked independently in areas as diverse as eastern India, the southeastern tropics of the Malay peninsula area, and the South American and African rainforests have published in very different journals but only rarely communicate. Nutrient analysis of edible wild species should be accelerated, information shared, and young scholars in different nations of the world encouraged and trained in botanical techniques—before loss of this important, critical biomass. A database should be developed of so-called famine foods and the information preserved for all generations to come—lest persons starve in the midst of food plenty, being unable to recognize potential foods in the surrounding environment. Would it not be a tragedy of extraordinary dimension to lose such information?

Unusual Plant Themes

A considerable number of interesting relationships have developed between humans, nonhuman animals, and plants. One curiosity that I described early in my Kalahari work was how baTlokwa pregnant women snacked on the nutmeats of *morula (Sclerocarya kaffra)*—but only after the kernels had been eaten by goats and had undergone "heating" in the goats' stomach/intestinal organs. Such kernels obtained in goat kraals were cleaned, the nutmeats dug out, and consumed with gusto. *Morula* kernels that had not transited the goats' digestive system were regularly consumed by other baTlokwa, but the "heated" kernels were the prerogative of pregnant women (Grivetti, 1976). Other such animal-plant relationships, whereby germination does not occur unless the seed transits the intestinal system of an animal, represents an interesting evolutionary process and is worthy of more careful inspection and study.

Study of animals as agents of seed dispersals also lies at the interface between botany and zoology. Cattle that feed on specific species of *Acacia* and other trees have been responsible for the expansion of plant boundaries within different regions of Africa. Many seeds, of course, remain viable throughout intestinal transit, and as cattle are herded from one geographical area to another plant distributions have expanded (Grivetti, 1976).

Plants in Magic and Mythology

It is common in 2005 to consider science as almighty and to scoff at older traditions when plants were adored or worshiped for specific characteristics. The stories of many plant species have been told, and their roles in ancient folklore traditions have been discussed (Baker, 1978; Bergen, 1899; Gordon, 1977; Lehner and Lehner, 1960, 1962; Maple, 1980; Northcote, 1971; Thiselton-Dyer, 1889). My undergraduate students rarely know of these wonderful tales, and such knowledge is being lost on a global scale. In 1977 I visited Avebury, England, and purchased numerous corn dolls, those wonderful geometric icons of woven wheat described by James George Frazer in his *Golden Bough* (1900). Once, these "spirits of the corn" were woven with precise designs that were characteristic of different geographical districts. But no more: on a recent trip to Avebury in 2001, corn dolls were no longer sold, and two of the three young, summer salespersons had never heard of them. Too bad. What might be done to preserve this knowledge?

CODA

Let me return to Botswana for a final comment. The two elderly men who taught me the Kalahari plants, Mr. Mphoeng Lekoko and Mr. Gaborone Sekgokgo, exhibited great patience with me. On many occasions when we walked past baTlokwa households I pointed out what I perceived to be patches of dry weeds, areas that in my mind represented potential fire hazards and potential habitats for dangerous Kalahari snakes. Both of my teachers would say: "Wait, Louis, be patient. Wait for the rains."

And when the rains arrived that second year of my field study, I remember to this day my amazement. What I identified as merely patches of dried weeds, in fact, were cultural gardens composed of Kalahari Desert species that had been transplanted by baTlokwa men, women, and children. The areas in front of the household walls were filled with blooms, and we stopped, viewed, and reflected upon the vibrant colors—the blues, magentas, oranges, reds, violets, whites, and yellows—all blossoms of wild desert species—interspersed with stunning green leaves of different shapes and patterns. At such times I recalled how Edgar Anderson had written that domestication of plants was not for food, but came about because of human attraction to aesthetics and beauty. Thinking back from the perspective of nearly 30 years of fieldwork, I still think that Anderson was correct.

REFERENCES

Anderson, E. (1952). *Plants, life, and man.* Boston: Little, Brown and Company.

Athenaeus (1927-1941). *The deipnosophists.* Translated by C.B. Gulick. 7 Vols. New York: G. P. Putnam's Sons.

Baker, M. (1978). *Gardener's magic and folklore.* New York: Universe Books.

Bergen, F.D. (1899). *Animal and plant lore: Collected from the oral tradition of English-speaking folk.* New York: American Folk-Lore Society.

Corlett, J.L., M.S. Clegg, C.L. Keen, and L.E. Grivetti (2001). Culinary and medicinal plant species cultivated by Hmong refugees in California. *International Journal of Food Sciences and Nutrition* 52: 1-12.

Corlett, J.L., E.A. Dean, and L.E. Grivetti (2003). Hmong gardens: Botanical diversity in an urban setting. *Economic Botany* 57: 365-379.

Dalsin, M.F., E.A. Laca, G. Abuova, and L.E. Grivetti (2002). Livestock-owning households of Kazakstan. Part 1. Food systems. *Ecology of Food and Nutrition* 41: 301-343.

Dillinger, T.L., P. Barriga, S. Escarcega, M. Jimenez, D.S. Lowe, and L.E. Grivetti (2000). Food of the gods—Cure for humanity? A cultural history of the medicinal and ritual use of chocolate. *Journal of Nutrition* 130 (Supplement): 2057S-2072S.

Doughty, J. (1979a). Dangers of reducing the range of food choices in developing countries. *Ecology of Food and Nutrition* 8: 275-283.

Doughty, J. (1979b). Decreasing variety of plant foods used in developing countries. *Qualitas Plantarum* 29: 163-177.

Frazer, J.G. (1900). *The golden bough: A study in magic and religion,* second edition. 3 volumes. London: Macmillan.

Gilliland, L.E. (1985). Proximate analysis and mineral composition of traditional California native American foods. Unpublished master's thesis, Department of Nutrition, University of California, Davis.

Gordon, L. (1977). *Green magic: Flowers, plants, and herbs in lore and legend.* New York: Viking Press.

Grivetti, L.E. (1976). Dietary resources and social aspects of food use in a Tswana tribe. Unpublished doctoral dissertation, Department of Geography, University of California, Davis.

Grivetti, L.E. (1978). Nutritional success in a semi-arid land: Examination of Tswana agro-pastoralists of the eastern Kalahari, Botswana. *American Journal of Clinical Nutrition* 31: 1204-1220.

Grivetti, L.E. (1979). Kalahari agro-pastoral-hunter-gatherers: The Tswana example. *Ecology of Food and Nutrition* 7: 235-256.

Grivetti, L.E. (1980a). *Agricultural development: Present and potential role of edible wild plants.* Part 1: *Central and South America and the Caribbean.* Report to the Department of State, Agency for International Development (USAID). Washington, DC: USAID.

Grivetti, L.E. (1980b). *Agricultural development: Present and potential role of edible wild plants.* Part 2: *Sub-Saharan Africa.* Report to the Department of State, Agency for International Development (USAID). Washington, DC: USAID.

Grivetti, L.E. (1981a). *Agricultural development: Present and potential role of edible wild plants.* Part 3: *India, East Asia, Southeast Asia, Oceania.* Report to the Department of State, Agency for International Development (USAID). Washington, DC: USAID.

Grivetti, L.E. (1981b). Geographical location, climate and weather, and magic: Aspects of agricultural success in the eastern Kalahari, Botswana. *Social Science Information: Human Societies and Ecosystems* 20: 509-536.

Grivetti, L.E., C.J. Frentzel, K.E. Ginsberg, K.L. Howell, and B.M. Ogle (1987). Bush foods and edible weeds of agriculture: Perspectives on dietary use of wild plants in Africa, their role in maintaining human nutritional status, and implications for agricultural development. In Akhtar, R. (Ed.), *Health and disease in tropical Africa: Geographical and medical viewpoints.* London: Harwood.

Grivetti, L.E. and B.M. Ogle (2000). Value of traditional foods in meeting macro- and micronutrient needs: The wild plant connection. *Nutrition Research Reviews* 13: 1-16.

Humphry, C., M.S. Clegg, C. Keen, and L.E. Grivetti (1993). Food diversity and drought survival. The Hausa example. *International Journal of Food Sciences and Nutrition* 44:1-16.

Johannessen, C.L. and A.Z. Parker (1989). Maize ears sculptured in 12th and 13th century A.D. India as indicators of pre-Columbian diffusion. *Economic Botany* 43: 164-180.

Johnson, N. and L.E. Grivetti (2002a). Environmental change in northern Thailand. Impact on wild edible plant availability. *Ecology of Food and Nutrition* 41: 373-399.

Johnson, N. and L.E. Grivetti (2002b). Gathering practices of Karen women: Questionable contribution to beta-carotene intake. *International Journal of Food Sciences and Nutrition* 53: 489-501.

Lehner, E. and J. Lehner (1960). *Folklore and symbolism of flowers, plants, and trees.* New York: Tudor Publishing.

Lehner, E. and J. Lehner (1962). *Folklore and odysseys of food and medicinal plants.* New York: Tudor Publishing.

Leopold, A.C. and R. Ardrey (1972). Toxic substances in plants and the food habits of early man. *Science* 176: 512-514.

Lockett, C., C.C. Calvert, and L.E. Grivetti (2000). Energy and micronutrient composition of dietary and medicinal wild plants consumed during drought: Study of rural Fulani, northeastern Nigeria. *International Journal of Food Sciences and Nutrition* 51: 195-208.

Lockett, C., and L.E. Grivetti (2000). Food-related behaviors during drought. A study of rural Fulani, northeastern Nigeria. *International Journal of Food Sciences and Nutrition* 51: 91-107.

Maple, E. (1980). *The secret lore of plants and flowers.* London: Robert Hale.

Merriam, C.H. (1918). The acorn: A possibly neglected food source. *National Geographic* 34: 129-137.

Nguyen, T.B. and M.D. Bui (1994). *Wild edible vegetables in Vietnam.* Hanoi: People's Army Publishing House.

Northcote, R. (1971). *The book of herb lore.* New York: Dover Publications.

Ogle, B.M. (2001). *Wild vegetables and micronutrient nutrition. Studies on the significance of wild vegetables in women's diets in Vietnam. Comprehensive summaries of Uppsala dissertations from the faculty of medicine.* Number 1056. Uppsala, Sweden: Acta Universitatis Upsaliensis.

Ogle, B.M. and L.E. Grivetti (1985a). Legacy of the chameleon. Edible wild plants in the kingdom of Swaziland, southern Africa. A cultural, ecological, nutritional study. Part 1: Introduction, objectives, methods, Swazi culture, landscape, and diet. *Ecology of Food and Nutrition* 16: 193-208.

Ogle, B.M. and L.E. Grivetti (1985b). Legacy of the chameleon. Edible wild plants in the kingdom of Swaziland, southern Africa. A cultural ecological, nutritional study. Part 2: Demographics, species availability and dietary use, analysis by ecological zone. *Ecology of Food and Nutrition* 17: 1-30.

Ogle, B.M. and L.E. Grivetti (1985c). Legacy of the chameleon. Edible wild plants in the kingdom of Swaziland, southern Africa. A cultural, ecological, nutritional study. Part 3: Cultural and ecological analysis. *Ecology of Food and Nutrition* 17: 31-40.

Ogle, B.M. and L.E. Grivetti (1985d). Legacy of the chameleon. Edible wild plants in the kingdom of Swaziland, southern Africa. A cultural, ecological, nutritional study. Part 4: Nutritional analysis and conclusions. *Ecology of Food and Nutrition* 17: 41-64.

Pauling, L.W. and L.E. Grivetti (1984). Importance of animals and forage sources within a rice cropping system, northern Luzon, Philippines. In Flora, C.B. and P.P. Nichols (Eds.), *Proceedings, Kansas State University's 1983 Farming Systems Research Symposium: Animals in the farming system.* Manhattan, Kansas: International Programs Office, Kansas State University.

Sauer, C.O. (1952). *Agricultural origins and dispersals.* New York: American Geographical Society.

Sauer, C.O. (1969). *Agricultural origins and dispersals: The domestication of animals and foodstuffs,* second edition. Cambridge: The Massachusetts Institute of Technology Press.

Smith, G.C., M.S. Clegg, C.L. Keen, and L.E. Grivetti (1995). Mineral values of selected plant foods common to southern Burkina Faso and to Niamey, Niger, West Africa. *International Journal of Food Sciences and Nutrition* 47: 41-53.

Smith, G.C., S.R. Dueker, A.J. Clifford, and L.E. Grivetti (1996). Carotenoid values of selected plant foods common to southern Burkina Faso, West Africa. *Ecology of Food and Nutrition* 35: 43-58.

Thiselton-Dyer, T.F. (1889). *The folk-lore of plants.* New York: D. Appleton and Company.

Washington, G. (1777). *General order dated June 9th, 1777. Washington's Headquarters, Middle-Brook.* Washington, DC: National Archives.

Chapter 2

Tibetan Foods and Medicines: Antioxidants As Mediators of High-Altitude Nutritional Physiology

Patrick L. Owen

INTRODUCTION

Procurement of adequate nutritional needs from extreme environments is of great significance for understanding fundamental adaptive capacities of human populations. Food habits of Arctic hunter-gatherers, for example, have revealed paradoxical patterns that challenge contemporary views of nutrition and health. Despite their almost exclusive dependence on meat, the Inuit have a lower incidence of atherosclerosis and coronary heart disease compared to nonnatives (Young et al., 1993). This difference in disease outcome is thought to be due to the high levels of omega-3 fatty acids in marine mammals and fish (Kuhnlein et al., 1991) that confer cardioprotective benefits such as fibrinolytic, vasodilating, and antiarrhythmic activity (Abeywardena and Head, 2001).

High altitude is another example of an extreme environment, characterized by cold temperatures, hypobaric hypoxia, increased exposure to solar radiation, aridity, and low biomass. Due to such stressors, travel to high altitude enhances oxidative stress, arising from maladaptive biological responses to low oxygen pressure and increased exposure to ultraviolet (UV) radiation (Askew, 2002). Reac-

The author is supported by the Natural Science and Engineering Research Council (NSERC) of Canada, le Fond Québecois de la Recherche sur la Nature et les Technologies, and the Society for Economic Botany Richard E. Schultes Award. The comments of Dr. E. W. Askew were highly helpful and appreciated.

tive oxygen species (ROS) and free radicals are key mediators in the pathogenesis of several chronic diseases, including cardiovascular disease (CVD). Similar to the Inuit, Tibetan highlanders have had to rely on a high-meat diet virtually devoid of fruits and vegetables due to poor plant-growing conditions. Unlike the Inuit, however, Tibetans rarely eat fish due to religious taboos, so are thus not exposed to the heart-protective benefits of omega-3 fatty acids. Instead, Tibetans rely on large mammals such as yaks, beef, and mutton, which are rich in saturated fats and cholesterol. Saturated fats have been linked to increased risk of CVD due to their ability to elevate serum levels of low-density lipoprotein (LDL) cholesterol. Elevated LDL, compounded with oxidative stress, paves the path toward atherosclerotic plaque formation and, ultimately, ischemic heart disease. Despite a saturated-fat–rich diet, low consumption of antioxidant-rich fruits and vegetables, and residence in a high-oxidative stress environment, Tibetan highlanders have a low incidence of ischemic heart disease (Fujimoto et al., 1989).

A hypothesis my colleague and I put forth (Owen and Johns, 2002) questioned the importance of antioxidants in Tibetan foods and medicines in conferring protection against diet and altitude-related CVD risk factors. Although fruit and vegetable consumption may be low, other commonly consumed plant foods that are imported from lower altitudes may provide antioxidants and other cardioprotective elements. Further benefits may be obtained from quantitatively less-significant items such as spices, condiments, and medicinal plants that may contribute functional phytochemicals able to mediate metabolism and physiology (Johns, 1996).

In the present review, our hypothesis is expanded and positioned within a behavioral evolutionary framework to explore subsistence strategies to sustain life and reproduction at high altitude. Considering the biological distinctiveness of the Tibetan highland population, the environmental conditions of high altitudes, and the cultural dietary behavior of Tibetan nomads, the interaction of food components and health outcomes is rendered considerably more complex. Human physiological and genetic responses to high altitude are first discussed to highlight the population's unique characteristics. Sources of oxidative stress at high altitude are then explored. Finally, Tibetan highland foods and medicines are discussed in relation to their effects on cardiovascular health.

ADAPTATIONS TO ALTITUDE

The cost of living is so severe at high altitudes that maintenance of normal metabolic function at 4,500 m requires more than twice the nutrient requirements of sea level (Marriot and Carlson-Newberry, 1996), while work capacity is greatly reduced (Moore et al., 1992). Cold temperatures can be circumvented easily enough by sociocultural measures such as insulating clothing and shelter. Hypoxia, however, is unavoidable and cannot be modified by behavior. Human long-term tolerance to low ambient oxygen pressure therefore required adaptation at the physiological and genetic level (Rupert and Hochachka, 2001). Consequently, high-altitude natives are biologically different from sea-level populations. Archaeological evidence places human occupation of the Tibetan plateau at 25,000 to 50,000 years ago (Zhimin, 1982)—longer than other high-altitude populations (Aldenderfer, 1999). If we assume that the length of time of residency is related to degree of acclimatization, then Tibetans would represent the most adapted population to hypoxic conditions. Some of the more clear-cut adaptations are seen in respiratory kinetics and hematology.

1. *Tibetans have a higher resting ventilation rate than Andeans and retain a sensitive hypoxic ventilatory response (HVR) similar to sea-level standards* (Beall et al., 1997). In order to maintain aerobic metabolic processes, a fundamental primary response to lower ambient oxygen concentrations is increased ventilation. The HVR is initiated by O_2 sensors in the carotid bodies and serves to increase O_2 uptake in the lung (Samaja et al., 1997). An acclimatized lowlander will eventually develop a blunted HVR, which may serve to counteract acid-base problems arising from hyperventilation (Samaja et al., 1997). This adaptation unfortunately enhances the risk of developing chronic mountain sickness (CMS, a.k.a. altitude sickness or Monge's disease), a condition that is rare among Tibetans (Monge et al., 1992).

2. *The hemoglobin concentration and hematocrit of Tibetans is elevated compared to sea-level standards, but less so than Andean natives* (Beall et al., 1990). This adaptation also serves to reduce the frequency of CMS. To maintain the oxygen-carrying capacity of blood, red blood cell (RBC) mass increases as a result of stimulated erythropoietin (EPO) expression (Goldberg et al., 1988). A hematocrit of 45 to 60 percent is typical for sea-level migrants to altitude; although

above 55 percent, blood viscosity increases in a curvilinear fashion, which raises the risk of thrombotic stroke (Altahan et al., 1998; Fujimaki et al., 1986). Additional CVD risk may result from increased levels of serum triglycerides and cholesterol that occur due to a reduced serum pool. Epidemiological studies support this, indicating a strong correlation between elevated hematocrit and serum cholesterol levels, indicating increased CVD risk at high altitude (Temte, 1996).

Among Tibetan highlanders, hematocrit levels do not usually reach levels that are detrimental to health (Beall et al., 1990), due in part to genetic influences that allow greater arterial hemoglobin O_2 saturation (Beall et al., 1994). Despite this, a high incidence of hypertension has been documented (Sun, 1986), a condition that is usually absent or rare in other high-altitude populations (Hanna, 1999). The explanation may lie in the diet: Tibetans consume large amounts of sodium, up to one kilogram a month, much of it added to their tea, and their potassium intake is low.

3. *Effects of altitude on birthweight in Tibetans are less pronounced,* providing support of a protective mechanism against altitude-associated fetal growth retardation (Zamudio et al., 1993). Altitude residency is associated with reduced birthweight compared to sea-level standards (Jensen and Moore, 1997) attributed to maternofetal oxygen insufficiency. As such, birthweight can be used as an indirect interpretation of the efficiency of adaptive responses to hypoxia through its effects on infant mortality (Wiley, 1994). Likewise, the differential reproductive success of women is affected by superior responses to hypoxia, which could have operated through generations of selective forces acting at high altitude (Hochachka et al., 1999). However, the condition is complicated by poor maternal nutrition and infectious diseases that commonly afflict impoverished highland populations (Giussani et al., 2001).

OXIDATIVE STRESS AND ANTIOXIDANTS

The oxidation of serum LDL is considered a key initiating step in atherosclerotic plaque formation, and supplementation with antioxidants has proven to increase LDL resistance to oxidation (Jialal and Grundy, 1992). Epidemiological evidence supports this, demonstrating a negative correlation between plasma antioxidant concentrations and CVD risk (Gey et al., 1993; Riemersma et al., 1991). Endogenous antioxidant enzymes are the first line of defense against ROS produced from mitochondrial respiration and are inducible in response to oxidative stress. Certain minerals are required as cofactors: selenium for glutathione peroxidase (GSH-Px), manganese for mitochondrial superoxide dismutase (SOD), zinc and copper for cytoplasmic SOD, and heme iron for catalase. These nutrients must be obtained from the diet. Since humans have low levels of endogenous antioxidants compared to other mammals, additional forms of oxidative defense must be acquired from the diet. Best known are vitamins C and E and beta-carotene, although a growing number of nonnutrients such as flavonoids, isoflavonoids, hydroxycinnamic acids, and other phenols are recognized as important contributors.

The multistressor environment of high altitudes has been shown to increase whole-body oxidative stress, as evidenced by increased erythrocyte peroxidation and breath pentane levels in humans at high altitude that is attenuated by vitamin E supplementation (Simon-Schnass, 1996). Hypobaric hypoxia increases levels of oxidized glutathione in rats (Chang et al., 1989) and malondialdehyde (MDA) levels are increased in plasma and tissues (Nakanishi et al., 1995; Sarada et al., 2002). In humans, exercise in hypoxic environments produced increased DNA strand breaks and oxidative DNA damage compared to exercise under normal conditions. The authors deduced that hypoxia depleted the antioxidant system of its capacity to withstand oxidative stress produced by exercise (Møller et al., 2001).

Askew (2002) explored possible sources of free radicals and ROS associated with high altitude. The majority of sources arise as a consequence of exercise in hypoxic conditions. For instance, exercise at high altitude may exacerbate ROS production from accelerated metabolism and increased serum catecholamine and hypoxanthine production. Reductive stress may also arise due to decreased availability of oxygen as terminal electron acceptors during mitochondrial respiration, which leads to the accumulation of reducing equivalents. Non-exercise-related sources of oxidative stress include photooxidation of the dermis and subcutaneous tissues due to greater UV exposure and a lack of dietary antioxidants.

Although oxidative stress is an unquestionable aspect of high-altitude travel, little is known on how high-altitude natives circumvent this to maintain free from ROS-mediated pathologies. A study in Andean highlanders indicated that erythrocyte GSH-Px levels were significantly reduced, while catalase and SOD levels were unchanged compared to sea-level controls (Agostoni et al., 1983). The authors deduced that low GSH-Px levels were due to selenium deficiency and concluded that high-altitude Andean residents were poorly protected from oxidative stress. In an in vivo animal study, Sarada and colleagues (2002) found that selenium supplementation reversed hypoxia-induced indices of oxidative stress. Selenium deficiency is also a significant problem in Tibet due to poor soil concentrations. Kashin-Beck disease (KBD), an endemic osteochondropathy that is mediated by ROS-induced damage to developing bone and cartilage (Peng et al., 1992), is caused in part by selenium deficiency (Suetens et al., 2001) and consequently diminished GSH-Px levels. Consuming foods that are rich in antioxidants has been suggested as a strategy to alleviate KBD prevalence.

Plants that grow at high altitudes are an excellent source of antioxidants. The increased light intensity at altitude has obliged plants to increase antioxidant defenses to offset the higher ROS production caused by hyperstimulation of the photosynthetic apparatus (Ren et al., 1999; Wildi and Lütz, 1996). As a result, plants produce more antioxidants as they spread and grow to higher elevations. Moreover, the abundance of nonstructural carbohydrates (sugars, starch, fructans), lipids, energy, flavonoids and related phenolics, anthocyanids, and carotenes is also greater in alpine plants (reviewed in Kröner, 1999). Herbivores are able to subsist on this vegetation, which in turn sustain carnivores. As omnivores, humans living at high altitudes depend primarily on animals and supplement their diet with endemic plants. However, the dwarf growth forms of most alpine plants, among other disadvantages, discourage their use as a major food source. Nonetheless, they may have been partially exploited during migrations to altitude to help offset increased oxidative stress. Use of alpine plant species as human food in the context of high altitude colonization has very limited mention in the literature. They are exploited for pharmacological applications, however, as reflected in the extensive herbals of Tibetan medicine.

TIBETAN HIGH-ALTITUDE FOOD SYSTEMS

Colonization of the Tibetan plateau likely occurred in several discrete stages that coincided with major paleoclimate fluctuations over the past 50,000 years (Brantingham et al., 2003). During the Upper Paleolithic era, hunter-gatherers journeyed to high altitude, although long-term habitation would have been hindered by low environmental carrying capacity. On the plateau, few plants other than artemesia, wild nettles, dwarf willows, and a variety of grasses are able to grow. Reliance on meat was therefore essential for survival. Domestication of the wild yak (*Bos grunniens* L.) and the practice of nomadic pastoralism during the middle Holocene era in Tibet were economic adaptations that enabled successful permanent residence.

In order to access greater dietary diversity, nomads needed to trade with lower-altitude regions, where growing conditions were more favorable. For centuries, Tibetan nomads have subsisted by harvesting products from their yaks, sheep, and goats, directly consuming some, such as yogurt, butter, and meat, and trading others for barley, wheat, and tea. *Tsamba,* roasted barley, is the staple of Tibet, and *chhatang,* salted butter tea, is the national beverage. The two are frequently mixed together in bowls, made into a paste with fingers, and consumed. Other major food items include colza, peas, beans, potatoes, and radishes. Flavorings usually include onions, garlic, and salt. Smaller-sized animals such as poultry and fish are rarely eaten due to Buddhist beliefs, which discourage the slaughter of several smaller animals, rather than a single large one, to obtain similar quantities of meat (Majupuria and Lobsang, 2000).

Diet varies seasonally, and much more calories are consumed in winter than in summer (Beall and Goldstein, 1993). In one nomadic group, tsamba provided 51 to 73 percent of calories during summer months and 30 to 40 percent in winter. Animal products were consumed throughout the year, with dairy products contributing 12 to 19 percent and 36 to 53 percent of total summer and winter calories, respectively. Accumulated body fat during the winters was assumed to buffer the summer periods of low intake (Beall et al., 1996). Body composition analysis of Tibetans, though, show that percent body fat, fat mass, and body weight were consistent with those reported for rural non-European men and women, which suggests that obesity was uncommon (Vaz et al., 1999).

Barley (Hordeum vulgare L.)

Whole-grain foods in general are considered beneficial for cardio-vascular health. A series of large cohort studies (reviewed in Trustwell, 2002) demonstrated a significant inverse association of cereal fiber or whole grains with coronary heart disease. Only a minor fraction of this protective effect was attributable to the cholesterol-lowering effect of soluble fiber. Additional factors may have been due to folate and/or vitamin-E contents, glucose/insulin responses, and/or hemostatic factors. Barley has confirmed hypocholesterolemic properties (McIntosh et al., 1995), demonstrated in a well-controlled 11-week crossover study in 21 mildly hypercholesterolemic men, where a diet high in barley fiber resulted in lower total and LDL cholesterol levels compared with wheat (McIntosh et al., 1991). Activity was attributed on one hand to the β-glucan component of soluble dietary fiber, which increases the meal bolus viscosity and delays absorption (Wursch and Pi-Sunyer, 1997), and on the other hand to tocotrienol and α-linolenic acid (18:3n-3) (Burger et al., 1984). Tocotrienol is proposed to influence cholesterol metabolism by inhibiting the rate-limiting enzyme, HMG-CoA reductase, in cholesterol synthesis. As a tocopherol, tocotrienol is also an antioxidant, along with other components of barley such as flavanols ([+]-catechin, [–]-epicatechin, and [+]-gallocatechin), other tocopherols (α, δ, and γ) and carotenoids (lutein and zeaxanthine) (Goupy et al., 1999). The roasting of barley as practiced in Tibet, however, significantly diminishes the antioxidant activity, a result of lower catechin, tocopherol, and lutein content (Duh et al., 2001). Nonetheless, regular consumption of roasted barley likely confers a cardiovascular benefit to Tibetans.

Brick tea (Camellia sinensis [L.] Kuntz.)

Tea and polyphenols contained therein have well-established antioxidant activity and consumption is attributed to numerous health benefits (Weisburger, 1999). Epigallocatechin gallate (EGCG) is a powerful antioxidant and the main component (>30 percent dry weight) of tea leaves. Epidemiological studies have shown that regular tea drinkers had lower risk of heart disease than nonusers when comparing populations with similar risk factors (Ishikawa et al., 1997; Hertog et al., 1995). This is supported by in vitro studies that demonstrate reduced LDL susceptibility to oxidation (deWhalley et al., 1990). Cross-cultural studies also show that tea consumption is associated with reduced serum cholesterol concentrations (Kono et al., 1992). However, Tibetans consume a tea variety made from old and coarse leaves and branches that are tightly pressed and shaped into bricks in order to facilitate transportation and storage. Such processing techniques may adversely affect the phenolic content. Moreover, brick tea usually includes leaves from other plants, most often those found growing alongside the tea when collected.

Tea selectively absorbs fluorine from soils and progressively accumulates it in the leaves, so that older leaves have higher concentrations (Jin et al., 2001). Fluoride levels in brick tea are extraordinarily high, up to 200 to 300 times higher than green or black tea, which causes high incidence of dental and skeletal fluorosis among Tibetans (Cao et al., 1996). Fluoride toxicity increases lipid peroxidation in murine livers (Shivashankara et al., 2002), kidney (Sharma and Chinoy, 1998), and human erythrocytes (Saralakumari and Rao, 1991), indicating ROS-mediated pathogenesis. Animal studies demonstrate that fluoride-toxicity–induced oxidative stress depletes intrinsic ascorbic acid and glutathione (Shivashankara et al., 2002). Moreover, studies involving antioxidants and fluoride compounds show that fluorides can adversely affect the action of antioxidants (Sztarbala et al., 1998). Therefore, the health benefits of ECGC may be severely compromised in tea leaves with high fluoride concentrations. In this regard, it is difficult to evaluate whether the antioxidant benefits of brick tea outweigh the hazards of fluorosis, since little is known of whether long-term cardiovascular health is affected.

Meat and Dairy Products

Implicit in dietary recommendations of most government health agencies is an overall pattern higher in plant foods and lower in animal foods (Health Canada, 1997; United States Department of Agriculture, 2000). This is supported by research that has consistently shown plant-based diets to be associated with lower risks of coronary heart disease (Krauss et al., 1996), cancer (American Cancer Society Advisory Committee, 1996), and type 2 diabetes mellitus (American Diabetes Association, 2000). Meats, on the other hand, are primary contributors of total fats, saturated fats, and cholesterol in the diet, and are associated with increased risk of chronic disease (Hu et al., 2000).

A diet high in protein and fat may seem to fulfill an ideal energy requirement to endure the cold, harsh, Tibetan climate. However, experiments show that both protein and energy intake is reduced during mountaineering expeditions (Zamboni et al., 1996), and a preference for carbohydrates usually develops. This may be due to metabolic reorganization of fuel substrates such that glucose is preferred over fatty acids as fuel for the heart and muscles, which improves the yield of adenosine triphosphate (ATP) per mole of O_2 consumed (Holden et al., 1995; Brooks at el., 1991). High-carbohydrate diets significantly improve oxygen tension and oxyhemoglobin saturation in arterial blood (Lawless et al., 1999) and increase lung-pulmonary diffusion capacity (Dramise et al., 1975). It would seem that carbohydrates, therefore, are the more efficient energy source for work at high altitude.

Although barley and wheat are significant carbohydrate sources, Tibetan highlanders rely on calorie-rich animal foods to meet their energy requirements. Yak has a thick layer of subcutaneous fat, and meat contains up to 20.84 and 23.6 percent fat and protein, respectively. Yak milk is 4.4 to 7.0 percent fat, up to twice the fat of Friesian cattle milk (3.5 percent), and has comparable protein content (Prasad, 1997). The cholesterol-raising effect of saturated fatty acids is believed to occur when the liver becomes enriched with myristic (14:0) and palmitic (16:0) acids, which shifts the regulatory pool of cholesterol esters to free cholesterol. This suppresses liver LDL receptor activity and drives circulatory levels up (Bergeron and Havel, 1997).

Despite a high–saturated-fat diet, Tibetan highlanders have a low serum cholesterol and serum apolipoprotein (apo) B and apoB/apoA-I ratio compared to Japanese controls (Fujimoto et al., 1989). Apolipoproteins are important in stabilizing and conferring specificity to the lipoprotein, allowing them to be recognized by specific receptors on cell surfaces. ApoB-100 is associated with LDL, and apoA-I with high-density lipoproteins (HDL). Since high HDL levels are associated with health benefits, and high LDL levels with health risks, it is desirable to have a low LDL/HDL (apoB/apoA-I) ratio in the interest of preventing CVD (Goodnight et al., 1982).

Despite low cholesterol levels, Tibetans have a serum lipid profile that shows a thrombogenic pattern: a high proportion of 16:0 and stearic acid (18:0) and a low proportion of linoleic acid (18:2, n-6)

(Fujimoto et al., 1989). Linoleic acid is a precursor for arachidonic acid (20:4, n-6) and eicosanoids such as prostaglandins and thromboxanes. Part of the mechanism by which diet, hypertension, and other stressors contribute to CVD development is through an imbalance between thromboxane A_2 (TXA_2), which promotes platelet aggregation and vasoconstriction, and prostaglandin I_2 (PGI_2), which has the opposite effects (Hirsh et al., 1981). Tibetans however, showed a discrepancy between serum total lipids and serum phospholipids: levels of 16:0 were low and levels of 18:2, n-6 were high. The fatty acid composition of serum phospholipids is considered important because of its influence on cell membrane structure and, ultimately, the function of membrane enzymes. Despite the thrombogenic fatty acid pattern in serum total lipids, the high proportion of unsaturated fatty acids in serum phospholipids may indicate a sort of defense mechanism in fatty acid metabolism against the development of atherosclerosis (Fujimoto et al., 1989). Not surprisingly, levels of eicosapentaenoic acid (20:5, n-3) (EPA), the omega-3 fatty acid responsible for the low incidence of CVD among the fish-consuming Inuit, was low in both serum total lipids and phospholipids (Fujimoto et al., 1989). This may be considered a disadvantage in preventing CVD development.

Lactose from milk consumption has been suspected as a possible risk factor for ischemic heart disease (Segall, 1994), as indicated by some epidemiological studies (Popham et al., 1983; Segall, 1980). The biological plausibility arises from calcium's ability to increase fecal excretion of lipids and hence elicit a hypolipidemic effect, but this is counteracted by lactose, which facilitates calcium absorption. This issue should not be of concern for Tibetans, however, since yak milk is made lactose-free via fermentation. As with other Asian populations, Tibetans are likely to be lactose intolerant. Lactose-free dairy products, such as butter and cheese, show no correlation with CVD (Segall, 1994).

TIBETAN MEDICINE

The impact of Tibetan medicine on CVD risks in Tibetan highlanders at first may seem ambiguous. The frequency that medicinal plants are ingested, if at all, among nomadic pastoralists is not certain. Wild garlic (*Allium cyaneum* Regel., Liliaceae), a Himalayan wildflower, is reportedly collected as a spice by the Hongyuan nomads of eastern Tibet (Blasum, 1997). Organosulfur compounds in the genus is well-known to reduce CVD risk by inhibiting platelet aggregation and reducing blood lipids (Bordia et al., 1998). Silverweed (*Potentilla anserina* L., Rosaceae) is also collected as food (Blasum, 1997). As a high-protein plant, it is encouraged as a supplement to prevent childhood malnutrition (Craig, 2003). Tibetans also use roseroot (*Rhodiola rosea* L., Crassulaceae) (E. W. Askew, personal communication, January 30, 2003), a well-studied Himalayan plant with numerous pharmacological properties, including powerful antioxidant activity attributed to its phenolic content. The plant is used traditionally as a powerful adaptogen to combat physical stress, toxins, cold, and high-altitude sickness (reviewed in Brown et al., 2002).

Whether ingested for their pharmacological effect or nutritive value, Tibetans have long recognized the medicinal properties of food and perceive them as important agents in therapy (Clark, 1995). The fundamental classic of Tibetan medicine, the *rGyud-bZhi*, or the *Four Tantras*, written in 1727, includes three chapters that address dietary principles for health maintenance and healing. In brief, health is maintained through the holistic harmony of the three humors: wind *(rlung)*, bile *(mKhris-pa)* and phlegm *(bad-kan)*, all of which are directly affected by diet. Understanding one's humoral disposition, the proper diet is prescribed as preventive medicine. So serious is the impact of diet that diseases in general are considered to have their roots in disorders of the digestive process.

According to Tibetan medical concepts, CVD is caused by mental depression, irregular meals, interrupted sleep, and violent anger. Seven types of CVD are recognized, each caused by an imbalance of a combination of different humors (*wind* heart pain, *wind* fever, *blood* heart pain, *blood* fever, etc.), each associated with specific symptoms and forms of treatment (Dorjee and Richards, 1985). In our search to explore Tibetan foods and medicines for antioxidants, we opted to study plants that were included most often (>30 percent) in compound medicines prescribed for all disorders of the cardiovascular system according to literature (Rinpoche, 1973; Tsarong, 1986; Dash, 1994). Fourteen plants (see Figure 2.1) were ultimately selected, collected, extracted, fractionated, and tested for their ability to scavenge free radicals and protect human LDL from in vitro oxida-

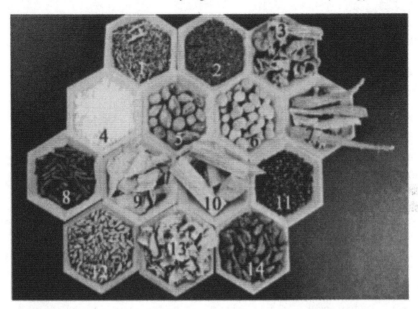

FIGURE 2.1. Plants most frequently occurring in Tibetan compound medicines prescribed for cardiovascular disorders. 1. Malabar nut, *Justicia adhatoda* Nees. (Acanthaceae); 2. Safflower, *Carthamus tinctorius* L. (Asteraceae); 3. Costus, *Saussaurea lappa* (Decne.) Sch. Bip. (Asteraceae); 4. Bamboo pith, *Bambusa arundinaceae* McClure. (Poaceae); 5. Myronbalan, *Terminalia chebula* Retz. (Combretaceae); 6. Nutmeg, *Myristica fragrans* Houtt. (Myristicaceae); 7. Elecampane, *Inula racemosa* Hook. f. (Asteraceae); 8. Long pepper, *Piper longum* L. (Piperaceae); 9. White sandalwood, *Santalum album* L. (Santalaceae); 10. Agarwood, *Aquilaria agallocha* Roxb. (Thymeliaceae); 11. Clove, *Syzygium aromaticum* (L.) Merr. & Perry. (Myrtaceae); 12. Cardamom, *Elletaria cardomomum* (L.) Maton. (Zingiberaceae); 13. Greater cardamom, *Hedychium spicatum* Ham. ex. Sm. (Zingiberaceae); 14. Spiked ginger lily, *Amomum sabulatum* Roxb. (Zingiberaceae).

tion. Interestingly, most were spices. Spices are common medicinal ingredients that are regarded as active elements in themselves or as facilitators and mediators of other bioactive compounds (Handa, 1998). Also included were the "Six Good Things" *(bzang-drug)*, which are considered essential for health maintenance and to "simply give happiness to people," according to Tibetan theory (Clifford, 1990). They are nutmeg, clove, greater cardamom, cardamom, saffron, and bamboo pith. It is therefore not surprising that such items are included in numerous compound medicines.

Most plants tested positive for free radical scavenging activity, particularly agarwood, greater cardamom, malabar nut, nutmeg, sandalwood, clove, and myrobalan. Myrobalan in particular had the strongest activity, comparable to vitamin C, catechin, epicatechin, and quercetin (Owen and Johns, 2002); a finding that is corroborated with previous studies (Vani et al., 1997; Maulik et al., 1996). The high concentration of tannins (up to 32 percent) in the fruit is assumed to be responsible, which may limit its use as an internal medicine since tannins bind readily to proteins (Okuda et al., 1991). Nonetheless, small amounts are absorbed and may elicit a therapeutic effect. Other antioxidants in myrobalan include vitamin C, vanillic acid, ferulic acid, caffeic acid and p-coumaric acid (Kim et al., 1993). Myrobalan has a special significance in Tibetan medicine: the Medicine Buddha is traditionally depicted holding the plant in his right hand in the gesture of giving (Clifford, 1990). Considered the "all-conquering king of medicines," legend maintains the tree grew from drops of nectar released from the gods (Rinpoche, 1977). Its potent antioxidant action may explain its use for the past 3,000 years in Ayurveda and its occurrence in hundreds of compound medicines prescribed for a variety of disorders.

Clove, another commonly occurring ingredient in Tibetan medicine, displayed extraordinary LDL-protective effects in our assay, almost fourfold greater than a water-soluble analog of vitamin E (Owen and Johns, 2002). The lipophilic phenylpropanoids eugenol and isoeugenol in the essential oil were likely able to infiltrate the lipoprotein membrane and thus were better positioned to inhibit peroxidation. Eugenol and isoeugenol also occur in nutmeg. According to Tibetan medical theory, clove is specifically used for the "life-vein, which is connected to the heart and where the subtle life force serving as a mount for consciousness resides" (Clifford, 1990). Consequently, clove is an almost universal ingredient of compound medicines prescribed for heart and cardiovascular disorders.

Additional benefits may have been obtained from plant ingredients that may not have had particularly strong antioxidant activity, but either have cardioprotective properties of their own or act synergistically or cumulatively with other bioactive elements. Long pepper serves as a good example: it has previously demonstrated hypocholesterolemic (Bao and Wu, 1992) and coronary vasodilating activity (Shoji et al., 1986b), and is also able to enhance the bioavailability of other bioactive principles of coingested medicines (Atal et al., 1981). Saffron (*Crocus sativus* L.) is able to increase oxygen diffusion in plasma and reduce cholesterol and triglyceride levels (Gainer and Jones, 1975). Epidemiological evidence also suggests that the low incidence of CVD in parts of Spain may be related to the liberal, almost daily consumption of saffron (Grisiola, 1974). Table 2.1 summarizes the pharmacology of these plants according to traditional Tibetan and biomedical concepts.

Clearly, antioxidants form the therapeutic basis for several indigenous drugs, which may explain the efficacy of Tibetan medicines used for ROS-mediated pathologies such as arthritis (Ryan, 1997), intermittent claudation (Sallon et al., 1998), and atherosclerosis (Gieldanowski et al., 1992). Similarly, combinations of different antioxidants confer greater protection from LDL peroxidation than when used singly (Knudsen et al., 1996). Such is the reasoning behind the use of compound medicines, which is the fundamental characteristic of Tibetan medicine. As a holistic therapeutic medical system, symptomatic treatment of individual organs is supplemented with medicines that increase drug efficacy and decrease toxicity while supporting other organs and body systems. Similar reasoning can be extended to the functional complexity of diets, such that isolated nutraceuticals often do not provide the health benefits derived from whole foods (Marchioli et al., 2001), particularly in the case for chronic-diseases prevention.

SUMMARY

A complex interplay between risk factors and protective elements results in low CVD prevalence among Tibetan highlanders, suggesting either genetic involvement or behavioral modifications to ingest functional dietary elements. In my attempt to review biotic and abiotic influences on CVD risks, the primary consideration remains the physiological distinctness of the population under study. The Tibetan highlander diet is unique in itself and, if considered independently, would facilitate interpretations concerning health and disease. However, dietary behavior has evolved in direct response to the environment, such that reliance on livestock, and not agricultural prod-

TABLE 2.1. Tibetan traditional and biomedical pharmacology of plants included in our analysis. Although plants usually possess more than one bioactive property, only those related to CVD indices are listed.

Family, English, and Tibetan name	Tibetan ethnopharmacology	Biomedical pharmacology
Acanthaceae Malabar nut Ba śa ka	Cures blood fevers (Clark, 1995)	Increases endogenous antioxidant enzyme activity and is a chemical chemopreventative (Singh et al., 2000)
Asteraceae Safflower Gur gum	Cures all types of liver diseases, closes rupture of blood vessels (Clark, 1995)	Unsaturated fatty acids can reduce cholesterol levels. Increases platelet linoleic acid levels associated with a change in thromboxane B_2 levels (Cox et al., 1998)
Asteraceae Costus Ru rta	Wind and blood regulator, cures angina (Tsarong, 1994)	Coronary vasodilating activity (Shoji et al., 1986a)
Asteraceae Elecampane Ma nu	Pain in upper body, analgesic (Tsarong, 1994)	Anti-ischemic activity and prevention of angina (Tripathi et al., 1984)
Combretaceae Myrobalan A ru ra	Cures all disease of wind, bile, and phlegm, wholesome for the body (Clark, 1995)	Reduces serum lipids and cholesterol in rats (Khanna et al., 1993)
Iridaceae Saffron Gur gum	Cures all types of liver diseases, closes rupture of blood vessels (Clark, 1995)	Crocetin increases oxygen diffusion in plasma. Decreases cholesterol and triglyceride levels (Gainer and Jones, 1975)
Myristicaceae Nutmeg Dza' ti	Removes wind disorders, cures heart disorders (Clark, 1995)	Eugenol inhibits prostaglandin synthesis and action, and inhibits platelet aggregation (Janssens et al., 1990)
Myrtaceae Clove Li śi	Cures disorders of life channel (e.g., aorta), cold wind disorders (Clark, 1995)	Eugenol inhibits prostaglandin biosynthesis and platelet aggregation (Rasheed et al., 1984); antithrombotic activity (Srivastava, 1993)
Piperaceae Long pepper Pi pi ling	Cures all cold and wind disorders (Clark, 1995)	Coronary vasodilating activity (Shoji et al., 1986b); Hypocholesterolemic in mice (Bao and Wu, 1992)

Family, English, and Tibetan name	Tibetan ethnopharmacology	Biomedical pharmacology
Poaceae Bamboo pith *Cu gan*	Cures all lung diseases, reduces fevers associated with wounds (Clark, 1995)	Bamboo pith is predominantly silica, which has an antiatheromatous effect in rabbits fed an atherogenic diet (Trinca et al., 1999)
Santalaceae White sandalwood *Tsan dan dkar po*	Cures fever of the heart (Clark, 1995)	Oil is a popular fragrance with little medicinal use. Diuretic and urinary antiseptic properties (Leung, 1980).
Thymeliaceae Agarwood *A ga ru*	Cures fevers of the heart and life channel (Clark, 1995)	Oil is a popular fragrance. Benzene extract has central nervous system depressant activity (Okugawa et al., 1993)
Zingiberaceae Greater cardamom *Ka ko la*	Cures cold disorders of stomach and spleen (Clark, 1995)	Main constituent, 1,8-cineole, has hypotensive effect in i.v.-treated normotensive rats (Lahlou et al., 2002)
Zingiberaceae Cardamom *Sug smel*	Cures cold kidney and wind disorders (Clark, 1995)	Reduces blood pressure in rats (Haranath et al., 1987)
Zingiberaceae Spiked ginger lily *Gah-kyah*	Destroys "cold" tumors, alleviates disorders of phlegm and wind, dissolves congealed blood (Tsarong, 1994)	Reduces blood pressure in i.v.-treated anesthetized dog (Shaw, 1980)

ucts, for sustenance has constituted a more practical subsistence alternative. A virtually unaddressed issue is whether Tibetan highlanders, whose adaptation to high altitude is well established, are equally adapted to their high saturated fat, low fruit and vegetable diet, particularly when faced with increased oxidative stress at altitude. Or, as proposed here, they have developed ingestive behaviors that incorporate foods and adjuncts that contain prophylactic elements. The issue is clearly complex and multifaceted, requiring further investigation.

REFERENCES

Abeywardena, M.Y. and R.J. Head (2001). Longchain n-3 polyunsaturated fatty acids and blood vessel function. *Cardiovascular Research* 52: 361-371.

Agostoni, A., G.C. Gerli, L. Beretta, G. Palazzini, G.P. Buso, H. Xusheng, and G. Moschini (1983). Erythrocyte antioxidant enzymes and selenium serum levels in an Andean population. *Clinica Chimica Acta* 133: 153-157.

Aldenderfer, M. (1999). The Pleistocene/Holocene transition in Peru and its effects upon human use of the landscape. *Quaternary International* 53/54: 11-19.

Altahan, A., J. Buchur, F. Elkhwsky, A. Ogunniyi, S. Alrajeh, E. Larbi, A. Daif, and E. Bamgboye (1998). Risk factors of stroke at high and low altitude areas of Saudi Arabia. *Archives of Medical Research* 29: 173-177.

American Cancer Society Advisory Committee (1996). Guidelines on diet, nutrition, and cancer prevention: Reducing the risk of cancer with healthy food choices and physical activity. *CA: A Cancer Journal for Clinicians* 46: 325-341.

American Diabetes Association (2000). Nutrition recommendations and principles for people with diabetes mellitus. *Diabetes Care* 19: S47-S49.

Askew, E.W. (2002). Work at high altitude and oxidative stress: Antioxidant nutrients. *Toxicology* 180: 107-119.

Atal, C.K., U. Zutshi, and P.G. Rao (1981). Scientific evidence on the role of Ayurvedic herbals on bioavailability of drugs. *Journal of Ethnopharmacology* 4: 229-232.

Bao, Z.T. and E. Wu (1992). Effects of unsaponifiable matter of the *Piper longum* oil on cholesterol biosynthesis in experimental hypercholesterolemic mice. *Chung Tsào Yao* 23: 197-199.

Beall, C.M., J. Blangero, S. Williams-Blangero, and M.C. Goldstein (1994). Major gene for percent of oxygen saturation of arterial hemoglobin in Tibetan highlanders. *American Journal of Physical Anthropology* 95: 271-276.

Beall, C.M., G.M. Brittenham, F. Macuaga, and M. Barragan (1990). Variation in hemoglobin concentration among samples of high-altitude natives in the Andes and the Himalayas. *American Journal of Human Biology* 2: 639-652.

Beall, C.M. and M.C. Goldstein (1993). Dietary seasonality among Tibetan nomads. *National Geographic Research and Exploration* 9: 475-479.

Beall, C.M., J. Henry, C. Worthman, and M.C. Goldstein (1996). Basal metabolic rate and dietary seasonality among Tibetan nomads. *American Journal of Human Biology* 8: 361-370.

Beall, C.M., K.P. Strohl, J. Blangero, S. Williams-Blangero, L.A. Almasy, M.J. Decker, C.M. Worthman, M.C. Goldstein, E. Vargas, M. Villena, R. Soria, A.M. Alarcon, and C. Gonzalez (1997). Ventilation and hypoxic ventilatory response of Tibetan and Aymara high-altitude natives. *American Journal of Physical Anthropology* 104: 427-447.

Bergeron, N. and R.J. Havel (1997). Assessment of postprandial lipemia: Nutritional influences. *Current Opinion in Lipidology* 8: 43-52.

Blasum, H. (1997). Ethnobotany of Hongyuan nomads. Available online at http://www.blasum.net/holger/wri/alpeg/mumin/nomadeng.html.

Bordia, A., S.K. Verma, and K.C. Srivastava (1998). Effect of garlic *(Allium sativum)* on blood lipids, blood sugar, fibrinogen and fibrinolytic activity in patients with coronary artery disease. *Prostaglandins, Leukotrienes and Essential Fatty Acids* 58: 257-263.

Brantingham, P.J., M. Haizou, J.W. Olsen, G. Xing, D.B. Madsen, and D.E. Rhode (2003). Speculation on the timing and nature of Late Pleistocene hunter-gatherer colonization of the Tibetan plateau. *Chinese Science Bulletin* 48 (14): 1510-1516.

Brooks, G.A., G.E. Butterfield, R.R. Wolfe, B.M. Groves, R.S. Mazzeo, J.R. Sutton, E.E. Wolfel, and J. T. Reeves (1991). Increased dependence on blood glucose after acclimatization to 4,300 m. *Journal of Applied Physiology* 70: 919-927.

Brown, R.P., P.L. Gerbarg, and Z. Ramazanov (2002). *Rhodiola roseus:* A phytochemical overview. *HerbalGram* 56: 40-52.

Burger, W.C., A.A. Qureshi, Z.Z. Din, N. Abuirmeileh, and C.E. Elson (1984). Suppression of cholesterol biosynthesis by constituents of barley kernel. *Atherosclerosis* 51: 75-87.

Cao, J., Y. Zhao, J.W. Liu, X.X. Bai, D.Y. Zhou, S.L. Fang, M. Jia, and J.S. Wu (1996). Fluorine intake of a Tibetan population. *Food and Chemical Toxicology* 34: 755-757.

Chang, S.W., T.J. Stelzner, J.V. Weil, and N.F. Voelkel (1989). Hypoxia increases plasma glutathione disulfide in rats. *Lung* 165: 269-276.

Clark, B. (1995). *The quintessence of Tibetan medicine.* Ithaca, NY: Snow Lion Publications.

Clifford, T. (1990). *Tibetan Buddhist medicine and psychiatry.* York Beach, ME: Samuel Weiser Inc.

Cox, C., W. Sutherland, J. Mann, S. deJong, A. Chrisholm, and M. Skeaff (1998). Effects of dietary coconut oil, butter and safflower oil on plasma lipids, lipoproteins and lathosterol levels. *European Journal of Clinical Nutrition* 52: 650-654.

Craig, S. (2003). Saving Tibet's children. *Kyoto Journal* 53: 15-17.

Dash, V.B. (1994). *Pharmacopoeia of Tibetan medicine.* Delhi: Sri Satguru Publications.

deWhalley, C.V., S.M. Rankin, J.R. Hoult, W. Jessup, and D.S. Leake (1990). Flavonoids inhibit the oxidative modification of low-density lipoproteins by macrophages. *Biomedical Pharmacology* 39: 1743-1750.

Dorjee, P. and E. Richards (1985). Cures and concepts of Tibetan medicine. *Tibetan Medicine* 2: 7-56.

Dramise, J.G., C.M. Inouye, B.M. Christensen, R.D. Fults, J.E. Canham, and C.F. Consolazio (1975). Effects of a glucose meal on human pulmonary function at 1600 m and 4300 m altitudes. *Aviation Space and Environmental Medicine* 46: 365-368.

Duh, P.D., G.C. Yen, W.J. Yen, and L.W. Chang (2001). Antioxidant effects of water extracts from barley (*Hordeum vulgare* L.) prepared under different roasting temperatures. *Journal of Agricultural and Food Chemistry* 49: 1455-1463.

Fujimaki, T., M. Matsutani, A. Asai, T. Kohno, and M. Koike (1986). Cerebral venous thrombosis due to high altitude polycythemia. Case report. *Journal of Neurosurgery* 64: 148-150.

Fujimoto, N., K. Matsubayashi, T. Miyahara, A. Murai, M. Matsuda, H. Shio, H. Suzuki, M. Kameyama, A. Saito, and L. Shuping (1989). The risk factors for ischemic heart disease in Tibetan highlanders. *Japanese Heart Journal* 30: 27-34.

Gainer, J.L. and J.R. Jones (1975). The use of crocetin in experimental atherosclerosis. *Experientia* 31: 548-549.

Gey, K.F., U.K. Moser, P. Jordan, H.B. Stähelin, M. Eichholzer, and E. Lüdin (1993). Increased risk of cardiovascular disease at suboptimal plasma concentrations of essential antioxidants: An epidemiological update with special attention to carotene and vitamin C. *American Journal of Clinical Nutrition* 57: 787S-797S.

Gieldanowski, J., T. Dutkiewicz, L. Samochowiec, and J. Wójcicki (1992). Padma 28 modifies immunological functions in experimental atherosclerosis in rabbits. *Archivum Immunologiae et Therapiae Experimentalis* 40: 291-295.

Giussani, D.A., P.S. Phillips, S. Anstee, and D.J.P. Barker (2001). Effects of altitude versus economic status on birth weight and body shape at birth. *Pediatric Research* 49: 490-494.

Goldberg, M.A., S.P. Dunning, and H.F. Bunn (1988). Regulation of the erythropoietin gene: Evidence that the oxygen sensor is a heme protein. *Science* 242: 1412-1415.

Goodnight, S.H., Jr., W.S. Harris, W.E. Connor, and D.R. Illingworth (1982). Polyunsaturated fatty acids, hyperlipidemia, and thrombosis. *Arteriosclerosis* 2: 87-113.

Goupy, P., M. Hugues, P. Boivin, and M.J. Amiot (1999). Antioxidant composition and activity of barley *(Hordeum vulgare)* and malt extracts and of isolated phenolic compounds. *Journal of the Science of Food and Agriculture* 79: 1625-1634.

Grisolia, S. (1974). Hypoxia, saffron and cardiovascular disease. *Lancet* 2: 41.

Handa, S.S. (1998). The integration of food and medicine in India. In Pendergast, H.D.V., N.L. Etkin, D.R. Harris, and P.J. Houghton (Eds.), *Plants for food and medicine* (pp. 57-68). Kew: Royal Botanical Gardens.

Hanna, J.M. (1999). Climate, altitude, and blood pressure. *Human Biology* 71: 553-582.

Haranath, P.S.R.K., M.H. Akther, and S.I. Sharif (1987). Acetylcholine and choline in common spices. *Phytotherapy Research* 1: 91-92.

Health Canada (1997). *Canada's food guide to healthy eating*. Ottawa: Minister of Supply and Services Canada.

Hertog, M.G.L., D. Kromhout, C. Aravanis, H. Blackburn, R. Buzina, F. Fidanza, S. Giampaoli, A. Jansen, A. Menotti, and S. Nedeljkovic (1995). Flavonoid intake and long-term risk of coronary heart disease and cancer in the Seven Countries Study. *Archives of Internal Medicine* 155: 381-386.

Hirsh, P.D., W.B. Campbell, J.T. Willerson, and L.D. Hillis (1981). Prostaglandins and ischemic heart disease. *American Journal of Medicine* 71: 1009-1021.

Hochachka, P.W., J.L. Rupert, and C. Monge (1999). Adaptation and conservation of physiological systems in the evolution of human hypoxia tolerance. *Comparative Biochemistry and Physiology Part A* 124: 1-17.

Holden, J.E., C.K. Stone, W.D. Brown, R.J. Nickles, C. Stanley, C.M. Clark, and P.W. Hochachka (1995). Enhanced cardiac metabolism of plasma glucose in high altitude natives: Adaptations against chronic hypoxia. *Journal of Applied Physiology* 79: 222-228.

Hu, F.B., E.B. Rimm, M.J. Stampfer, A. Ascherio, D. Spiegelman, and W.C. Willett (2000). Prospective study of major dietary patterns and risk of coronary heart disease in men. *American Journal of Clinical Nutrition* 72: 912-921.

Ishikawa, T., M. Suzukawa, T. Ito, H. Yoshida, M. Ayaori, M. Nishiwaki, A. Yonemura, Y. Hara, and H. Nakamura (1997). Effect of tea flavonoid supplementation on the susceptibility of low-density lipoprotein to oxidative modifications. *American Journal of Clinical Nutrition* 66: 261-266.

Janssens, J., G.M. Laekeman, L.A. Pieters, J. Totte, A.G. Herman, and A.J. Vlietinck (1990). Nutmeg oil: Identification and quantification of its most active constituents as inhibitors of platelet aggregation. *Journal of Ethnopharmacology* 29: 179-188.

Jensen, G.M. and L.G. Moore (1997). The effect of high altitude and other risk factors on birthweight: Independent or interactive effects? *American Journal of Public Health* 87: 1003-1007.

Jialal, I. and S. Grundy (1992). The effect of dietary supplementation with alpha-tocopherol on the oxidative modification of low-density lipoprotein. *Journal of Lipid Research* 33: 899-906.

Jin, C., Z. Yan, and L. Jianwei (2001). Processing procedures of brick tea and their influence on fluorine content. *Food and Chemical Toxicology* 39: 959-962.

Johns, T. (1996). Phytochemicals as evolutionary mediators of human nutritional physiology. *International Journal of Pharmacognosy* 34: 327-334.

Khanna, A.K., R. Chander, N.K. Kapoor, C. Singh, and A.K. Shrivastava (1993). Hypoglycemic activity of *Terminalia chebula* in rats. *Fitoterapia* 64: 351-356.

Kim, J.S., G.D. Lee, J.H. Kwon, and H.S. Joon (1993). Identification of phenolic antioxidant components in *Terminalia chebula* Retz. *Journal of Korean Agricultural and Chemical Society* 36: 239-243.

Knudsen, C.A., A.L. Tappel, and J.A. North (1996). Multiple antioxidants protect against heme protein and lipid oxidation in kidney tissue. *Free Radical Biology and Medicine* 20: 165-173.

Kono, S., K. Shinchi, N. Ikeda, F. Yanai, and K. Imanishi (1992). Green tea consumption and serum lipid profiles: A cross-sectional study in northern Kyushu, Japan. *Preventive Medicine* 21: 526-531.

Krauss, R.M., R.J. Deckelbaum, N. Ernst, E. Fisher, B.V. Howard, R.H. Knopp, T. Kotchen, A.H. Lichtenstein, H.C. McGill, T.A. Pearson, et al. (1996). Dietary guidelines for healthy American adults: A statement for health professionals from the Nutrition Committee, American Heart Association. *Circulation* 94: 1795-1800.

Kröner, C. (1999). *Alpine plant life: Functional plant ecology of high mountain ecosystems.* Berlin: Springer-Verlag Berlin Heidelberg.

Kuhnlein, H.V., S. Kubow, and R. Soueida (1991). Lipid components of traditional Inuit foods and diets of Baffin Island. *Journal of Food Composition and Analysis* 4: 227-236.

Lahlou, S., A.F. Figueiredo, P.J. Magalhaes, and J.H. Leal-Cardoso (2002). Cardiovascular effects of 1,8-cineole, a terpenoid oxide present in many plant essential oils, in normotensive rats. *Canadian Journal of Physiology and Pharmacology* 80: 1125-1131.

Lawless, N.P., T.A. Dillard, K.G. Torrington, H.Q. Davis, and G. Kamimori (1999). Improvement in hypoxia at 4600 meters of simulated altitude with carbohydrate ingestion. *Aviation, Space and Environmental Medicine* 70: 874-878.

Leung, A.Y. (1980). *Encyclopedia of common natural ingredients used in food, drugs and cosmetics.* New York: J. Wiley and Sons.

Majupuria, I. and D. Lobsang (2000). *Tibetan cooking.* Bangkok: Crafsman Press.

Marchioli, R., C. Schweiger, G. Levantesi, L. Tavazzi, and F. Valagussa (2001). Antioxidant vitamins and prevention of cardiovascular disease: Epidemiological and clinical trial data. *Lipids* 36: S53-S63.

Marriot, B.M. and S.J. Carlson-Newberry (1996). *Nutritional needs in cold and high-altitude environments: Applications for military personnel in field operations.* Washington, DC: National Academy Press.

Maulik, G., V.E. Kagam, S. Pakrashi, N. Maulik, and D.K. Das (1996). Extracts of some Indian plants with potent antioxidant properties. In Packer, L., M.G. Traber, and W. Xin (Eds.), *Proceedings of the International Symposium on Natural Antioxidants: Molecular mechanisms and health effects* (pp. 90-98). Champaign, IL: AOS Press.

McIntosh, G.H., R.K. Newman, and C.W. Newman (1995). Barley foods and their influence on cholesterol metabolism. *World Review of Nutrition and Dietetics* 77: 89-108.

McIntosh, G.M., J. Whyte, R. McArthur, and P.J. Nestel (1991). Barley and wheat foods: Influence on plasma cholesterol concentrations in hypercholesterolemic men. *American Journal of Clinical Nutrition* 53: 1205-1209.

Møller, P., S. Loft, C. Lunby, and N.V. Olsen (2001). Acute hypoxia and hypoxic exercise induce DNA strand breaks and oxidative DNA damage in humans. *FASEB Journal* 15: 1181-1186.

Monge, C.C., A. Arregui, and F. Leon-Velarde (1992). Pathophysiology and epidemiology of chronic mountain sickness. *International Journal of Sports Medicine* 13: S79-S81.

Moore, L.G., L. Curran-Everett, T.S. Droma, B.M. Groves, R.E. McCullough, R.G. McCullough, S.F. Sun, J.R. Sutton, S. Zamudio, and J.G. Zhuang (1992). Are Tibetans better adapted? *International Journal of Sports Medicine* 13: S86-S88.

Nakanishi, K., F. Tajima, A. Nakamura, S. Yagura, T. Okawara, H. Yamashita, K. Suzuki, N. Taniguchi, and H. Ohno (1995). Effects of hypobaric hypoxia on antioxidant enzymes in rats. *Journal of Physiology* 489: 869-876.

Okuda, T., T. Yoshida, and T. Hatano (1991). Chemistry and biological activity of tannins in medicinal plants. In Wagner, H. and N.R. Farnsworth (Eds.), *Economic and Medicinal plant research*, Volume 5 (pp. 389-419). London: Academic Press.

Okugawa, H., R. Ueda, K. Matsumoto, K. Kawanishi, and A. Kato (1993). Effect of agarwood exracts on the central nervous system in mice. *Planta Medica* 59: 32-36.

Owen, P.L. and T. Johns (2002). Antioxidants in medicines and spices as cardioprotective agents in Tibetan highlanders. *Pharmaceutical Biology* 40: 346-357.

Peng, A., C. Yang, H. Rui, and H. Li (1992). Study on the pathogenic factors of Kashin-Beck disease. *Journal of Toxicology and Environment Health* 35: 79-90.

Popham, R.E., W. Schmidt, and Y. Israel (1983). Variation in mortality from ischaemic heart disease in relation to alcohol and milk consumption. *Medical Hypotheses* 12: 321-329.

Prasad, S.K. (1997). The yak: A valuable genetic resource of alpine region. *Indian Journal of Animal Sciences* 67: 517-520.

Rasheed, A., G. Laekeman, J. Totte, A.J. Vlietinck, and A.G. Herman (1984). Eugenol and prostaglandin biosynthesis. *New England Journal of Medicine* 310: 50-51.

Ren, H.X., Z.L. Wang, X. Chen, and Y.L. Zhu (1999). Antioxidative response to different altitudes in *Plantago major*. *Environmental and Experimental Botany* 42: 51-59.

Riemersma, R.A., D.A. Wood, C.C.A. Macintyre, R.A. Elton, K.F. Gey, and M.F. Oliver (1991). Risk of angina pectoris and plasma concentration of vitamins A, C, and E and carotene. *Lancet* 337: 1-5.

Rinpoche, R. (1973). *Tibetan medicine*. Berkeley: University of California Press.

Rupert, J.L. and P.W. Hochachka (2001). Genetic approaches to understanding human adaptation in the Andes. *Journal of Experimental Biology* 204: 3151-3160.

Ryan, M. (1997). Efficacy of the Tibetan treatment for arthritis. *Social Science and Medicine* 44: 535-539.

Sallon, S., G. Beer, J. Rosenfeld, H. Anner, D. Volcoff, G. Ginsberg, O. Paltiel, and Y. Berlatzky (1998). The efficacy of Padma 28, a herbal preparation, in the treatment of intermittent claudation: A controlled double-blind pilot study with the objective assessment of chronic occlusive arterial disease patients. *Journal of Vascular Investigations* 4: 129-136.

Samaja, M., C. Mariani, A. Prestini, and P. Cerretelli (1997). Acid-base balance and O_2 transport at high altitude. *Acta Physiologia Scandanavia* 159: 249-256.

Sarada, S.K.S., M. Sairam, P. Dipti, B. Anju, T. Pauline, A.K. Kain, S.K. Sharma, S. Bagawat, G. Ilavazhagan, and D. Kumar (2002). Role of selenium in reducing hypoxia-induced oxidative stress: An in vivo study. *Biomedicine and Pharmacotherapy* 56: 173-178.

Saralakumari, D. and P.R. Rao (1991). Erythrocyte glutathione metabolism in human chronic fluoride toxicity. *Biochemistry International* 23: 349-357.

Segall, J.J. (1980). Hypothesis: Is lactose a dietary risk factor for ischaemic heart disease? *International Journal of Epidemiology* 9: 271-276.

Segall, J.J. (1994). Dietary lactose as a possible risk factor for ischaemic heart disease: Review of epidemiology. *International Journal of Cardiology* 46: 197-207.

Sharma, A. and N.J. Chinoy (1998). Role of free radicals in fluoride-induced toxicity in liver and kidney of mice and its reversal. *Fluoride* 31: S26.

Shaw, B.P. (1980). Effect of kapur kachari *(Hedychium spicatum)* on the blood pressure and respiration of the anesthetized dog. *Nagarjun* 24: 7-9.

Shivashankara, A.R., Y.M. Shivarajashankara, P.G. Bhat, and S.H. Rao (2002). Lipid peroxidation and antioxidant defense systems in liver of rats in chronic fluoride toxicity. *Bulletin of Environmental Contamination and Toxicology* 68: 612-616.

Shoji, N., A. Umeyama, N. Saito, T. Takemoto, A. Kajiwara, and Y. Ohizumi (1986a). Vasoactive substance from *Saussurea lappa. Journal of Natural Products* 49: 1112-1113.

Shoji, N., A. Umeyama, N. Saito, T. Takemoto, A. Kajiwara, and Y. Ohizumi (1986b). Dehydropipernonaline, an amide possessing coronary vasodilating activity, isolated from *Piper longum* L. *Journal of Pharmaceutical Sciences* 75: 1188-1189.

Simon-Schnass, I. (1996). Oxidative stress during exercise at high altitude and effects of vitamin E. In Marriott, B.M. and S.J. Carlson (Eds.), *Nutritional needs in cold and high altitude environments* (pp. 393-418). Washington, DC: National Academy Press.

Singh, R.P., B. Padmavathi, and A.R. Rao (2000). Modulatory influence of *Adhatoda vesica (Justicia adhatoda)* leaf extract on the enzymes of xenobiotic metabolism, antioxidant status and lipid peroxidation in mice. *Molecular and Cellular Biology* 213: 99-109.

Srivastava, K.C. (1993). Antiplatelet principles from a food spice clove (*Syzygium aromaticum* L.). *Prostaglandins, Leukotrienes and Essential Fatty Acids* 48: 363-372.

Suetens, C., R. Moreno-Reyes, C. Chasseur, F. Mathieu, F. Begaux, E. Haubuge, M.C. Durand, J. Nève, and J. Vanderpas (2001). Epidemiological support for a multifactorial aetiology of Kashin-Beck disease in Tibet. *International Orthopaedics* 25: 180-187.

Sun, S.F. (1986). Epidemiology of hypertension on the Tibetan plateau. *Human Biology* 58: 507-515.

Sztarbala, T., R. Gos, J. Kedziora, J. Blaszczyk, E. Sibinska, and M. Goralczyk (1998). Changes in the antioxidant system of the vitreous in rabbits after administration of sulfur hexafluoride. *Klinika Oczna* 100: 69-71.

Temte, J.L. (1996). Elevation of serum cholesterol at high altitude and its relationship to hematocrit. *Wilderness and Environmental Medicine* 7: 216-224.

Trinca, L., O. Popescu, and I. Palamaru (1999). Serum lipid picture of rabbits fed on silicate-supplemented atherogenic diet. *Revista Medico—Chiruricala A Societatii de Medici si Naturalisti Din Iasi* 103: 99-102.

Tripathi, S.N., B.N. Upadhyaya, and V.K. Gupka (1984). Beneficial effect of *Inula racemosa* (Pushkarmoola) in angina pectoris: A preliminary report. *Indian Journal of Physiology and Pharmacology* 28: 73-75.

Trustwell, A.S. (2002). Cereal grains and coronary heart disease. *European Journal of Clinical Nutrition* 56: 1-14.

Tsarong, T.J. (1986). *Handbook of traditional Tibetan drugs.* Kalimpong: Tibetan Medical Publications.

Tsarong, T.J. (1994). *Tibetan medicinal plants.* Kalimpong: Tibetan Medical Publications.

United States Department of Agriculture (2000). *Nutrition and your health: Dietary guidelines for Americans.* Home and Garden Bulletin no. 232. Washington, DC: Government Printing Office.

Vani, T., M. Rajani, S. Sarkar, and C. J. Shishoo (1997). Antioxidant activity of the Ayurvedic formulation Triphala and its constituents. *International Journal of Pharmacognosy* 35: 313-317.

Vaz, M., T.T. Ukyab, R. Padmavathi, R. Kuriyan, S. Muthayya, B. Diffey, and A.V. Kurpad (1999). Body fat topography in Indian and Tibetan males of low and normal body mass index. *Indian Journal of Physiology & Pharmacology* 43: 179-185.

Weisburger, J.H. (1999). Tea and health: The underlying mechanisms. *Proceedings of the Society for Experimental Biology and Medicine* 220: 271-275.

Wildi, B. and C. Lütz (1996). Antioxidant composition of selected high alpine plant species from different altitudes. *Plant, Cell and Environment* 19: 138-146.

Wiley, A.S. (1994). Neonatal and maternal anthropometric characteristics in a high altitude population of the Western Himalaya. *American Journal of Human Biology* 6: 499-510.

Wursch, P. and F.X. Pi-Sunyer (1997). The role of viscous soluble fiber in the metabolic control of diabetes. A review with special emphasis on cereals rich in beta-glucan. *Diabetes Care* 20: 1774-1780.

Young, T.K., M.E.M. Moffatt, and J.D. O'Neil (1993). Cardiovascular diseases in a Canadian Arctic population. *American Journal of Public Health* 83: 881-887.

Zamboni, M., F. Armellini, E. Turcato, R. Robbi, R. Micciolo, T. Todesco, R. Mandragona, G. Angelini, and O. Bosello (1996). Effect of altitude on body composition during mountaineering expeditions: Interrelationships with changes in dietary habits. *Annals of Nutrition and Metabolism* 40: 315-324.

Zamudio, S., T. Droma, K.Y. Norkyel, G. Acharya, J.A. Zamudio, S.N. Neirmeyer, and L.G. Moore (1993). Protection from intrauterine growth retardation in Tibetans at high altitude. *American Journal of Physical Anthropology* 94: 215-224.

Zhimin, A. (1982). Paleoliths and microliths from Shenja and Shuanghu, Northern Tibet. *Current Anthropology* 23: 493-499.

Chapter 3

Wild Food Plants in Farming Environments with Special Reference to Northeast Thailand, Food As Functional and Medicinal, and the Social Roles of Women

Lisa Leimar Price

INTRODUCTION

I had my first encounter with nondomesticated wild plant foods in 1986, while conducting research in Northeast Thailand for my master's degree in anthropology. I had originally planned a time-and-labor allocation study on vegetable gardening. I was amazed that I saw virtually nothing that I could recognize as a garden and wondered about the origin of the strange and various vegetables that I saw people eating in the small village of my study. As I followed women around in their daily activities, it then became clear: women gathered plant foods from every imaginable location, most often in association with other tasks, such as irrigating rice fields that held seedlings, on their way to cultivate their more distant cassava fields, or collecting a bit of this or that in the general village surroundings. For the total observations of food procurement/production activities, women spent 4.35 percent of their time on actual vegetable gardens but 31.88 percent of their time on the collection of wild foods (collection of plants and small protein items such as frogs, freshwater crabs, and insects) (Leimar, 1987). Since this first encounter, my interest in and research on wild plant foods has continued and grown with field research in a number of regions in Thailand and the Philippines.

This chapter represents some of my findings over the years, some of the important themes, and some of the questions that have emerged for me. The research of others who have published on wild plant foods has been critical to enhancing my understanding of patterns of gathering, marketing, and use. I also look at what researchers have reported from other regions of Asia and the world that I believe point to important questions or indicate that patterns or issues I put forth are of a cross-cultural nature. I do not claim that this chapter reviews all the literature on wild food plants from agricultural environments, but it does set forth some of the themes of concern regarding gender, availability, use, and management of plants from disturbed environments and the overlap of wild plant foods with medicine and as functional foods.

With regard to gathering rights and management, I attempt to explore the role of multiuse value and perceived rarity beyond what I have previously published. It is at this juncture that the overlap of food, functional food, and medicine has a special consideration. Of particular concern are the factors that act as a stimulus to the protection and conservation as well as the privatization of these resources. The links to the physical environment, environmental change, and marketing of these plant foods are critical to our understanding of availability and use of these plant foods as well. Intimately intertwined with these issues are the specific roles played by women and gender. Women farmers are at the center of wild plant food use and management in Northeast Thailand and appear to be so in numerous studies of communities around the globe.

WILD PLANT FOODS
IN THE FARMING ENVIRONMENT

Among researchers, interest in wild plant foods has been increasing over the past two decades as a growing number of studies document the collection and consumption of wild plant foods from agricultural environments (see Scoones et al., 1992). As a result, it has become increasingly clear that semiwild or wild-managed, nondomesticated plant foods in food-production environments and other rural settings disturbed by human activity are a primary feature of farming systems.

The gathering of these food plants by farmers is in evidence among the range of subsistence orientations around the globe. Particularly important locations for these foods are fallow fields and field boundaries. For example, Vainio-Mattila (2000) found that wild green leafy vegetables consumed by the Sambaa people in Tanzania include 73 species of wild plant foods, most of which are ruderal, growing by the roadsides, and weeds on arable land. Ogle and Grivetti (1985a) identified more than 200 wild edible species used by the Swazi of Swaziland and further note that 56 percent of the 211 informants reported agricultural fields as their usual collection sites (Ogel and Grivetti, 1985b). Dufour and Wilson (1994) found that 41 percent of the 130 food plants used by the indigenous populations of Amazonia were trees, of which over half were reported from garden fallows. They note that successional vegetation is an important source of food (Dufour and Wilson, 1994, pp. 117-118). Vickers found that one of the few greens consumed by the Siona-Secoya of the Amazon in Ecuador is a weedy herb that grows in secondary growth (Vickers, 1994, p. 147).

Among agriculturalists in heavily populated and intensively farmed areas of the Hausa in northern Nigeria, Etkin and Ross (1994) discovered that about 50 percent of all food plants consumed in their study community were collected from the local environment. They documented 39 wild food plant species from the farm, 6 species from farm borders, and 16 species from public lands. Among rainfed paddy rice farmers in northeastern Thailand, Price (1993, 1997) documented 77 wild food plant species, 44 of which occurred in agricultural fields and 12 in gardens behind houses or in general village environments such as roadsides. In the same village where Price (1993, 1997) worked, Moreno-Black and colleagues (1996) documented that women in 88 percent of the households had nondomesticated food plants in their home gardens. Wilken (1970) documented their use among farmers in Mexico who sell their domesticated produce but eat the plants foraged from disturbed environments. Farmers in Europe also consume this class of wild plant: Galt and Galt (1976) documented the gathering of wild plant foods from unhoed fields, roadsides, and field boundary walls in Sicily, and 133 species (belonging to 48 families) are documented as being collected in northwest Tuscany in central Italy (Pieroni, 1999). Fallow fields and field borders are sites where rural women in Central Anatolia in Turkey gather wild food plants for domestic consumption and market sale (Ertug, 2003).

Defining the Wild

One of the important features of wild plant foods among agriculturalists is their existence in environments disturbed by human activity rather than undisturbed or pristine environments. Farmers may use species from both disturbed and pristine environments, depending on the natural environment available to them and access possibilities and rights. Many of the plant foods in most disturbed environments used by farmers are, however, opportunistic commensals to domesticates and agricultural practices, as the numerous case studies previously noted illustrate.

These plant communities change and differ in species diversity, subject to influencing factors such as the age and cultivation status of the field or whether the plant community is found within open fields or along the periphery of fields bordering roads or canals. These communities are comprised of species other than the original colonizers, and the communities change due to the nature of agricultural practices, which bring selection pressures on the communities. For example, practices such as winnowing and weeding, as well as mechanization and the application of chemical herbicides, all influence plant communities. It is also proposed that these pressures and their effects are greater with more intensive, rather than shifting, cultivation (Barrett, 1983).

Wild and semidomesticated plant foods in the system may receive less human management attention than the dietary staple, but many of the wild species may still receive attention, which can include selective harvesting, transplanting, or propagation. A wild food plant can be cultivated without becoming a domesticate, and the transition from cultivation to domestication never occurs for most species.

Dufour and Wilson (following Clement, 1990 and Harlan, 1975) attempt to help distinguish plants along this continuum. They use the terms domesticated, semidomesticated, cultivated, managed, and wild. Citing Clement (1990), Dufour and Wilson define these terms as follows:

- A *domesticated* plant is a genetically modified species completely dependent on humans for survival.

- A *semidomesticated* plant has been significantly modified but is still not completely dependent on humans for survival.
- A *cultivated* plant has been introduced into human agroecosystems and is nurtured in a prepared seed bed.
- A *managed* plant is protected from human actions that might harm it, is liberated from competition with other species, or is planted in areas other than prepared seedbeds.
- A *wild* plant may be used but is neither managed nor cultivated (Dufour and Wilson, 1994, p. 115).

For the purposes of this chapter I am concerned with anthropogenic microenvironments in the general agricultural setting with a focus on those plants that are in more highly disturbed environments. I believe that Dufour and Wilson's definitions are useful for understanding the multiple ways we need to think about wild food plants. These are the definitions of the terms I will use when speaking specifically about management. It should also be understood, however, that I use the term wild in a general sense to refer to semidomesticated and wild managed as well as truly wild, unless otherwise stipulated.

Abundance: The Botanical-Dietary Paradox

A number of studies indicate that managed horticultural and agricultural environments can be favorably compared to natural forests in terms of species composition (Conklin, 1961; Kunstader, 1978; Heckman, 1979). It is also proposed that folk inventories of wild plant taxa among agriculturists may be richer in species diversity than those of hunter gatherers (Meilleur, 1994). As noted earlier, plant communities change with changes in human behavior.

In Ogle and Grivetti's (1985c) study in Swaziland, three different zones were identified and studied for changes in gathered plant food species. Their study was the first to name the "botanical-dietary paradox" of agriculturalists. Species loss in less intensively cultivated areas was less; the high veld had a mean loss of 4.5 species and low veld a mean loss of 2. Their informants reported a mean loss of ten species in the middle veld area. Respondents attributed this loss of more species in the middle veld to expanded agricultural development. However, middle veld respondents had increased availability and use of agricultural weeds as plant foods:

The Middleveld, despite its population and extensive botanical disruption presents a botanical-dietary paradox. Here, more varieties of edible wild leaves are consumed than elsewhere in Swaziland. . . . Such vigorous herbaceous species associated with agriculture thrive in the same fields as domesticated crops or in fields left fallow; their presence at these localities, however, makes gathering easier. . . . The Middleveld population, rather than halting the practice of gathering when specific indigenous wild species became scarce, or when time constraints prevented longer collection journeys, have changed their plant focus and have turned to more easily accessible, but non-cultivated weeds of agriculture. (Ogle and Grivetti, 1985c, p. 59)

The concept of the botanical-dietary paradox is critical to our understanding that while selected species in the diet of those dependant on forest resources may decline, the impact on any given farming population may not be the same. As the Ogle and Grivetti study indicates, new gathered plant foods are brought into the diet. Given the extensive literature that has emerged on farmer's consumption of agricultural weeds and other commensals to agriculture cited in this chapter as well as this volume, it clearly is a pattern that occurs across cultures. To date, we have no knowledge of what the actual processes are of incorporating these commensals into the diet. Who in a community experiments with new plants, how does it occur, and what are the social, cultural, and agricultural parameters that foster this switch? We also do not know how and under what conditions farmers simultaneously develop a botanical-medicinal paradox and how this process may differ from incorporating new species as food.

What happens to these wild food plants of agriculture once selected species start to decline in the agricultural environments? For this question, my research in Northeast Thailand provides evidence that rare, valued species come under a system of protection that includes limiting gathering rights and privatization (Price, 1997). This is discussed further and in more detail in the section Multiple-Use Value, Rarity, and Privatization (pp. 89-91).

The continued consumption of wild food plants that are not particularly desirable in taste and that are used primarily as famine foods may also have important implications for availability. It has been proposed that regular use of some species is important to assure sufficient human protection so that species density does not fall below sustainability (Etkin, 1994).

Discovery of New Edible Species

We have some indication that the discovery of the edibility of new species is a product of women's and children's experimentation. Such experimentation, while serving the long-term good of the population, is not without its risks. Scudder (1971) documents this experimentation process among African savanna cultivators during a relocation program. There was a high incidence of female and child death in the relocated community that was not reflected in the surrounding indigenous population. After much medical and anthropological research, the deaths were attributed to poisoning due to test consumption of unfamiliar wild plant foods.

WOMEN'S ROLES, WOMEN'S WORK, AND WOMEN'S KNOWLEDGE

Investigating gender roles in general, and women's roles in particular, is a crucial aspect of understanding both farming and gathering behavior. In general, gathering, because it is the work of women and children, has received less attention than the activities of men (Etkin, 1994; Price, 2000). This is further complicated by the fact that much of women's gathering is for domestic consumption on a daily basis and can be easily overlooked by outside observers (Dufour and Wilson, 1994). Fortunately, this situation is increasingly being remedied (for example, see Daniggelis, 2003; Ertug, 2003; Howard, 2003; Malaza, 2003; Pieroni, 2003; Price, 2003; Turner, 2003).

Gender Division of Labor and Knowledge

It is well-known that households and communities organize production and resource management around the gender division of labor and responsibilities. Among contemporary horticulturalists and agriculturalists, gathering for domestic consumption is women's work. Wild food plant collection from disturbed environments under consideration in this paper is further linked to contemporary farm

women's work in their weeding and seed management of domesticated plant foods (Ertug, 2003; Price, 2003). Women's work and
knowledge are the link between food production/procurement and
food preparation for family consumption (Daniggelis, 2003; Ertug,
2003; Price, 2003).

Within the context of Northeast Thailand, women are the plant
gatherers (Price, 1997, 2000, 2003; Somnasang et al., 1998) while
men engage in deep-water fishing and hunting (Somnasang et al.,
1998). Northeastern Thai farm women and girls are more likely to
correctly identify wild food plants than boys and men (Somnasang,
1996). Girls acquire gender-based knowledge about plants—how
to identify them; when, where, and how to collect them; and how to
cook and preserve them. Boys, by the same token, obtain knowledge
of fishing and hunting by working with their fathers (Somnasang et
al., 1998). The role of daughters learning from their mothers has also
been documented for Turkey, where Ertug (2003) observed that
mothers teach daughters how to identify wild food plants and their locations on active gathering trips.

Actual management of this class of food plants is also gender
based in Northeast Thailand, with women predominating not only in
collection but also in protection and transplanting in fields and gardens in Thailand (Moreno-Black and Somnasang, 2000; Price, 1997,
2003).

Marketing

Northeastern Thai farm women are also engaged in the small-scale
marketing of these plants, providing a source of food not only for urban populations (provincial capitals) but also for other women farmers, who buy them from the market for the purpose of either consuming them or planting them on their own land (Moreno-Black and
Price, 1993; Price, 1997, 2000, 2003; Somnasang et al., 1998).

A market study I conducted with Moreno-Black of wild food sellers in Kalasin Province in Northeast Thailand showed that 78 percent
of the sellers were farm women who did the gathering themselves and
55 percent of what they sold came from agricultural fields, while only
18 percent came from forested areas. Women were the sole marketers
of these foods, which included primarily wild food plants and occasionally small wild protein foods such as snails, crabs, frogs, and in-

sects (Moreno-Black and Price, 1993). This pattern was echoed in another market study that covered 11 early morning markets where farmers predominate as sellers in the three Northeastern provinces of Kalasin, Roi Et, and Khon Kaen. At these 11 markets, 5,909 vendors were recorded, of which 94 percent were women selling 110 non-domesticated plant species and 130 domesticated plant food species (Moreno-Black et al., 1996). Women farmers' marketing of wild plant foods has also been documented in Turkey, where there are "women's areas" in daily markets (Ertug, 2003). In both Thailand and Turkey the market earnings belong to the women who can spend it as they deem appropriate (Ertug, 2003; Moreno-Black and Price, 1993).

The markets of local towns of Northeast Thailand act not only as a place where women can sell these plant foods and earn money but, as noted previously, they are also places were women farmers as consumers can purchase selected species for consumption or transplanting onto their own land. Women not only transplant wild species they obtain from the market, they in fact more commonly move selected species from public lands to their own land, from one field to the next, and from field to garden area around their homes in the village. In addition to buying plants from markets to plant, they obtain plants from neighbors, friends, and kin to transplant onto their own lands (Moreno-Black et al., 1996; Price, 1993, 1997, 2000, 2003). This implies a number of linked areas that deserve further systematic investigation. First is the role of the market in making selected species available to a larger geographic area. Second is the role of social networks of women in species maintenance. Third is gender-based gathering and knowledge transmission. Finally, the role marketing plays in putting pressure on the plant resources and how communities, particularly women in communities, cope with these pressures regarding gathering entitlements.

Agricultural policy and market demand can also impact the cultivation status of wild plant food species. A study conducted by Pemberton and Lee (1996) examines the market sale of wild food plants gathered from field and forest in South Korea. This study represents a level of consumer demand and intensive marketing of wild plant foods not documented for Thailand to date. According to their knowledge and observations regarding gender roles (although their article did not discuss gender roles), they communicated to me that Korean women have traditionally predominated in both gathering and marketing of wild plant foods and still predominate in the market. Selling wild plant foods continues as a female-only occupation in both large urban and small rural markets (Pemberton and Lee, personal communication).[1] We do not know, however, what shifts in gender labor, knowledge, and authority outside of market selling may have taken place as the wild plant foods moved increasingly under cultivation for market sale, as described following.

The article by Pemberton and Lee (1996) documents 112 species in 82 genera and 40 families in the markets. Green leafy vegetables made up 73.2 percent of the total. The next most abundant were fruits at 25 species (22.3 percent). They document the trend from 1989 to 1992 as one of increasing cultivation of wild-type food plants. Of the 14 species cultivated in both 1989 and 1992, 12 had increased areas of cultivation during these three years and cultivation of 7 of these species increased many fold. As of 1992, approximately 25,000 households in South Korea grew these plants, and 8,000 households had them in actual cultivation. The trend from 1989 to 1992 was an increase in the number of species under cultivation and the area of cultivation (Pemberton and Lee, 1996, p. 64).

CONSUMPTION AND NUTRITION

Wild plant foods from disturbed environments also hold diverse positions in the diet (daily, seasonal, or famine consumption). Women not only gather them for daily meals, but in some regions they also engage in their preservation through drying and storage for later consumption and in transplanting and nurturing activities to ensure continued availability of these foods to counteract seasonal and famine food stress (Moreno-Black and Somnasang, 2000; Ogle and Grivetti, 1985b).

Our knowledge on the actual contribution of these plant foods to the nutritional status of farmers is growing. The important contribution of wild plants to the diet in meeting macro- and micronutrient needs of groups at risk (infants, children, the elderly, and pregnant and lactating women) are revealed by numerous studies, although the literature is scattered (Grivetti and Ogle, 2000). Dietary diversity is a close correlate to dietary sufficiency, and dietary diversity obtained from these wild plant foods has been deemed critical to dietary sufficiency, particularly for women and children (Huss-Ashmore and Curry, 1991; Nesamvuni et al., 2001; Nordeide et al., 1996; Ogle and Grivetti, 1985c; Ogle, Hung, and Tuyet, 2001; Somnasang et al., 1987). Ogle and Grivetti discuss dietary diversity in their Swaziland study and conclude that the 59 different species gathered made a considerable contribution to maintaining the nutritional adequacy of the local diet (Ogle and Grivetti, 1985c, p. 59).

A number of studies on wild greens (including those in agricultural fields) have discovered they contain vitamins A and C, riboflavin, calcium, and thiamine (Begum and Pereira, 1977; Bye, 1981; Caldwell and Enoch, 1972; Mwajumwa et al., 1991; Nesamvuni et al., 2001; Nordeide et al., 1996). Wild food plants contributed significantly to the overall micronutrient intake of rural women in two agro-ecological settings in Vietnam (Ogle, Dao, et al., 2001).

The role of the mother is important in adequate nutrition and child survival. A number of the authors cited previously also emphasize the role and knowledge of women by using women as informants on the consumption of wild plant foods (Campbell, 1987; Huss-Ashmore and Curry, 1991; Nesamvuni et al., 2001; Nordeide et al., 1996; Somnasang et al., 1987). Women's diets are also used as a "proxy for household diet because women have primary control over the preparation and distribution of food within the household. Further, women's central roles in food production make it important to identify inadequacies for this portion of the population" (Huss-Ashmore and Curry 1991, pp. 170-171).

Numerous studies also stress the importance of these foods as a regular part of the diet. Primary harvesting occurs when the cultivated staple is in shortest annual supply. In addition to peak gathering seasons, more regular consumption is documented as well. Nesamvuni and colleagues (2001) found in their interviews of 412 women from multiple districts in Venda, South Africa, that among the ten plants they studied in-depth, the frequency of consumption was once per week, per plant. Women also engaged in the storage of surplus in a dried form (either cooked or raw) for at least six months.

A study done in Northeast Thailand in the rainy season documents that wild foods (plants and small protein items such as frogs) made up 50 percent of the farmer's diet (Somnasang et al., 1987). Even at the national level in Thailand, wild vegetables were found to play a significant role in the diet, especially in rural areas (Ngarmsak, 1987). In the Mekong Delta of Vietnam, 90 percent of the women in the Ogle, Dao, and colleagues study (2001) ate wild food plants (naturally occurring vegetables), which made up between 72 and 75 percent of the total vegetables consumed in the wet season (Ogle, Dao, et al., 2001).

It is further suggested that cash income when used to purchase foods does not necessarily replace this diversity. Farmers of Central Thailand (high-input, high-productivity, rice-growing area) lost most of their wild plant foods with land modifications for direct, dry-seeded rice that removed paddy dikes and increased changes in production methods that resulted in greater herbicide use—the traditional foods were not replaced due to their unavailability on the market or their high price; instead, the dietary diversity consumed was reduced (Price, 2000). In a study of unconventional foods in the Thai diet for the whole nation, Ngarmsak (1987, p. 40) concludes that the nutritional status of mothers in the population decreased with the move from traditional foods (accompanied by the use of "more ready to eat" purchased foods) and it is nutritionally better for villagers to obtain their food from their surroundings or from what they have grown.

Wild Plant Food Consumption and Social Stigma

These plant foods vary in taste, abundance, and resilience to biotic stresses, which in turn is related to which species are consumed as a regular part of the diet and which are consumed only in times of extreme food shortage. The degree to which wild plant foods are incorporated into the diet of agriculturalists depends also in part on whether any social status restrictions on the consumption of these foods (or selected species) exists; that is, if they are considered peasant food or foods of poverty and are infrequently consumed by the more prosperous. The greater the social stigma, the more likely these foods will be used as a buffer in times of stress and shortage rather than daily consumption. Wilken (1970), in his work among farmers in Tlaxcala, Mexico, highlights the role of social stigma in the consumption of wild plant foods the farmers regularly harvested from fallow fields and along irrigation canals:

> Social status restricts the use of a group of foods that could supplement an otherwise limited diet. This is unfortunate. As in other economically depressed farming regions, Tlaxzcalan farm-

ers cannot afford to consume the dietary diversity and abundance they produce [for the market]. (Wilken, 1970, p. 294)

Evidence that wild plant foods are somewhat stigmatized has also been found in Swaziland. Ogle and Grivetti (1985b) document that, despite the high use and appreciation of these foods, 29 percent of the adult respondents would hesitate to serve wild foods to guests in their homes because gathered plant foods can be symbolic of poverty and could cause the host embarrassment. However, Ogle and Grivetti's informants expressed pleasure in the consumption of these foods as everyday foods (Ogle and Grivetti, 1985b, p. 39).

In a field study conducted in Swaziland, Malaza (2003) compares the Swazi diet to the findings of Ogle and Grivetti (1985a, b, c). She documents a decline in the consumption of many wild species that were gathered and eaten prior to the growth of intensive agricultural and cash-crop production. Several reasons are given for this decline, including an increase in social stigma of wild plant foods in rural areas, which reflects growing distaste of wild plant foods in urban areas.

One gauge of the level of acceptance of wild plant foods (truly wild, managed, or semidomesticated) is their presence in the marketplace and the varying degree to which social classes above farmers consume them (Leimar, 1987; Malaisse and Parent, 1985; Pemberton and Lee, 1996; Price, 1993; Wilken, 1970).

OVERLAPS: MEDICINAL AND FUNCTIONAL FOOD

Medicinal Food

In their study of medicinal plants in Nigeria, Etkin and Ross (1994) found that 10 percent were cultivated and the rest were semi-wild. They listed 235 noncultigen medicinal plants, 82 of which grew in farm areas (39 of which were also consumed as food); 36 grew in farm border areas (six of which were also used as food); and 56 grew on public lands (of which 16 were also used as food). Ultimately, 26 percent of what Etkin terms "local semi-wild plants" used as medicine were also consumed to meet dietary needs (Etkin, 2002, p. 81). She further makes the important point that we should not conceptualize the category medicinal food to mean that people do not distinguish between food and medicine or that people select food based on its therapeutic effect. The same species can in one circumstance simply be food, yet in the context of treating an illness be a medicine.

The concept that food can also be used as medicine was documented for 16 wild-gathered food plants among the Karen in Northern Thailand. Of the 11 species discussed in detail, four were from rice-paddy and fallow areas, three from riverbank areas, and one from a transition area. Only three of the 11 were from forested areas (Johnson and Grivetti, 2002).

Among farmers in Vietnam, Ogle and colleagues (2003) uncovered 94 wild-gathered plant species used as food; 46 percent of these were also used for medicine. They state,

> From a nutrition viewpoint it is important to pay attention to this group of traditional foods for several reasons. Their direct nutritional contribution is often significant but neglected. Very little is known about the health benefits of regular consumption of small quantities of medicinal foods. (p. 103)

Functional Foods

Health benefits from the consumption of food and dietary diversity are not only associated with the nutrient content of the food. Other specific functional properties are recognized. Some of the health-related functions of food plants include antioxidant, immunostimulation, anti-inflammatory, and antibiosis properties. The benefits of nonnutrient functional properties may exceed those attributed to nutrients. As Johns (2001) states,

> Vegetable diets that make modest contributions to improving vitamin A status result in significant increases in serum levels of lutein (de Pee et al., 1998), an antioxidant for which protective benefits in relation to ocular disease (Brown et al., 1999; Sommerburg et al., 1998), as well as cardiovascular disease and cancer, are increasingly recognized. (p. 6)

Thus, wild food plants can be functional foods; that is, consumed as food but acting beyond their basic nutritional function as food by providing protection or reducing the risk of chronic disease. Pieroni and Quave (see Chapter 4, this volume) note that a great number of the gathered weedy species from disturbed environments in the agricultural setting consumed by south Italians fit into "folk functional foods," in that people think they are healthy to eat but with a general rather than a unique specification of the benefiting action.

Pieroni and colleagues (2002) have evidence that gathered plant foods exist on a continuum of food—food medicine—medicine as linked to indigenous perceptions and classifications of taste. Mild and mildly bitter-tasting greens were considered food, those gathered plants with increased bitterness were in the overlapping category of both food and medicine, and plants perceived as very bitter were consumed as medicines.

MEDICINAL AND FUNCTIONAL FOOD: WILD PLANTS OF NORTHEAST THAILAND

In Northeast Thailand, trees in paddy fields as well as herbaceous species provide both food and medicine. Young leaves and flowers are consumed as vegetables and can also serve as medicine. Grandstaff and colleagues (1986) documented 54 species of trees in paddy fields (on dikes and hillocks), of which 32 species were naturally occurring and 4 species could be either naturally occurring or planted. They note that "many tree species both naturally occurring and planted, provide food and medicine. Young leaves and flowers of *Cassia siamea* frequently are used in making a type of curry and, in more concentrated form, a laxative" (Grandstaff et al., 1986, p. 285). Eighteen of the 32 naturally occurring tree species they documented serve as food and medicine. It is unclear from their publication, however, the extent to which the various species serve both functions (food or medicine versus food and medicine).

In my village field research in Northeast Thailand (Price, 1997) I identified 77 gathered plant foods. Fifty-five, of which 36 have the scientific name identified, were clearly from the agricultural environment. A recent attempt to examine which of these 36 food plants have medicinal value using secondary botanical and other sources reveals that 15 of these food species also have important medicinal uses, and 13 of these 15 were sold as vegetables by farming households for cash income at markets. These 15 species are described in the next sections and shown in Table 3.1.

TABLE 3.1. Wild food plants with medicinal value gathered from disturbed environments in Northeast Thailand, market sale, and rights to gather plants from privately owned property.

Scientific name	Local name (Northeast Thailand)	Market sale	Gathering restriction for eating	Gathering restriction for sale
Alpina malaccensis	Kaa paa	Y	R P	F
Amaranthus spinosus	Phak hom (phak khom)	Y	N	N
Azadirachta indica	Phak kadao	Y	R P	F
Barringtonea acutangula	Phak kradon [naam]	Y	N	F
Capparis tennera	Bak lep maeo	N	N	N
Cassia siamea	Phak kheelek	Y	N	F
Coccinia wightiana	Phak tam luang (phak tam nin)	Y	N	N
Eclipta prostrata	Phak liang (phak kariang)	N	N	N
Ipomoena aquatica	Phak bung	Y	N	N
Limnophila aromatica	Phak kayaeng	Y	N	N
Lindernia crustacean	Phak leum pua	Y	N	N
Monochoria hastate	Phak tob (phak top)	Y	R	F
Nymphaea pubescens	Sai bua	Y	N	F
Oroxylum indicum	Phak lin faa	Y	R P	F
Tiliacora triandra	Yaa naang (bai yaa naag)	Y	N	N

Source: Author's data.

Notes: Alternate local name is in parentheses. Variety qualifier is in brackets.

Market sale: Y = plants sold on the market; N = plants not sold on market.

Gathering restriction for eating: N = no restrictions on amount collected from property of others; R = restricted in the amount you can gather; P = restricted and you must first have permission to gather from the landowner.

Gathering restriction for selling: N = no gathering restrictions from private property; F = forbidden to gather from the land of others for marketing purposes.

Although the knowledge of the informants about the overlap of medicinal or functional foods was not specifically investigated during my numerous research trips to the Northeast, they were asked if they thought wild foods were better, worse, or the same for health. The majority thought they were better for health (Moreno-Black and Price, 1993). Similarly, throughout Northeast Thailand gathered plant foods are thought to have "health promoting or medicinal qualities" (Moreno-Black et al., 1996, p. 112).

Despite this assessment, however, these food plants may fall into what Pieroni and Quave (see Chapter 4, this volume) termed "folk functional foods." The people of Northeast Thailand, like those of Southern Italy, seem to think these foods are healthy to eat but with a general rather than a unique specification of the benefiting action. This also seems to be substantiated by the species-specific ethnobotanical elicitations conducted (Price, 1997), in which no medicinal properties were mentioned. More detailed (ethno) botanical research is needed in the area of botanical identification, since local names can vary within the region. More detailed anthropological, nutritional, and (ethno) medicinal investigations are also called for of domestic healing (rather than specialist healing) given the increasing recognition of the important overlap of food—functional food—medicine. In this regard, women's roles, work, knowledge, and entitlements are the links between the environment and the table and a healthy family. Functional foods, by the very fact that they are consumed as food rather than medicine, are intimately interwoven with the local cuisine and the kitchen. Thus, women must figure prominently as informants.

GATHERED FOOD PLANTS OF NORTHEAST THAILAND WITH MEDICINAL VALUE

In the language of Northeast Thailand, Thai-Lao, the word *phak* indicates a vegetable and the word *yaa* indicates medicine. Interestingly, one of the most common vegetables consumed is *yaa naang,* where in food preparation the leaves are crushed in water and provide a viscous green base for soups locally known in the village as curry. The term *bak* identifies a fruit and *kaa* identifies a rhizome (such as ginger), *bai* indicates leaf (a more unusual prefix).

Alpina malaccensis *(Burm. f.) Roscoe: Kaa paa*

English vernacular name: None

Plant: Robust herb, 2 to 3 cm tall, that is strongly aromatic when bruised.

Ecology: Prefers shady conditions and is often found in secondary growth, rarely in primary forest. At the research site, informants said it was found in forested areas beyond village and fields and transplanted to village and home areas.

Part eaten as food: Young shoot (leaves and stem) and root (rhizome)

Medicinal: The dichloromethane and methanol extracts of *A. malaccensis* showed essential oil (yield of up to 0.2 percent) consisting of 75 percent methyl cinnamate. Rhizome yielded 0.3 percent essential oil. Exact use of *A. malaccensis* is not known; however, the rhizome of medicinally used Alpina have been documented throughout Southeast Asia, including Thailand, as being taken for a large array of ailments.

Marketing: Yes

Source: Van Valkenburg and Bunyapraphatsara, 2001

Amaranthus spinosus *L.: Phak hom*

English vernacular name: Spiny amaranth, prickly amaranth, spiny pigweed

Plant: Annual erect herb up to 100 cm tall, much branched

Ecology: Optimal growth in areas with moderate moisture, very common at roadsides, waste places, cropped land, gardens, and other disturbed areas throughout Southeast Asia.

Part eaten as food: Whole young plants and new shoots (young leaves and stems) if plant is old

Medicinal: Roots are known as an effective diuretic and a remedy using the root is used to treat gonorrhea in Thailand. Rutin (flavonoid) has been found in the aboveground matter. Dried leaves found to contain up to 4.5 percent potassium.

Marketing: Yes

Source: De Padua et al., 1999

Azadirachta indica: *Phak kadao*

English vernacular name: None
Plant: Tall tree
Ecology: Grows on rice paddy hillocks, in the village and house areas.
Part eaten as food: Shoot (young leaves and stems) flowers
Medicinal: Yes (no detail)
Marketing: Yes
Sources: Siemonsma and Piluek, 1993

Capparis tennera: *Bak lep maeo*

Capparis L.: 40 species in mainland Southeast Asia.
English vernacular name: None
Plant: (*C. tennera*) erect to climbing shrub, branches overhanging. Wild, never transplanted.
Ecology: (*C. tennera*) found in hedges and forest borders that meet fields.
Part eaten as food: (*C. tennera*) ripe (sour) and unripe fruit (sweet). Fruit ripe in October/November. Fruits are a source of vitamin C.
Medicinal: Most species seem to have some antibacterial activity.
Marketing: No
Source: Van Valkenburg and Bunyapraphatsara, 2001

Barringtonea acutangula: *Phak kradon naam*

English vernacular name: None
Plant: Wild tree, 10 to 30 m high
Ecology: Found near water (rivers and depressions that remain as small lakes/swamps after annual rains. Village informants, however, note that there are two types of kradon (*Careya sphaerica* Roxb.) and it is the "naam" variety (*Barringtonea acutangula*) that grows at swamp and field boundaries. Thus exact identification of the species is not yet certain and needs further botanical identification.

Part eaten as food: Shoots (young leaves and stems) and flowers are eaten raw.

Medicinal: Has a very high antioxidative potency, containing more than 100 mg butylated hydroxyanisole equivalent (BHA eq.) in 100 g fresh vegetable (Trakoontivakorn and Saksitpitak, 2000).

Marketing: yes

Sources: Brenner, 2003; Trakoontivakorn and Saksitpitak, 2000

Cassia siamea *Britt.: Phak kheelek*

English Vernacular name: Cassod tree
Plant: Wild tree, 4 to 8 m high; wild but also transplanted
Ecology: Found along river banks or ditches
Part eaten as food: Young leaves and flower buds; bitterness reduced through boiling
Medicinal: Leaves and flowers are diuretic and mild laxative (bark also).
Marketing: Yes
Sources: Jacquat, 1990

Coccinia wightiana: *Phak tam luang*

English vernacular name: Ivy gourd
Plant: Herbaceous climber
Ecology: Occurs wild in grassland, on roadsides, and in light forests and brushwood. It grows along fences and with trees, according to informants. Gathered wild in the study village, other villages are said to transplant it.
Part eaten as food: Young shoots, young leaves, and stem
Medicinal: Numerous medicinal applications, including poultice, antipyretics
Marketing: Yes
Sources: Siemonsma and Piluek, 1993

Eclipta prostrata: *Phak liang; phak kariang*

English vernacular name: False daisy, ink plant; Central Thai vernacular: *Kameng*
Plant: Annual or short-lived perennial herb

Ecology: Anthropogenic species found in the rice paddy and around water courses, swampy areas, and roadsides. Common weed in rice.

Part eaten as food: Young shoots (leaves and stems)

Medicinal: Widely used in traditional medicine throughout Southeast Asia and China. Crushed leaves used against skin diseases (eczema as well as leprosy, ringworm, and mycosis of fingers and feet). Leaves or flower heads used internally for colic, constipation, and also against diarrhea. Aerial parts generally known for their antibiotic and hemostatic properties (treating blood in the urine, nose and wound bleeding, and ulcers).

Marketing: No

Source: Van Valkenburg and Bunyapraphatsara, 2001

Ipomoena aquatica *Forsskal: Phak bung (Thai)*

English vernacular name: Water convolvulus; water spinach

Plant: Perennial, fast-growing herb 2 to 3 cm long, trailing or floating; stem hollow or spongy. Two types of *phak bung* (also called *kangkong* on other areas of Southeast Asia) are distinguished. A plant with green/purple stems, dark green leaves, and light purple to white flowers is the *phak bung* Thai gathered wild. The cultivated type has green/white stems and white flowers and is referred to as *phak bung chin.*

Ecology: On paddy dikes at rice field edges, ditches, irrigation canals, and other moist, marshy, or inundated locations

Part eaten as food: Stems and leaves, young tops or plants

Medicinal: Eating *phak bung* Thai can be used against sleeplessness, headache, and stress, as it has a nerve-calming effect. The leaves can be used in a remedy for cough.

Marketing: Yes

Sources: Siemonsma and Piluek, 1993; Van Valkenburg and Bunyapraphatsara, 2001

Limnophila aromatica: *Phak kayaeng*

English vernacular name: None

Plant: Fleshy annual to perennial herb, 30 to 100 cm tall, aquatic/semiaquatic herb

Ecology: Found along riversides, marshy areas, and is a common "weed" in flooded rice fields

Part eaten as food: Young shoots (leaves and stalk)

Medicinal: Plant used as a cooling agent in fevers and given to nursing mothers as a galactagogue. Thought to calm the stomach after eating durian.

Marketing: Yes

Sources: Siemonsma and Piluek, 1993; Van Valkenburg and Bunyapraphatsara, 2001

Lindernia crustacea: *Phak leum pua*

English vernacular name: None

Plant: Small annual to short-lived perennial herb, 5 to 20 cm tall.

Ecology: Grows in rice fields (nonflooded) and on paddy dikes, riverbeds, ditches, and disturbed soils. Never transplanted.

Part eaten as food: Whole plant, including the roots

Medicinal: A remedy made of the leaves is given after childbirth. Shown also to have good results in treating bilious disorders, dysentery, amenorrhea, and hepatitis. One of the most common plants in Chinese pharmacies in Indonesia and Malaysia.

Marketing: Yes

Sources: Van Valkenburg and Bunyapraphatsara, 2001

Monochoria hastata: *Phak tob*

English vernacular: Pondweed

Plant: Rhizomatous perennial with strong stem, can attain a height of up to 2 m during the rain, adjusting height to water depth.

Ecology: Weed in flooded rice fields, grows in swamps, along ditches, and canal banks.

Part eaten as food: Young stalk and young flower

Medicinal: Juice of leaves used for curing coughs and pulverized rhizome is applied to relieve itching.

Marketing: Yes

Sources: Siemonsma and Piluek, 1993

Nymphaea pubescens *Willd.: Sai bua*

English vernacular name: Water lily, lotus lily

Plant: Nymphaea species is a perennial aquatic herb; rhizome cone-like, tuberous. Flowers solitary, 8 to 18 cm in diameter, held 5 to 20 cm above the water. Flowers are slightly fragrant.

Ecology: N. Pubescens found in deeper ponds and swamps

Part eaten as food: N. Pubescens, stem

Medicinal: Screening of *N. pubescens* Willd. leaf extract showed antifungal activity that causes 85 percent inhibition of spore germination in *Fusarium solani.* In Southeast Asia, Nymphaea species are considered astringent, in Thailand the flowers are taken as a cardiotonic.

Marketing: Yes

Sources: Van Valkenburg and Bunyapraphatsara, 2001

Oroxylum indicum: *Phak lin faa*

English vernacular name: Midnight horror

Plant: Semideciduous tree up to 27 m tall and trunk up to 40 cm in diameter. Bark is gray.

Ecology: Nongregarious, short-lived, encountered in secondary growth and thickets, widespread and common in disturbed areas throughout Southeast Asia. At the research site it is found on paddy field dikes, in upland fields, and around the village.

Part eaten as food: Leaves, shoots, flowers; the young long flat pods (fruit) are eaten cooked as vegetables.

Medicinal: In Thailand the root and root bark are used for diarrhea and dysentery; stem bark is applied to ulcers and abscesses. Seed is used as a laxative and antidiarrheal. The flavonoids and lapachol isolated show pharmacological activities in virus inhibition and anti-inflammatory activity. Among the flavonoids found, the leaves, stem and root bark, and seed contain baicalein.

Marketing: Yes

Sources: Van Valkenburg and Bunyapraphatsara, 2001

Tiliacora triandra: *Yaa naang; bai yaa naag*

English vernacular name: None
Plant: Woody vine; climbing with support (liane)
Ecology: Common in scrub vegetation in lowland areas and
    other clearings. Commonly transplanted to house garden ar-
    eas.
Part eaten as food: Leaves crushed in water. Leaves then dis-
    carded and the leaf extract used as a green and viscous base
    for soup locally called "curry."
Medicinal: Aerial parts widely used as an antipyretic in Thai-
    land. Little is known about the pharmacological properties.
Marketing: Yes
Sources: Siemonsma and Piluek, 1993; Lemmens and Bunya-
    praphatsara, 2003

INVESTIGATIONS OF WILD PLANT FOODS
AS FUNCTIONAL /MEDICINAL FOODS IN THAILAND

The Institute of Food Research and Product Development at
Kasetsart University in Bangkok has been working since 1998 on the
notion that local Thai vegetables can be used to prevent diseases.
Their researchers have been conducting studies on the antioxidant activity and antimutagenicity of indigenous gathered vegetables (of the
northern and northeastern regions) and have studied approximately
200 species they collected from local markets. Their results indicate
that many plant species possess great potential as functional foods
(Trakoontivakorn, 2003). A number of traditional vegetables tested
are to be found in my Thailand research. *Barringtonea acutangula
(phak kradon naam), Cassia siamea (phak keelek),* and *Azadirachta
indica (phak kadao)* are among the group of vegetables they classify
as "very high potency," containing more than 100 mg BHA eq. in
100 g fresh vegetable. *Amaranthus spinosus (phak hom)* was classified in the "high potency" range, containing antioxidant substances
25 to 100 mg in 100 g fresh vegetable (Trakoontivakorn and Saksitpitak, 2000).

In a study done on 134 edible Thai plants for anti-tumor-promot-
ing activity, 17 species exhibited strong inhibitory activity, 21 species

were moderately active, and 33 species were slightly active. One gathered wild vegetable from the village study, *Oroxylum indicum (phak lin faa),* has been noted as having exceptionally high potential in cancer prevention (Suratwadee et al., 2002). Nakahara and colleagues (2001) have also studied *Oroxylum indicum* and note that the tests on the edible part of the plant exhibited antimutagenic properties.

MULTIPLE-USE VALUE, RARITY, AND PRIVATIZATION

An overlap in food and medicine may be an important indicator of multiple-use value for selected species and thus act to stimulate indigenous prohibitions on overexploitation of rarer species for market sale. Such considerations are important not only in protecting the biodiversity of wild plants as food but also medicines and functional foods. Such multiple-use value was briefly noted by Cunningham (1995, p. 3): "The widespread practice in Africa of conserving edible wild fruit-bearing trees for their fruits or shade also ensures availability of some traditional medicines as several are multiple-use species."

Northeast Thailand

Currently, there is little empirical evidence of how wild plant foods come under a system of protection, management, and privatization. Based on research in Northeast Thailand, it has been proposed that factors such as the reduction of common-property forests, population pressures (Grandstaff et al., 1986), and proximity to towns and cities (Ngarmsak, 1987) may each have a bearing on the availability and management of wild plant foods.

My research in Northeast Thailand (Price, 1997) illustrates that intensive management (including propagation) of wild plant food species is species specific and applies to species that have multiple-use value and are perceived as rare. This is also supported by the research results of Stoffle and colleagues (1990), whose work among the Paiute and Shoshone Native American groups in Nevada document the importance of perceived rarity with the development of special management techniques to encourage protection and propagation of wild plants. Cunningham (1995, p. 3) provides an appropriate summary of decisive factors for plant management to take place. He states:

> For any society to institute intentional resource management controls, certain conditions have to be fulfilled: the resource must be of value to the society; the resource must be perceived to be in short supply and vulnerable to over-exploitation by people; the socio-political nature of the society must include the necessary structures for resource management.

In the study I conducted in Northeast Thailand among rice farmers (Price, 1993, 1997), restrictions on gathering were due to a combination of three factors: (1) perceived rarity, (2) desirability of the taste of the plant food, and (3) the market value of the species.

Twenty-five of 77 species fit these criteria. This placed them in a category where gathering from private property (such as agricultural fields) was forbidden for nonowners. The usufruct rights for gathering for consumption of these "forbidden species" varied but remained species specific. In no case was there a restriction on gathering for consumption that did not have a corresponding prohibition on gathering for market sale. In some cases one could gather with permission, while in other cases one could gather enough just to eat on the spot without permission, or one could gather enough for a family meal without permission. Of the 15 food plants from my study that also had medicinal value, seven were forbidden for collection for market sale and, of these seven, four had restrictions on gathering for consumption (see Table 3.1). In no case, however, was the health or functional food/medicinal value mentioned or implied as a value of consideration in restricting gathering rights on privately owned land. The values were rarity, taste, and marketability. The functional and medicinal values of these plant foods deserve further investigation into their relationship to management and protection.

In an attempt to test the role of the market in relationship to human management of wild plant food species in disturbed environments, I discovered that plants might be managed even if the plant species was not sold on the market, but that management was a critical aspect of "forbidden species" (Price, 1997). Also critical to placing a species in the category of "forbidden" was the centrality of women in the local sociocultural context of the village: it was they who came to consensus on a given species' status. Women were the owners of the resource (matrilineal inheritance of land); spent their whole lives in the village (matrilocal residence); and were thus intimately familiar with the ecology and were the gatherers, marketers, and preparers of these wild plants for domestic consumption in their kitchens (Price, 2003).

Although the village women farmers in this study may not recognize or consider the specific benefiting actions of the plant foods (as functional or medicinal), nonetheless the conservation for food inadvertently conserves the plants for their general folk function of "healthy to eat."

CONCLUSIONS

Defining what wild plant foods are in the farming environment and the important role they play in farmer's diets around the world and particularly in Northeast Thailand has been one of the tasks of this chapter. This study points to some important linkages that come from a combination of the literature and my own research interests in the fields; it also points to some knowledge gaps. What we still understand very little about is the process of bringing these "weeds of agriculture" and other plant foods from disturbed environments into the diet. What we can propose is that a movement away from dependence on plants from forests as food and medicine appears to be accompanied by an increase in consumption of plant foods and medicines gathered from the farming environment, and that this occurs as a cross-cultural phenomenon. Thus, as agriculture grows and old forest growth declines and is farther and farther from the dwellings (and gatherers) there is a growing reliance on plant foods from the environments disturbed by human activity, including fields, border areas, along foot paths, and so on. Undoubtedly, species composition changes with land-use changes and agronomic practices. New species are brought into the diet through a process of experimentation, but not without difficulty. The only study we have on the discovery of plants and incorporating new species into the diet is by Scudder (1971), who discovered that women (and children) experiment in consuming wild plant foods unknown to them, with the accompanying higher incidence of poisoning from this consumption.

Dietary diversity, with regard to the number of different species in the diet, seems to increase with this shift from wild forest species to the species of agriculture. This has been labeled the botanical-dietary paradox (Ogle and Grivetti 1985c).

This chapter has provided significant evidence from a number of important studies that gathered plant foods from agricultural environments also act as medicine. Indeed, within the context of my own research in Northeast Thailand, out of 36 species gathered from agricultural environments, 15 were shown to have important medicinal properties through the examination of secondary source material. Thirteen of these 15 species were sold by women at local markets as food. The relationship between food as functional and food as medicinal in the minds of the farmers themselves is less clear. The gathered food plants are thought to have health-promoting qualities but may be along the lines of "folk functional foods" (see Chapter 4 by Pieroni and Quave, this volume), in that they are thought of as healthy to eat but are without specifically identified benefiting actions. This, of course, would be quite different for plants clearly within the folk medical system. In the case of the vegetable *phak lin faa* (*Oroxylum indicum*), for example, the roots and bark are used as medicine in Thailand but the leaves are used as a vegetable. Although farmers may distinguish between the use of different plant parts for different purposes and only indicate that the vegetable parts are "healthy to eat," extensive biopharmacological research conducted by Nakahara and colleagues (2001) has shown that the edible parts (not just the roots) of *Oroxylum indicum* exhibited antimutagenic properties. It is not only farmers, however, who may lack an understanding of the specific benefits of eating foods with medicinal properties (or functional foods). As noted earlier, scientific knowledge is still lacking on the benefits to human health from eating small quantities of these plant foods that also have medicinal properties.

The extent to which farmers use and are able to continue to use the wild food plants of agriculture depends on a number of factors. Social stigma attached to eating wild plant foods among farmers is an important factor deserving further investigation. Not only may this affect the consumption within households but it also may certainly have an impact on the valuation of plant species and desires to participate in conservation strategies, be these indigenous or introduced from outside the community. The stigma on wild plant foods seems to be their association with poverty. In contexts where these plant foods are not stigmatized, a greater possibility exists of not only culinary pride and indigenous conservation management but also opportunities to market these foods on a local or even national or international level.

Why and how selected wild plant food species come under a system of protection and privatization among farmers is an area that desperately needs further in-depth investigation. Evidence from my research in Thailand and the research of others suggests that more conscious and intensive management of wild food plants in agricultural environments begins with resource pressure and perceived rarity, coupled with multiple-use value, on a species basis. Because many of these plants actually occur on agricultural land, their privatization begins to occur. Collection for market sale appeared in my research as serving as one "use" in the multiuse criteria. A rare species that was also very desirable in taste and fetched a good market price became forbidden to gather for market sale from the land of others. This also has an impact on general gathering rights of community members for domestic consumption where prohibitions existed, but to a lesser degree (such as gathering only what could be eaten on the spot, taking only enough for a meal, and so on). Although the women farmers in the research area in Northeast Thailand may not recognize or consider the specific benefiting actions of plant foods (as functional or medicinal) in their considerations to protect a given species from overexploitation, conservation of foods for their general folk function of being "healthy to eat" inadvertently conserves the plants that have specific beneficial properties.

Overall, the role of women in the gathering, use, and management of wild plant foods from disturbed rural environments appears to be critical in sustaining these foods. Their work in gathering and managing the various species is intrinsically linked to their gender role as food preparers. It is also linked to their daily routine, as women collect these foods generally on a daily basis for meal preparation.

Women as gatherers, managers, and marketers of these resources are also the ones with the knowledge of the status of a particular species. I have documented them as the key to the process of developing gathering restrictions and privatization, while at the same time being sensitive to usufruct rights for domestic consumption of the larger community. This was, however, documented in a context where women are the owners of agricultural land and reside matrilocally.

They have both the gender-based knowledge of resources and each other on a lifelong basis, as well as authority. It is indeed probable that women are also the ones that brought the new species of agriculture into the local diet and cuisine through experimentation.

We do not yet know how such species-level systems of increasing protection and privatization function in contexts where women are lacking the authority over agricultural land, long-term social networks, and female kinship networks, nor do we grasp the different valuations men versus women place on selected species and where conflict and cooperation may emerge.

NOTE

1. Dr. Robert Pemberton is currently at the Invasive Plant Research Laboratory, USDA Agricultural Research Service in Ft. Lauderdale, Florida. Dr. Nam Sook Lee is in the Department of Biology, Ewha Womans University in Seoul, Korea.

REFERENCES

Barrett, S.C.H. (1983). Crop mimicry in weeds. *Economic Botany* 3:255-282.

Begum, A. and S.M. Pereira (1977). The beta-carotene content of Indian edible green leaves. *Tropical and Geographic Medicine* 29:74-50.

Brenner, V. (2003). *Utilization of floodplain vegetation in Northeastern Thailand: Compilation of survey results from Ban Pak Yam, a village in the Songkhram River Basin.* SEFUT Working Paper No. 8. Working Group Socio-Economics of Forest Use in the Tropics and Sub-Tropics. Freiburg, Germany: University of Freiburg.

Brown, L., E.B. Rimm, J.M. Seddon, E.L. Giovannucci, L. Chasan-Taber, D. Spiegelman, W.C. Willet, and S.E. Hankinson (1999). A prospective study of carotenid intake and risk of cataract extraction in U.S. men. *American Journal of Clinical Nutrition* 70:517-524.

Bye, R.A. (1981). Quelites—Ethnoecology of edible greens—Past, present, and future. *Journal of Ethnobiology* 1:109-123.

Caldwell, M.J. and T.C. Enoch (1972). Riboflavin content of Malaysian leafy vegetables. *Ecology of Food and Nutrition* 1:309-312.

Campbell, B.M. (1987). The use of wild fruits in Zimbabwe. *Economic Botany* 3:375-385.

Clement, C.R. (1990). Fruit trees and the origin of agriculture in the neotropics. Paper presented at the Second International Congress of Ethnobiology, Yunnan, People's Republic of China.

Conklin, H. (1961). The study of shifting cultivation. *Current Anthropology* 1:27-61.

Cunningham, A.B. (1995). *African medicinal plants: Setting priorities at the interface between conservation and primary healthcare.* People and Plants Working Paper 1, People and Plants Online. Available online at www.rbgkew.org.uk/peopleplants/index.html.

Daniggelis, E. (2003). Women and "wild" foods: Nutrition and household security among Rai and Sherpa forager-farmers in Eastern Nepal. In Howard, P.L. (Ed.), *Women and plants.* New York: Zed and St. Martin's Press.

De Padua, L.S., N. Bunyapraphatsara, and R.H.M.J. Lemmens (Eds.) (1999). *PROSEA 12 (1): Medicinal and poisonous plants 1.* Leiden: Backhuys Publishers.

De Pee, S., C.E. West, D. Permaesih, D. Martuti, and J.G. Hautvast (1998). Orange fruit is more effective than are dark-green, leafy vegetables in increasing serum concentrations of retinol and beta-carotene in schoolchildren in Indonesia. *American Journal of Clinical Nutrition* 68:1058-1067.

Dufour, D.L. and W.M. Wilson (1994). Characteristics of "wild" plant foods used by indigenous populations in Amazonia. In Etkin, N.L. (Ed.), *Eating on the wild side* (pp. 114-142). Tucson: University of Arizona Press.

Ertug, F. (2003). Gendering the tradition of plant gathering in central Anatolia (Turkey). In Howard, P.L. (Ed.), *Women and plants.* New York: Zed and St. Martin's Press.

Etkin, N.L. (1994). The cull of the wild. In Etkin, N.L. (Ed.), *Eating on the wild side.* Tucson: University of Arizona Press.

Etkin, N.L. (2002). Local knowledge of biotic diversity and its conservation in rural Hausaland, northern Nigeria. *Economic Botany* 56(1):73-88.

Etkin, N. and P.J. Ross (1994). Pharmacological implications of "wild" plants in the Hausa diet. In Etkin, N.L. (Ed.), *Eating on the wild side.* Tucson: University of Arizona Press.

Galt, A.H. and J.W. Galt (1976). Peasant use of some wild plants on the island of Pantelleria, Sicily. *Economic Botany* 31:20-26.

Grandstaff, S., T.B. Grandstaff, P. Rathakette, D.E. Thomas, and J.K. Thomas (1986). Trees in paddy fields in Northeast Thailand. In Marten, G.E. (Ed.), *Traditional Agriculture in Southeast Asia.* Boulder: Westview Press.

Grivetti, L.E. and B.M. Ogle (2000). Value of traditional foods in meeting macro- and micronutrient needs: The plant connection. *Nutrition Research Reviews* 1:31-46.

Harlan, J.R. (1975). *Crops and man.* Madison, WI: American Society of Agronomy.

Heckman, C.W. (1979). *Rice field ecology in Northeast Thailand: The effect of wet and dry seasons on a cultivated aquatic ecosystem.* Monographiae Biologicae volume 34 . Illies, J. (Ed.). The Hague: Dr. W. Junk bv Publishers.

Howard, P.L. (2003). Women and the plant world: An exploration. In Howard, P.L. (Ed.), *Women & plants: Gender relations in biodiversity management and conservation.* New York: Zed and St. Martin's Press.

Huss-Ashmore, R. and J.J. Curry (1991). Diet, nutrition, and agricultural development in Swaziland. 2. Patterns of food consumption. *Ecology of Food and Nutrition* 26:167-185.

Jacquat, C. (1990). *Plants from the markets of Thailand.* Bangkok: Editions Duank
Kamol.

Johns, T. (2001). Dietary diversity, global change, and human health. In *Proceedings of the symposium "Managing Biodiversity in Agricultural Ecosystems,"*
Montreal, Canada, November 8-10.

Johnson, N. and L. Grivetti (2002). Gathering practices of Karen women: Questionable contribution of beta-carotene intake. *International Journal of Food Sciences and Nutrition* 53: 489-501.

Kunstader, P. (1978). Ecological modification and adaptation: An ethnobotanical
view of Lua' swiddeners in northwestern Thailand. In Ford, R. (Ed.), *The nature
and status of ethnobotany.* Ann Arbor: University of Michigan Museum of Anthropology.

Leimar, L. (1987). *Wild foods in an agricultural context: An exploratory study of
time and labor allocations of peasant women in Northeast Thailand.* Master of
arts thesis, Department of Anthropology, University of Kentucky, Lexington,
Kentucky.

Lemmens, R.H.M.J. and N. Bunyapraphatsara (2003). *PROSEA 12(3): Medicinal
and poisonous plants 3.* Leiden: Backhuys Publishers.

Malaisse, F., and G. Parent (1985). Edible wild vegetable products in the Zambezian woodland area. *Ecology of Food and Nutrition* 18:43-42.

Malaza, M. (2003). Modernization and gender dynamics in the loss of agrobio-
diversity in Swaziland's food system. In Howard, P.L. (Ed.), *Women & plants:
Gender relations in biodiversity management and conservation* (pp. 243-257).
New York: Zed and St. Martin's Press.

Meilleur, B.A. (1994). In search of "keystone societies." In Etkin, N.L. (Ed.), *Eating on the wild side.* Tucson: University of Arizona Press.

Moreno-Black, G. and L.L. Price (1993). The marketing of gathered food as an economic strategy of women in Northeast Thailand. *Human Organization* 52:398-
404.

Moreno-Black, G. and P. Somnasang (2000). In times of plenty and times of scarcity: Nondomesticated food in northeastern Thailand. *Ecology of Food and Nutrition* 38:563-586.

Moreno-Black, G., P. Somnasang, and S. Thamathawan (1996). Cultivating continuity and creating change: Women's home garden practices in Northeast Thailand. *Agriculture and Human Values* 3:3-11.

Mwajumwa, L.B.S., E.M. Kahangi, and J.K. Imungi (1991). The prevalence and nutritional values of some Kenyan indigenous leafy vegetables from three locations of Machokos District. *Ecology of Food and Nutrition* 2:275-280.

Nakahara, K., M. Onishi-Kameyama, H. Ono, M. Yoshida, and G. Trakoontivakorn (2001). Antimutagenic activity against Trp-P-1 of the edible Thai plant, *Oroxylum indicum* vent. *Bioscience, Biotechnology, and Biochemistry* 65: 2358-2560.

Nesamvuni, C., N.P. Steyn, and M.J. Potgieter (2001). Nutritional value of wild, leafy plants consumed by the Vhavenda. *South African Journal of Science* 97:51-54.

Ngarmsak, T. (1987). *Status and nutritional importance of unconventional food crops in Thai diets.* Report submitted to the Regional Office for Asia and the Pacific, Food and Agriculture Organization of the United Nations, Bangkok, Thailand.

Nordeide, M.B., A. Hatloy, M. Folling, E. Lied, and A. Oshaug (1996). Nutrient composition and nutritional importance of green leaves and wild food resources in an agricultural district, Koutiala, in southern Mali. *International Journal of Food Sciences and Nutrition* 6:455-468.

Ogle, B.M., H.T.A. Dao, G. Mulokozi, and L. Hambraeus (2001). Micronutrient composition and nutritional importance of gathered vegetables in Vietnam. *International Journal of Food Sciences and Nutrition* 52:485-499.

Ogle, B.M. and L.E. Grivetti (1985a). Legacy of the chameleon: Edible wild plants in the kingdom of Swaziland, southern Africa. A cultural, ecological, nutritional study. Part I: Introduction, objectives, methods, Swazi culture, landscape and diet. *Ecology of Food and Nutrition* 16:193-208.

Ogle, B.M. and L.E. Grivetti (1985b). Legacy of the chameleon: Edible wild plants in the kingdom of Swaziland, southern Africa. A cultural, ecological, nutritional study. Part II: Demographics, species availability and dietary use, analysis by ecological zone. *Ecology of Food and Nutrition* 17:1-30.

Ogle, B.M. and L.E. Grivetti (1985c). Legacy of the chameleon: Edible wild plants in the kingdom of Swaziland, southern Africa. A cultural, ecological, nutritional study. Part III: Cultural ecological analysis. *Ecology of Food and Nutrition* 17:31-40.

Ogle, B.M., P.H. Hung, and H.T. Tuyet (2001). Significance of wild vegetables in micronutrient intakes of women in Vietnam: An analysis of food variety. *Asia Pacific Journal of Clinical Nutrition* 10(1):30-40.

Ogle, B.M., H.T. Tuyet, H.N. Duyet, and N.N.X. Dung (2003). Food, feed or medicine: The multiple functions of edible wild plants in Vietnam. *Economic Botany* 57(1):103-117.

Pemberton, R.W. and N.S. Lee (1996). Wild food plants in South Korea: Market presence, new crops, and exports to the United States. *Economic Botany* 1:57-70.

Pieroni, A. (1999). Gathered wild food plants in the upper valley of the Serchio River (Garfagnana), central Italy. *Economic Botany* 3:327-341.

Pieroni, A. (2003). Wild food plants and Arberesh women in Lucania, Southern Italy. In Howard, P.L. (Ed.), *Women & plants: Gender relations in biodiversity management and conservation.* New York: Zed and St. Martin's Press.

Pieroni, A., S. Nebel, C. Quave, H. Munz, and M. Heinrich (2002). Ethnopharmacology of *Liakra:* Traditional weedy vegetables of the Arbeshe of the Vultura area in southern Italy. *Journal of Ethnopharmacology* 81:165-185.

Price, L.L. (1993). Women's wild plant food entitlements in Thailand's agricultural Northeast. Doctoral dissertation, Anthropology Department, University of Oregon.

Price, L.L. (1997). Wild plant food in agricultural environments: A study of occurrence, management and gathering rights in Northeast Thailand. *Human Organization* 2:209-221.

Price, L.L. (2000). The fields are full of gold: Women's marketing of wild foods from rice fields in Southeast Asia and the impacts of pesticides and integrated pest management. In Spring, A. (Ed.), *Women farmers and commercial ventures: Increasing food security in developing countries.* Boulder: Lynne Rienner Publishers.

Price, L.L. (2003). Farm women's rights and roles in wild plant food gathering and management in Northeast Thailand. In Howard, P.L. (Ed.), *Women & plants: Gender relations in biodiversity management and conservation.* New York: Zed and St. Martin's Press.

Scoones, I., M. Melynik, and J. Petty (1992). *The hidden harvest: Wild foods and agricultural systems, a literature review and annotated bibliography.* London: Sustainable Agriculture Program, IIED.

Scudder, T. (1971). *Gathering among African woodland savannah cultivators: A case study: The Gwembe Tonga.* Zambian papers, number 5. Manchester: Manchester University Press, [for] University of Zambia, Institute for African Studies.

Siemonsma, J.S. and K. Piluek (Eds.) (1993). *PROSEA 8: Vegetables.* Leiden: Backhuys Publishers.

Sommerburg, O.E., J.E. Keunen, A.C. Bird, and F.J. van Kuijk (1998). Fruits and vegetables that are sources for lutein and zeaxanthin: The macular pigment in human eyes. *British Journal of Opthalmology* 82:907-910.

Somnasang, P. (1996). Indigenous food use: Gender issues in rural Northeast Thailand. Doctoral dissertation, Department of Anthropology, University of Oregon.

Somnasang, P., G. Moreno-Black, and K. Chusil (1998). Indigenous knowledge of wild food hunting and gathering in Northeast Thailand. *Food and Nutrition Bulletin* 19:359-365.

Somnasang, P., P. Rathakette, and S. Rathanapanya (1987). The role of natural foods in Northeast Thailand. In Subhadira, S., G. Lovelace, and S. Simarap (Eds.), *Rapid Rural Appraisal in Northeast Thailand: Case Studies.* KKU-FORD Rural Systems Research Project. Khon Kaen, Thailand: Khon Kaen University.

Stoffle, R.W., D.B. Halmo, M.J. Evans, and J.E. Olmsted (1990). Calculating the cultural significance of American Indian plants: Paiute and Shoshone ethnobotany of Yucca Mountain Nevada. *American Anthropologist* 2:416-432.

Suratwadee, J., V. Santisopasri, A. Murakami, O. Kim, H.W. Kim, and H. Ohigashi (2002). Suppressive effects of edible Thai plants on superoxide and nitric oxide generation. Research Communication: Potential of edible Thai plants as chemopreventive agents. *Asian Pacific Journal of Cancer Prevention* 3:215-223.

Trakoontivakorn, G. (2003). Value-addition to agricultural products. In Mori, Y., T. Hatashi, and E. Highley (Eds.), *Value-addition to agricultural products,* JIRCAS International Symposium Series No. 11. Tsukuba, Japan: Japan International Center for Agricultural Sciences.

Trakoontivakorn, G. and J. Saksitpitak (2000). Antioxidative potential of Thai indigenous vegetable extracts. *Food* 8(3):164-176 [in Thai with English title and abstract].

Turner, N. (2003). Passing on the news: Women's work, traditional knowledge and plant resource management in indigenous societies of North-western North America. In Howard, P.L. (Ed.), *Women & plants: Gender relations in biodiversity management and conservation.* New York: Zed and St. Martin's Press.

Vainio-Mattila, K. (2000). Wild vegetables used by the Sambaa in the Usambara Mountains, NE Tanzania. *Annales Botanici Fennici* 37:57-67.

Van Valkenburg, J.L.C.H. and N. Bunyapraphatsara (Eds.) (2001). *PROSEA 12 (2): Medicinal and Poisonous Plants 2.* Leiden: Backhuys Publishers.

Vickers, W.T. (1994). The health significance of wild plants for the Siona and Secoya. In Etkin, N.L. (Ed.), *Eating on the wild side.* Tucson: University of Arizona Press.

Wilken, G. (1970). The ecology of gathering in a Mexican farming region. *Economic Botany* 24:286-295.

Chapter 4

Functional Foods or Food Medicines?
On the Consumption
of Wild Plants Among Albanians
and Southern Italians in Lucania

Andrea Pieroni
Cassandra L. Quave

INTRODUCTION

In the past decade, the food-medicine continuum has come to the forefront of ethnobiological and ethnopharmacological research (Johns, 1990; Etkin, 1994, 1996; Prendergast et al., 1998). Plants may be used both as medicine and food, and it can often be difficult to draw a line between the two groups: food may be used as medicine and vice versa.

Many studies in the past twenty years have stressed the ethno-biological and food aspects of gathering activities worldwide and the consumption of noncultivated botanicals in Africa (Etkin and Ross, 1982; Ogle and Grivetti, 1985a, b, c, d; Johns and Kokwaro, 1991; Humphry et al., 1993; Bukenya-Ziraba, 1996; Johns, Mhoro, and San-aya, 1996; Johns, Mhoro, and Usio, 1996; Hillocks, 1998; Schackleton et al., 1998; Lockett and Grivetti, 2000; Vainio-Mattila, 2000; Asfaw and Tadesse, 2001; Marshall, 2001; Mertz et al., 2001; Ogoye-Ndegwa and Aagaard-Hansen, 2003), in America (Bye, 1981; Lepofski et al., 1985; Kuhnlein, 1992; Turner, 1995, 1997; Ladio and Lozada, 2000,

Special thanks are due to all of the people of the Vulture and Dolomiti Lucane area for their marvelous hospitality during the past four years. We want to dedicate this chapter to all of them and to the young: present and future Lucanian generations.

2001, 2003; Ladio, 2001; Vierya-Odilon and Vibrans, 2001; Turner, 2003), and Asia (Moreno-Black et al., 1996; Pemberton and Lee, 1996; Price, 1997; Khasbagan and Stuart, 1999; Tukan et al., 1998; Khasbagan and Pei, 2000; Johnson and Grivetti, 2002a; Ogle et al., 2003).

Correlations between diet and community health status have been of particular interest in the Mediterranean (Matalas et al., 1999; Kafatos et al., 2000; Holdsworth et al., 2000). This interest has certainly been reinforced by the discovery of links between the dietary tradition of these populations and lower rates of coronary heart diseases, cancer, diabetes, and increased population longevity (Trichopoulou et al., 2000).

Relatively few studies, however, have taken an ethnobotanical approach in trying to analyze the anthropological and ethnopharmacological aspects of the consumption of noncultivated food plants in the Mediterranean (Forbes, 1976; Paoletti et al., 1995; Bisio and Minuto, 1999; Pieroni, 1999, 2000, 2003; Ertug, 2000; Pieroni, Nebel, et al., 2002; Bonet and Vallès, 2002; Guarrera, 2003), even though the consumption of olive oil and vegetables has been epidemiologically correlated with many of the previously described health benefits, as, for example, in the discussion about the "Albanian paradox" (Gjonça and Bobak, 1997).

However, most ethnobotanical and ethnopharmacological studies in Europe have primarily addressed popular pharmaceutical remedies and have often ignored noncultivated food plants. From an ethnopharmacological perspective, the dietary contribution of wild vegetables and their potential health benefits is now regarded as an important area of research for human dietary health (Guil et al., 1997; Chapman et al., 1997; Sena et al., 1998; Johns et al., 1999; Sundriyal and Sundriyal, 2001; Grivetti and Ogle, 2000; Lockett et al., 2000; Ogle, Hung, and Tuyet, 2001; Ogle, Johansson, et al., 2001; Ogle, Dao, et al., 2001; Corlett et al., 2002; Johnson and Grivetti, 2002b; Owen and Johns, 2002).

While weeds have been found to represent a central component of indigenous pharmacopoeias (Stepp and Moerman, 2001), very little attention has been paid to the medicinal character associated with the consumption of wild greens under an emic perspective, concentrating on the diverse degrees of perception of foods/medicines among cultures.

The aim of this chapter is to investigate the cross-cultural use of noncultivated plants (especially weedy greens) in the traditional diet of ethnic Albanian (Arbëreshë) and autochthonous southern Italians in southern Italy, as well as their indigenous perception and the cultural practices associated with their use, including the gathering, processing, cooking, and consuming of plants as part of the daily diet. In addition, we address some of the potential health benefits associated with the consumption of a few of these plants in an attempt to assess their potential value in preventing age-related diseases (ARDs).

As a premise, a clarification is needed here concerning the terms "traditional" and "traditionally," which are frequently abused in the terminology of many ethnobotanists. We will use these terms here for defining something that has been an *integrated part of a culture for more than one generation* (similar to that written recently by Ogoye-Ndegwa and Aaagaard-Hansen, 2003).

ETHNOGRAPHIC BACKGROUND

In the present study, we compared two territories located in the Basilicata region (also historically named Lucania, which is how the local population refers to their territory) of southern Italy (see Figure 4.1). The Italian National Statistical Institute (ISTAT, 2000) reports that Basilicata represents the Italian region having the lowest percentage of urban population (17 percent, calculated for the period 1997-1999) and the highest male life expectancy (75.7 years, calculated for the period 1991-1995).

We decided to compare two areas in Lucania that have similar socio-economic and demographic characteristics but different ethnic origins: the Vulture area in northern Lucania, inhabited by Arbëreshë (ethnic Albanians), and the Dolomiti Lucane area, in the central part of Lucania, inhabited by autochthonous South Italians (see Figure 4.1).

The Arbëreshë in Lucania

The Arbëreshë are descendants of Albanians who migrated to southern Italy in several migration flows to various central and southern inland regions of Italy in the fifteenth to eighteenth centuries

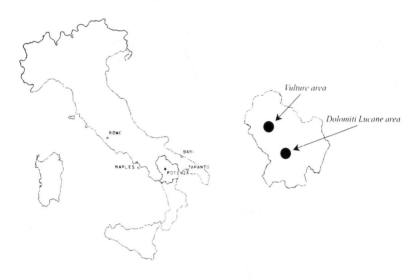

FIGURE 4.1. The location of the studied areas.

(Dessart, 1982). It is estimated that less than 80,000 people in Italy today are bilingual in Arbëreshë and Italian. The Arbëresh Albanian language belongs to the Albanian language group, which in turn represents the only surviving language ensemble from the Paleo-Balkan group (Illyrian, Messapic, and Thracian) of the Indo-European family (Grimes, 2000). Arbëresh Albanian presents features of archaic Albanian, Greek, and Southern Italian, and has been classified as an endangered language in the UNESCO *Redbook of Endangered Languages* (Salminen, 1999). The Italian Arbëreshë obtained official recognition as a historical ethnic minority by the Italian Parliament in 1999.

Our study took place in the Arbëresh communities of the Vulture area, which were founded after fifteenth-century migration flows to that area. These communities are unique in the fact that they have remained isolated from other Arbëresh communities concentrated in Calabria and Sicily, as well as a few other ethnic isles in southern Lucania, Apulia, Campania, Molise, and Abruzzo. Steps to maintain ethnic tradition in the village are also evident, as local events celebrating their ethnic food and culture are held annually, attracting many tourists in the vacation month of August.

This territory of the Arbëreshë was originally sustained by pastoralism and agriculture. Nowadays the cultivation of olive trees *(Olea europaea)*, a local variety of grape vine that gives its name to the local wine *(Vitis vinifera* var. Aglianico), durum wheat *(Triticum durum)*, and, for about ten years, labor in a nearby car factory represent the main economic sources of the local inhabitants.

Nowadays, the majority of the middle-aged (35 to 55 years) population can recall some words and basic customs of their Arbëresh history but do not incorporate these facets of traditional life into their present daily life. This group, for the most part, has abandoned the traditional agropastoralist way of life as a principal source of income and is sustained instead primarily by labor in factories.

Autochthonous Italians of the Dolomiti Lucane

The autochthonous South Italians of the Dolomiti Lucane live in small communities bordering the Basento River Valley and are isolated by the mountainous geography of the region. The economy is still primarily based on small-scale agriculture, including the management of sheep and the *Podolica* breed of cattle for making cheese. The region is best known for its old ties to "magic," brought into the spotlight by the works of the Italian anthropologist De Martino (1959), and even by an old television documentary broadcast of the famous witch/healer Mago Ferramosca (Giuseppe Calvello from Pietrapertosa, who died in 1968). The area is also well-known for the annual ritual feast of "il Maggio," traditionally organized in two villages (Accettura and Pietrapertosa), in which the old ritual "marriage" of two trees is celebrated. The history of the area has been characterized by Norman (starting from the eleventh century AD), Swabian (starting from the thirteenth century AD), and Spanish Bourbon (ca. the fifteenth century AD) domination.

Small-scale agricultural and animal-breeding activities have played a key role in this area for centuries. Durum wheat cultivation and *Podolica* cow[1] breeding particularly represent distinctive characters of the local economy and have been very important in building cultural identity. Today, most of the young people of Castelmezzano travel for work every day to the main Lucanian center of Potenza (mainly as service employees), while small agricultural and pastoral activities are mainly carried out by the older generations.

FIELD METHODS

Over a series of field studies from 2000 to 2003, we have collected data on the traditional use and consumption of wild food and medicinal plants in Lucania. These studies were conducted in three Arbëresh communities (Pieroni, Nebel, et al., 2002) and two autochthonous Italian communities of the Dolomiti Lucane area (Pieroni et al., 2004, 2005). Each of the selected communities were of a relatively small population size (ranging from ca. 700 to 3,000 inhabitants), and the majority of community members had until very recently a strong tie to the environment through agropastoral activities (durum wheat, olive trees, wine grapes; sheep and goat breeding) and small-scale home gardening.

Traditional knowledge regarding plants was assessed using standard ethnobiological and cognitive anthropological analyses for a better understanding of the folk-taxonomical hierarchies and systems, and for studying the most frequently quoted plants by free-listing, triad tests and pile sorts, and constructing a consensus index (Berlin et al., 1966; Rommey, 1989; Berlin, 1992; D'Andrade, 1995; Atran, 1999). This information was gathered through consented interviews with 247 randomly selected members of the studied communities.

In the first phase of the study, participants were asked to freely recall all medicinal food plants used both on a regular basis and used in the past. During the interviews, several fresh and dried plant specimens stocked in a transportable field herbarium were presented to the participants. Participants were asked to identify the local name, preparation, and use of the plant samples. Participation-observation techniques were also utilized to better understand the cultural implications of plant gathering, preparation and cooking of foods, and distribution of shared foods in the community. Round-table focus groups (Price, 1997) with local gatherers and women took place in the second phase of the study in order to discuss and elaborate details concerning the information collected.

Voucher specimens of all the nondomesticated and most uncommon cultivated ethnobotanicals were collected and identified following the standard botanical work for Italian flora (Pignatti, 1982). Voucher specimens and more than 150 hours of video and sound recordings of interviews are stored at the first author's address.

WILD FOOD AND MEDICINAL PLANTS IN LUCANIA

Wild Food Plants and the Lucanian
Cuisine: An Anthropological Perspective

Today, communities of the Dolomiti Lucane mountain range can be reached from the Arbëresh communities of Mount Vulture by roughly an hour-and-a-half drive on the highway. This distance and lack of convenient transportation between the two regions in the past has allowed for a distinct separation of contact between these two cultures and presented us with the opportunity to observe and compare the similarities (and differences) in the traditional use of plants in these two unique cultural groups.

Unfortunately, in both cultural subsets, it is apparent that traditional knowledge concerning the collection and preparation of wild vegetables for consumption is quickly disappearing as new trends in culture overcome both ethnic Albanian and traditional Italian practices. The community- and family-based roles of men and women in these areas are changing with the economy. Whereas in the past the economic role of young men was based in local agriculture, they are now expected to find and maintain a job in the larger cities outside of the village. Most go to work in automobile factories, where rotating work shifts assign men to work throughout the day some weeks and throughout the night on others. Little time is left for home gardening and gathering of wild vegetables—this has especially affected the consumption of such vegetables as tassel hyacinth (*Leopoldia comosa*), Spanish salsify (*Scolymus hispanicus*) and wild oregano (*Origanum heracleoticum*), which are located far from the central village and, along with mushrooms, are traditionally collected only by men.

These shifts in the socioeconomic status of the region have not only affected the men but also women and, thus, the family structure. Previously, the primary role of women in the family was as the caregiver in the home: raising the children, caring for older or disabled family members, home gardening, collecting local wild vegetables, and preparing food. Today, however, women also often join the workforce through factory labor and rely on older women in their family (mothers, aunts, grandmothers) to care for their children while at work and on Eastern European women that are hired to come to live with and care for the older disabled family members. These young women also have little time or, in many cases, desire to carry on the traditional ways of gathering, growing, or preparing wild and culti-vated vegetables, instead buying nearly all foodstuffs for the family from supermarkets and local vegetable vendors and relying on gifts of traditionally prepared dishes from older relatives and friends in the community.

For both sexes of the younger generation, trends toward leaving the "old" ways of living behind in the search for other lifestyles (reli-ant on electronic goods and premade meals) have played a detrimen-tal role in the transmission and perpetuation of traditional knowledge regarding the inclusion of wild edible botanicals in the diet. The abil-ity to identify a plant decreases dramatically among both men and women under age 50, though the women seem to be much more af-fected. Younger men, it seems, are more exposed to other people in the community (especially older men that gather in the local piazza), and as a result of this they have a slightly higher level of knowledge regarding plant identification than their female counterparts.

Thus, today, only the oldest women and men (who are physically able) continue in the collection of wild weedy greens and the care of home gardens. They often collect more than is needed for themselves and give many of the vegetables to younger family members and friends in either the raw form or, more commonly, as a prepared dish.

Food and/or Medicine? Diverse Degrees of Interrelations

Among both ethnic Albanians and southern Italians we recorded diverse ways of perceiving the degree of correlation between food and medicinal value of botanicals. We tried to schematize these find-ings in Figure 4.2:

1. Diverse plants are used in a multifunctional way, both for food and medicines, but without any kind of relationship between these two fields of uses (see Table 4.1).
2. A great number of plants (generally weedy species) are con-sumed and thought to be "healthy," but without any unique spec-ification for their assumed health-benefiting action. They are generally defined "depurative"; "good for blood turnover"; are consumed especially in spring (and, less frequently, in autumn); and fit completely in a kind of "folk functional foods" (see Table 4.2). Although there is no universally accepted definition, func-

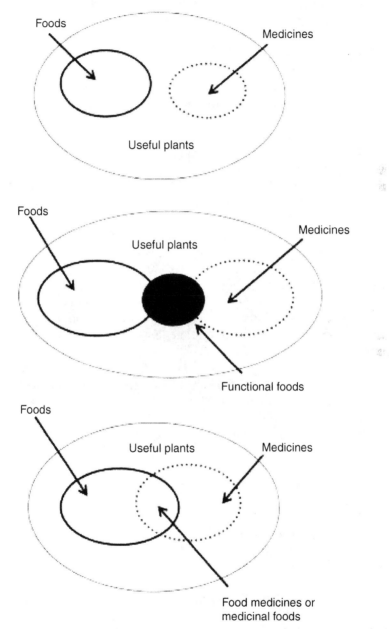

FIGURE 4.2. Scheme of three models of perception of the relation between plant foods and medicines in southern Italy.

tional foods can be described as foods that "have besides their main nutritional or delight purposes still other effects on body function" (Preuss, 1999) and occupy a third space between food and medicine.

3. A few species are consumed (ingested in a "food context"), in order to obtain a specific medicinal action (see Table 4.3); for them we will use the terms *medicinal foods* or *food medicines.*

A few botanical taxa are perceived and categorized in more than one field, and the whole picture can actually be extremely complex.

Differences in the Perception of Wild Plant Foods and Medicines Between Arbëreshë and Autochthonous Italian Communities

Culture strongly influences the preference and consumption of food/medicinal species. Between Arbëreshë and autochthonous Italian communities in Lucania, it is possible to point out a stronger role of weedy folk functional foods among ethnic Albanians. Moreover, a few food weedy species are not common in the two cuisines, and further analysis among Albanian communities in contemporary Albania and Kosovo could eventually relate these differences to specific cultural peculiarities.

The major role of functional folk foods among ethnic Albanians (see Figure 4.3) could be due to a slightly different geographical location, meaning a few differences in the ecology/availability of certain botanical species (although officially the flora of the two areas are considered identical), but also to more general differences in cultural aspects. The folk pharmacopoeia of the Arbëreshë is much more restricted than that of the southern Italians (Pieroni and Quave, 2005), which is also indicated by a minor number of food medicines (Table 4.1) and wild medicinal plants having food uses (Table 4.3). This could be compensated by a more complex system of preventive medicine (functional foods), which is exactly where the weedy greens fit in. Cultural adaptation phenomena could, for example, have played a role in these dynamics during the past four centuries.

Cultural Changes and Adaptation

Both in the Vulture and Dolomiti Lucane areas, emigration (mainly of the male subpopulation of the communities) to northern Italy or

TABLE 4.1. Wild botanical species utilized in the studied areas *as food and as medicines*, without any correlation between these two uses.

Botanical taxon and family	English name	Uses in the local medicine	Use in the local cuisine	Albanians	Italians
Clematis vitalba (Ranunculaceae)	Traveller's joy	Decoction, in gargles, to heal mouth in-flammations[fr]	Boiled and then fried with eggs[sh]	–	+
Cynara cardunculus (Asteraceae)	Wild artichoke	Decoction (together with cinquefoil *[Potentilla reptans]* and figwort *[Scrophularia canina]*), then in compress as antirheumatic[ap]	Eaten cooked[rec,st,ro]	–	+
Diplotaxis tenuifolia (Brassicaceae)	Wild rocket	Oleolite, in topical application to heal muscular pains[le]	Eaten raw in salads[le]	–	+
Ficus carica (Moraceae)	Fig	Dried, then in decoction with other herbs (generally including aerial parts of mallow *[Malva sylvestris]* and barley *[Hordeum vulgare]* seeds), to heal sore throats[pf]; topical application, to heal insect bites and against warts[sa]	Eaten raw or dried[pf]	+	+
Laurus nobilis (Lauraceae)	Bay tree	Decoction, with other herbs, to heal sore throats and as digestive[le]	Aromatizing diverse dishes[le]	+	+
Morus alba and *M. nigra* (Moraceae)	Mulberry tree	Decoction, to heal sore throats[le]	Eaten raw[pf]	–	+
Origanum heracleoticum (Lamiaceae)	Wild oregano	Fumigation on hot coke, to cure cough or toothache[ft]	Aromatizing a few dishes[ft]	+	+
Papaver rhoeas. (Papaveraceae)	Corn poppy	Decoction, as mild sedative for children[fl]	As wild vegetables, (cooked)[fl]	+	–

TABLE 4.1. *(continued)*

Botanical taxon and family	English name	Uses in the local medicine	Use in the local cuisine	Albanians	Italians
Prunus dulcis (Rosaceae)	Almond tree	Cold macerate, to heal intestinal pains (children)[se]; in mixture with other herbs, to heal sore throats[ep]	Eaten raw, fresh or dried[uf,se]	+	+
Prunus spinosa (Rosaceae)	Sloe	Decoction, as a "hepato-protector"[fr]	Eaten raw after the first frost, as snack[fr]	–	+
Rosa canina (Rosaceae)	Dog rose	Ground and topically applied, to heal insect bites[le]; stuffing for a little bag attached to clothing as an amulet against the evil eye[pf]	Eaten raw as snack[pf]	–	+
Rubus ulmifolius (Rosaceae)	Blackberry	Decoction (together or without rhizomes of couchgrass), as diuretic[le]; heated and then topically applied, to cure purulent skin abscesses[le]	Eaten raw; jam[pf]	+	+
Sonchus asper and *S. oleraceus* (Asteraceae)	Sow thistle	Cold macerate applied externally in the mouth, to cure afta[ap]	Eaten raw or cooked, as wild vegetables[ap]	+	–
Sorbus domestica (Rosaceae)	Service tree	Decoction, to heal diarrhea[fr]	Eaten raw after natural fermentation[fr]	–	+
Veronica beccabunga (Scrophulariaceae)	Broomkline	Decoction, as diuretic[ap]	Eaten raw in mixed salads[ap]	–	+
Ziziphus jujuba (Rhamnaceae)	Jujube	Decoction, mixed with other herbs, to heal sore throats and cough[fr]	Eaten raw as snack[fr]	–	+

Part(s) used: ap: aerial part; fl: flowers; fr: fruits; ft: flowering tops; le: leaves; pf: pseudo-fruits; re: flower receptacles; ro: root/tuber; se: seeds; sh: shoots; st: stems; uf: unripe fruits.

TABLE 4.2. Wild botanical species utilized in the studied areas as *folk functional foods*.

Botanical taxon and family	English name	Part(s) used	Culinary uses	Albanians	Italians
Allium ampeloprasum (Liliaceae)	Wild leek	bu	Cooked and condiment	+	+
Amaranthus retroflexus (Amaranthaceae)	Pigweed	le	Cooked	+	+
Apium nodiflorum (Apiaceae)	Fool's watercress	ap	Raw and cooked	+	–
Asparagus acutifolius (Liliaceae s.l.)	Wild asparagus	sh	Cooked	+	+
Bellavalia romana (Liliaceae s.l.)	Bellavalia	bu	Cooked	–	+
Beta vulgaris ssp. *maritima* (Chenopodiaceae)	Sea beat	ap	Cooked	+	+
Borrago officinalis (Boraginaceae)	Borage	le	Cooked	+	+
Capsella bursa-pastoris (Brassicaceae)	Shepherd's purse	wh	Cooked	+	–
Carlina acaulis (Asteraceae)	Stemless carline thistle	re	Cooked	–	+
Centaurea calcitrapa (Asteraceae)	Star thistle	wh	Cooked	+	–
Chenopodium album (Chenopodiaceae)	Fat hen	le	Cooked	+	+
Chondrilla juncea (Asteraceae)	Naked weed	wh, sh	Raw and cooked	+	–
Cichorium intybus (Asteraceae)	Wild chicory	wh	Raw and cooked	+	+
Clematis vitalba (Ranunculaceae)	Traveller's joy	sh	Cooked	+	+

113

TABLE 4.2. *(continued)*

Botanical taxon and family	English name	Part(s) used	Culinary uses	Albanians	Italians
Crepis vesicaria (Asteraceae)	Beaked hawksbeard	wh	Cooked	+	+
Cynara cardunculus ssp. *cardunculus* (Asteraceae)	Wild artichoke	st, re	Cooked	–	+
Diplotaxis tenuifolia (Brassicaceae)	Wild rocket	le	Raw	+	–
Foeniculum vulgare ssp. *piperitum* (Apiaceae)	Wild fennel	ap, fr	Raw, cooked, and condiment	+	+
Humulus lupulus (Cannabaceae)	Wild hops	sh	Cooked	+	–
Lactuca serriola spp. (Asteraceae)	Wild lettuce	ap	Raw and cooked	+	–
Leontodon (Asteraceae)	Hawkbit	wh	Raw and cooked	–	+
Leopoldia comosa (syn. *Muscari comosum*, Liliaceae s.l.)	Tassel hyacinth	bu	Cooked	+	+
Lycium europaeum (Solanaceae)	Boxthorn	sh	Cooked	+	–
Muscari atlanticum and *M. botryoides* (Liliaceae s.l.)	Grape hyacinth	bu	Cooked	+	+
Nasturtium officinale (Brassicaceae)	Watercress	le	Raw and cooked	+	–
Onopordum illyiricum (Asteraceae)	Cotton thistle	ro, st	Cooked	–	+
Origanum heracleoticum (Lamiaceae)	Wild oregano	ft	Condiment	+	+
Papaver rhoeas (Papaveraceae)	Poppy corn	wh, le	Cooked	+	+
Picris echioides (Asteraceae)	Bristly ox-tongue	wh	Cooked	+	+
Portulaca oleracea (Portulacaceae)	Green purslane	ap	Raw	+	+
Reichardia picroides (Asteraceae)	French scorzonera	wh	Raw and cooked	+	+

Species	Common name	Part(s) used	Preparation		
Ruscus aculeatus (Liliaceae s.l.)	Butcher's broom	sh	Cooked	–	+
Scolymus hispanicus (Asteraceae)	Spanish salsify	ls	Cooked	+	–
Silybum marianum (Asteraceae)	Milk thistle	st, ro	Cooked	–	+
Sinapis arvensis (Brassicaceae)	Wild mustard	ap	Cooked	+	+
Sisymbrium officinale (Asteraceae)	Hedge mustard	wh	Cooked	+	–
Sonchus asper and S. oleraceus (Asteraceae)	Sow thistle	wh	Raw and cooked	+	+
Stellaria media (Caryophylaceae)	Chickweed	ap	Raw and cooked	+	–
Tamus communis (Dioscoreaceae)	Black bryony	sh	Cooked	+	–
Taraxacum officinale (Asteraceae)	Dandelion	wh	Cooked	+	+
Tordylium apulum (Apiaceae)	Roman pimpernel	wh	Cooked, condiment	+	–
Urtica dioica (Urticaceae)	Nettle	le	Cooked	+	–
Valerianella carinata (Valerianaceae)	Keeled-fruited cornsalad	wh	Raw	+	–
Veronica beccabunga (Scrophulariaceae)	Brooklime	ap	Raw	–	+

Part(s) used: ap: aerial part; fl: flowers; fr: fruits; ft: flowering tops; le: leaves; ls: leaf stalks; pf: pseudo-fruits; re: flower receptacles; ro: root/tuber; se: seeds; sh: shoots; st: stems; uf: unripe fruits; wh: whorls.

TABLE 4.3. Wild botanical species utilized in the studied areas as foods consumed as proper medicines (*medicinal foods* or *food medicines*).

Botanical taxa and family	English name	Part(s) used	Culinary preparation	Medicinal use	Albanians	Italians
Asparagus acutifolius (Liliaceae s.l.)	Wild asparagus	sh	Boiled and consumed alone or with scrambled eggs and fresh cheese	Diuretic	–	+
Borago officinalis (Boraginaceae)	Borage	le	Soup	Postpartum reconstituent and galactagogue	+	–
			Soups with onions, dried sweet pepper, served on bread	Galactagogue	–	+
Cichorium intybus (Asteraceae)	Wild chicory	le	Soup	Laxative	–	+
Leopoldia comosa (Liliaceae s.l.)	Tassel hyacinth	bu	Cut, macerated in water, then fried	Antifever	+	–
Malva sylvestris (Malvaceae)	Mallow	le	Soup	To enhance uterine contractions during birth; galactagogue	+	–
Ruscus aculeatus (Liliaceae s.l.)	Butcher's broom	sh	Boiled and traditionally consumed with bread and sour cream from *Podolica* cow milk	Hepatodepurative	–	+
Sonchus oleraceus (Asteraceae)	Sow thistle	wh	Raw in salad	Antigastritis	–	+
Sorbus domestica (Rosaceae)	Service tree	fr	Eaten dried or boiled	Antidiarrhea	–	+
Veronica beccabunga (Scrophulariaceae)	Brooklime	ap	Eaten raw in salads	Diuretic	–	+

Part(s) used: ap: aerial parts; bu: bulbs; fr: fruits; le: leaves; sh: shoots; wh: whorls.

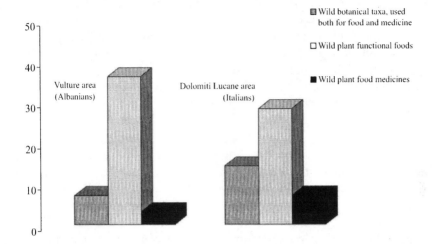

FIGURE 4.3. Wild plants perceived to be related with the three models of food medicines among Albanians and Italians.

Central Europe had its major peaks at the end of the 1960s and the beginning of the 1970s. This phenomenon certainly contributed greatly to the cultural change in both territories. The men who returned back home after a few years of well-paid labor in factories or in building trades began to work in similar sectors rather than in agriculture. They have played a certain role—especially among Albanians—in the positive internalization of the acculturation process and in the adoption of the mainstream Italian/European cultural models. These are the same people who generally began to reject Arbëresh cultural practices; in contrast to this group of men, elderly women try to actively maintain most of the original expression of their unique culture through continued involvement in gathering weedy greens and preparing traditional meals.

Another factor that has certainly played a role in this matter is represented by the emigrated families of the middle generation (those who left southern Italy during the 1980s to move to northern Italy), who normally come back to visit their parents or relatives in the summer. Among these people, perhaps because of the negative images portrayed by the media concerning the recent immigrant flows from Albania, the rejection of traditional culture is very strong. A man from this group of migrants tried to convince his interviewer that traditional Albanian culture is something that has be to hidden, because "Albanians, after all, are like *gypsies*" (gypsy has a strongly negative connotation among ethnic Italians), which strongly denies his roots.

There has surely been an exchange over time of Arbëresh and southern Italian women's knowledge of the culinary use of wild vegetables. A strong acculturation process took place in the Arbëresh centers from the 1960s onward, when streets were improved and exchanges with nearby southern Italian communities became very intense. Italian-speaking officers and civil servants arrived in the villages as local elementary schools and postoffices were established and when electricity and a sewage system was installed. This process began to slowly affect local cuisine. Today's daily Arbëresh diet doesn't differ substantially from that of neighboring Italian communities. When comparing traditional Arbëresh women's cuisine in the Vulture area with that of southern Italian women living in the Dolomiti Lucane area, only minor differences are evident (see Figure 4.4).

"Liakra" and "Foglie": Wild Functional Foods Among Albanians and Italians

Traditions related to gathering and cooking wild food greens are very popular in the Vulture area and, a little bit less, in the Dolomite Lucane. The Arbëreshë clearly distinguish between *liakra* (*edible* weedy vegetables) and *bara* (*nonedible* grasses and herbs). Liakra, used by the Arbëreshë as a synonym for "weedy greens," has an Albanian origin (*lakër* means "cabbage" in modern Albanian), even though the term no longer exists in the modern Tosk Albanian language. In the South-Italian dialects *foglie* ("leaves") is the term used to indicate the Albanian *liakra*.

"Food touches everything. It is a central pawn in political strategies of states and households. Food marks social differences, boundaries, bonds, and contradictions" (Counihan and Van Esterik, 1999). Social changes and modernization also affect food processing, storage, cooking, food habits, and social relations. Food, then, is not only nourishment; in the Vulture area, wild food botanicals represent central elements of the most important religious procession of the Catholic Holy Friday, the *processione della zingara in Barile* (procession

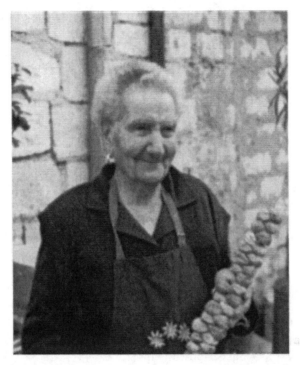

FIGURE 4.4. Zia Giovannina (from Ginestra) has collected figs *(Ficus carica)* on a thin piece of giant reed *(Arundo donax)*. Oftentimes, an almond (fruit of *Prunus dulcis)* is also inserted into the fig before drying. These fruits are used to make a decoction with diverse herbs for the prevention and treatment of sore throat during the winter months. Photo reprinted with permission

of the gypsy of Barile/Barilli). In this traditional procession, which is witnessed by all Arbëreshë (and southern Italians) in the Vulture area, a few typical Arbëresh characters are present alongside the classical representations of the Christian tradition. Among them, the most important is the "gypsy lady" *(la zingara),* who is dressed in traditional costume, covered by all the (real!) gold jewels previously collected from each family in the village. She symbolizes the temptations of Christ and, in the procession, everyone throws dried and roasted chickpeas *(Cicer arietinum)* at her. In Arbëresh symbolism, the chickpea is considered to be "negative" because it is believed that the sounds of its pods shaking led to the discovery of Jesus Christ during his flight to Egypt. The crown that adorns Christ's head in the procession is made with dried stems of boxthorn *(Lycium europaeum),* whose young shoots are consumed cooked and fried with other wild vegetables in the spring by the Albanians (a similar use has never been reported in the ethnobotanical studies in Europe) (Pieroni, Nebel, et al., 2002).

In the past, however, both *liakra* among Albanians and *foglie* among southern Italians were often eaten as snacks during fieldwork. More often, they were brought home, washed at the village fountain, and then boiled in the traditional terra-cotta pot. In the poorest families they were eaten raw with bread, without oil and salt. Nowadays, only very few wild greens are eaten raw. Commonly, both among Albanians and southern Italians, they are lightly boiled and then fried in olive oil together with garlic and, sometimes, a few hot chili peppers. The cooked greens are then added to boiled pasta as a kind of green vegetable sauce. In some cases, these weedy greens are boiled together with the pasta, and the entire preparation is fried in olive oil with garlic. Pasta with greens is often considered to be a main dish. In some other cases, the wild species are cooked and consumed with bean soup. This is the case with the traditional Albanian preparations *luljëkuq e fazuljë* (corn poppy leaves *[Papaver rhoeas],* and beans), or *bathë e çikour* (mashed fava beans *[Vicia faba]* and wild chicory *[Cichorium intybus]*), or they are eaten in a kind of soup prepared with mixtures of more than ten wild herbs (a similar recipe is also found among southern Italians). *Liakra* are only rarely used among Albanians to prepare special meals for feast days. On Christmas Eve, anchovies or dried fish are traditionally served with boiled and fried shoots of broccoli raab that are semicultivated in the area *(çim de rrapë, Brassica rapa* ssp. *rapa* [DC.] Metzg. [Group Ruvo Bailey], syn.: *Brassica rapa* L. Broccoletto Group), or of wild mustard *(sënap, Sinapis* spp.). During Easter, a kind of pie *(verdhët)* is prepared with eggs, lamb, ricotta, sheep cheese, and (previously boiled) leaf stalks of *Scolymus hispanicus* while, in the village of Maschito/ Masqiti, the young aerial parts of wild fennel *(Foeniculum vulgare* spp. *piperitum)* are used instead.

Among southern Italians, the *foglie* are traditionally eaten with a bean-based soup and pig lard, while wild fennel aerial parts are preferred on mashed green broad beans *(Vicia faba).* Among this group, we could not record any traditions of consuming special feast dishes with wild greens.

If southern Italian cuisine has had a strong influence on the Arbëresh diet, very few traces of the inverse trend (Italians living in the Vulture area adopting Arbëresh dishes) can be found: the use of the already mentioned *verdhët* (*verdhët* from the Albanian *verdhë*, in English "yellow," perhaps due to the large amount of eggs used in this festival dish) is, for example, also popular in the nearby Italian villages (Rionero, Ripacandida, Venosa). A *mutual* exchange of experiences and culinary knowledge between Arbëresh and Italian women has been hindered due to the dominance of mainstream Italian culture.

A special processing method is used for tassel hyacinth bulbs (*Leopoldia comosa,* syn.: *Muscari comosum*). The consumption of these bitter bulbs is a common factor in the Lucanian diet and, among the communities in our study, it is most predominantly used in the Arbëresh villages. The wild bulbs are usually gathered by men and are cleaned and prepared by women. In the cleaning process, women remove the outermost layer of "skin" with a knife and carve a small "x" onto the top of the bulb before placing it into a bowl of cool water to soak overnight, in order to decrease their bitterness. The next day, the bulbs are placed into a small terra-cotta pot with some water and are left to slowly roast throughout the day on the embers of a fire. When the bulbs are softened, they may be fried with some olive oil and sweet pepper *(Capsicum annuum)* or are stored in a jar of olive oil for future consumption as an appetizer. Bulbs of *Leopoldia* are also consumed in other areas of southern Italy (Casoria et al., 1999).

PHARMACOLOGY OF WILD FUNCTIONAL FOODS CONSUMED IN SOUTHERN ITALY

The consumption of wild plant functional foods plays a central role in the diet of Albanians and Italians in southern Italy, but very few phytopharmacological studies have dealt exhaustively with potential health benefits of such dietary supplements (Uiso and Johns, 1995; Chapman et al., 1997; Johns et al., 1999; Trichopoulou et al., 2000). Surveys on aromatic species of the traditional Mediterranean cuisine have recently demonstrated their significant health benefits (Lionis et al., 1998; Cervato et al., 2000; Martinez-Tome et al., 2001). Since reactive oxygen species (ROS) production and oxidative stress have been shown to be linked to aging-related diseases (ARDs,

Finkel and Holbrook, 2000) and a large number of other illnesses, the number of studies on antioxidant properties of plant foods and their phenolic constituents has become very impressive. For example, antioxidant activity was recently studied in relation to CNS disorders (Perry et al., 2001; Bastianetto and Quirion, 2002).

Our research group recently studied weedy food plants traditionally consumed among the Albanians of the Vulture area (Pieroni, Janiak, et al., 2002). The aim of the study was to evaluate the antioxidant activity of the most commonly consumed noncultivated vegetables of the traditional Arbëresh diet. In order to correlate the antioxidant activity of the plant extracts with their potential effects on ARDs, CNS-disorders, hyperuricaemia, and gout, selected extracts were evaluated for antioxidant activity using DPPH (1,1-diphenyl-2-picrylhydrazil radical) as well as the in vitro inhibition of bovine brain lipid peroxidation and of xanthine oxidase (XO).

Many noncultivated food species gathered in Lucania have shown remarkable antioxidant activity (Pieroni, Janiak, et al., 2002). Although the antioxidant properties of *Origanum* spp. (aerial parts) have been studied relatively well over the past years (Dapkevicius et al., 1998; Milos et al., 2000; Cervato et al., 2000), nothing was known of the relevant antioxidant properties of *Leopoldia, Centaurea,* and *Tordylium* spp. before our bioevaluation tests. The antioxidant activity of bulbs of *Leopoldia comosa* (syn.: *Muscari comosum*) and of young whorls of *Centaurea calcitrapa,* both in the prescreening DPPH and in the lipid peroxidation inhibition assays, are very interesting, and both species should be investigated phytochemically and biochemically focusing on these properties. The local processing and cooking procedures should also be taken into consideration.

The young whorls of *Centaurea calcitrapa* are boiled and fried in mixtures with other weedy noncultivated "greens." Aerial parts of *Centaurea calcitrapa* and *Tordylium apulum* are still poorly investigated phytochemically.

Moreover, the strong XO-inhibiting activity shown by extracts of aerial parts of *Cichorium intybus, Chondrilla juncea,* and *Stellaria media* in our recent studies could merit further investigation, focusing on natural products with potential effects on hyperuricaemia and gout. Very little has been reported about bioactive compounds from *Chondrilla juncea* and *Stellaria media.*

Mediterranean noncultivated weedy vegetables, which we have called in this chapter wild *"folk functional foods,"* represent then a neglected group of plants that offer an exciting challenge to modern phytotherapeutical researchers bridging the gap between pharmaceuticals and nutraceuticals.

CONCLUSION

We have presented here a variety of wild plants that have been commonly used in the recent past as a central portion of the daily diet in two cultures of southern Italy. They are still used sometimes in southern Italy as food or medicine, as functional food, or as medicinal foods (food medicines).

Research on the medicinal or nutraceutical value of many of these plants has demonstrated high antioxidant activity and potential as therapeutic agents for the management and prevention of chronic disease such as diabetes, stroke, and coronary heart disease. The presence of high levels of antioxidants in the human diet may be especially important in the prevention and management of ARDs.

Thus, recording and conserving traditional knowledge regarding the use of plants is of utmost importance, not only for the biocultural conservation of the communities/environments studied but also for future medical advancements in the prevention and management of chronic, diet-related diseases. An anthropological analysis of the socioeconomic shifts and their effects on cultural integrity, however, specifically concerning the transmission of these knowledge systems, has demonstrated that they likely will not survive forthcoming generations if efforts to restore their prominence in communities are not undertaken soon.

NOTE

1. This cow race is a descendant of the *Bos primigenius podolicus,* the very large, long-horned cattle thought to have been domesticated in the Middle East during the fourth century BC. It is bred in Lucania in a semidomesticated way, letting the animal roam free in the forest for most of the year and milking it only during April and May.

REFERENCES

Asfaw, Z. and M. Tadesse (2001). Prospect for sustainable use and development of wild food plants in Ethiopia. *Economic Botany* 55: 47-62.

Atran, S. (1999). Itzaj Maya folk biological taxonomy: Cognitive universals and cultural particulars. In Medin, D.L. and S. Atran (Eds.), *Folkbiology*. Cambridge, MA: The MIT Press.

Bastianetto, S. and R. Quirion (2002). Natural extracts as possible protective agents of brain aging. *Neurobiology of Aging* 23(5): 891-897.

Berlin, B. (1992). *Ethnobiological classification*. Princeton: Princeton University Press.

Berlin, B., D.E. Breedlove, and P.H. Raven (1966). Folk taxonomies and biological classification. *Science* 154: 273-275.

Bisio, A. and L. Minuto (1999). The Prebuggiun. In Pieroni, A. (Ed.), *Erbi Boni, Erbi degli Streghi—Good weeds, witches' weeds*. Cologne: Experiences Verlag.

Bonet, M.A. and J. Vallés (2002). Use of non-crop vascular plants in Montseny biosphere reserve (Catolonia, Iberian Peninsula). *International Journal of Food Sciences and Nutrition* 53: 225-248.

Bukenya-Ziraba, R. (1996). *The non-cultivated edible plants of Uganda*. Addis Ababa, Ethiopia: NAPRECA.

Bye, R.A. (1981). Quelites—Ethnoecology of edible greens—Past, present, and future. *Journal of Ethnobiology* 1: 109-123.

Casoria, P., B. Menale, and R. Muoio (1999). *Muscari comosum*, Liliaceae, in the food habits of south Italy. *Economic Botany* 53: 113-117.

Cervato, G., M. Carabelli, S. Gervasio, A. Cittera, R. Cazzola, and B. Cestaio (2000). Anti-oxidant properties of oregano *(Origanum vulgare)* leaf extracts. *Journal of Food Biochemistry* 24: 453-456.

Chapman, L., T. Johns, and R.L.A. Mahunnah (1997). Saponin-like in vitro characteristics of extracts from selected non-nutrient wild plant food additives used by Maasai in meat and milk based soups. *Ecology of Food and Nutrition* 36: 1-22.

Corlett, J.L., M.S. Clegg, C.L. Keen, and L.E. Grivetti (2002). Mineral content of culinary and medicinal plants cultivated by Hmong refugees living in Sacramento, California. *International Journal of Food Sciences and Nutrition* 53: 117-128.

Counihan, C. and P. Van Esterik (Eds.) (1999). *Food and culture: A reader*. New York: Routledge.

D'Andrade, R. (1995). *The development of cognitive anthropology*. Cambridge, UK: Cambridge University Press.

Dapkevicius, A., R. Venskutonis, T.A. van Beek, and J.P.H. Linssen (1998). Antioxidant activity of extracts obtained by different isolation procedures from some aromatic herbs grown in Lithuania. *Journal of the Science of Food and Agriculture* 77(1): 140-146.

De Martino, F. (1959). *Sud e Magia*. Milan: Feltrinelli.

Dessart, F. (1982). The Albanian ethnic groups in the world: A historical and cultural essay on the Albanian colonies in Italy. *East European Quarterly* 4: 469-484.

Ertug, F. (2000). An ethnobotanical study in central Anatolia (Turkey). *Economic Botany* 54: 155-182.

Etkin, N.L. (Ed.) (1994). *Eating on the wild side.* Tucson: The University of Arizona Press.

Etkin, N.L. (1996). Medicinal cuisines: Diet and ethnopharmacology. *International Journal of Pharmacognosy* 34: 313-326.

Etkin, N.L. and P.J. Ross (1982). Food as medicine and medicine as food: An adaptive framework for the interpretation of plant utilisation among the Hausa of northern Nigeria. *Social Science and Medicine* 16: 1559-1573.

Finkel, T. and N.J. Holbrook (2000). Oxidants, oxidative stress and the biology of ageing. *Nature* 408: 239-247.

Forbes, M.H.C. (1976). Gathering in the Argolid: A subsistence subsystem in a Greek agricultural community. *Annals of the New York Academy of Science* 268: 251-264.

Gjonça, A. and M. Bobak (1997). Albanian paradox, another example of protective effect of Mediterranean lifestyle? *The Lancet* 350: 1815-1817.

Grimes, B.F. (Ed.) (2000). Ethnologue [CD-ROM]. Dallas: Summer Institute of Linguistics.

Grivetti, L.E. and B.M. Ogle (2000). Value of traditional foods in meeting macro- and micronutrients needs: The wild plant connection. *Nutrition Research Review* 13: 31-46.

Guarerra, P.M. (2003). Food medicine and minor nourishment in the folk traditions of Central Italy (Marche, Abruzzo and Latium). *Fitoterapia* 74: 515-544.

Guil, J.L., I. Rodríguez-García, and E. Torija (1997). Nutritional and toxic factors in selected wild edible plants. *Plant Foods for Human Nutrition* 51: 99-107.

Hillocks, R.J. (1998). The potential benefits of weeds with reference to small holder agriculture in Africa. *Integrated Pest Management Reviews* 3: 155-167.

Holdsworth, M., M. Gerber, C. Haslam, J. Scali, A. Beradsworth, M.H. Avallone, and E. Sherrat (2000). A comparison of dietary behavior in central England and a French Mediterranean region. *European Journal of Clinical Nutrition* 54: 530-539.

Humphrey, C.M., M.S. Clegg, C.L. Keen, and L.E. Grivetti (1993). Food diversity and drought survival. The Hausa example. *International Journal of Food Science and Nutrition* 44: 1-16.

ISTAT (2000). *Servizio Popolazione e Cultura.* Rome: ISTAT.

Johns, T. (1990). *With bitter herbs they shall eat it.* Tucson: The University of Arizona Press.

Johns, T. and J.O. Kokwaro (1991). Food plants of the Luo of Siaya District, Kenya. *Economic Botany* 45: 103-113.

Johns, T., R.L.A. Mahunnah, P. Sanaya, L. Chapman, and T. Ticktin (1999). Saponins and phenolic content in plant dietary additives of a traditional subsistence community, the Bateni of Ngorongoro District, Tanzania. *Journal of Ethnopharmacology* 66: 1-10.

Johns, T., E.B. Mhoro, and P. Sanaya (1996). Food plants and masticants of the Batemi of Ngorongoro District, Tanzania. *Economic Botany* 50: 115-121.

Johns, T., E.B. Mhoro, and F.C. Usio (1996). Edible plants of Mara Region, Tanzania. *Ecology of Food and Nutrition* 35: 71-80.

Johnson, N. and L.E. Grivetti (2002a). Environmental change in Northern Thailand: Impact on wild edible plant availability. *Ecology of Food and Nutrition* 41: 373-399.

Johnson, N. and L.E. Grivetti (2002b). Gathering practices of Karen women: Questionable contribution to beta-carotene intake. *International Journal of Food Sciences and Nutrition* 53: 489-501.

Kafatos, A., H. Verhagen, J. Moschandreas, I. Apostolaki, and J.J.M. van Westerop (2000). Mediterranean diet of Crete: Foods and nutrient content. *Journal of the American Diabetic Association* 100: 1487-1493.

Khasbagan, H.-Y.H. and S.J. Pei (2000).Wild plants in the diet of Arhorchin Mongol herdsmen in inner Mongolia. *Economic Botany* 54: 528-536.

Khasbagan, Narisu and K. Stuart (1999). Ethnobotanical overview of *gogd* (*Allium ramosum* L.): A traditional edible wild plant used by Inner Mongolians. *Journal of Ethnobiology* 19: 221-225.

Kuhnlein, H.V. (1992). Change in the use of traditional foods by the Nuxalk native people of British Columbia. *Ecology of Food and Nutrition* 27: 259-282.

Ladio, A.H. (2001). The maintenance of wild edible plant gathering in a Mapuche community of Patagonia. *Economic Botany* 55: 243-254.

Ladio, A.H. and M. Lozada (2000). Edible wild plant use in a Mapuche community on northwestern Patagonia. *Human Ecology* 28: 53-71.

Ladio, A.H. and M. Lozada (2001). Nontimber forest product use in two human populations from northwestern Patagonia: A quantitative approach. *Human Ecology* 29: 367-380.

Ladio, A.H. and M. Lozada (2003). Comparison of wild edible plant diversity and foraging strategies in two aboriginal communities of northwestern Patagonia. *Biodiversity and Conservation* 12: 937-951.

Lepofski, D., N.J. Turner, and H.V. Kuhnlein (1985). Determining the availability of traditional wild food plants: An example of Nuxalk foods, Bella Coola, British Columbia. *Ecology of Food and Nutrition* 16: 223-241.

Lionis, C., Å. Faresjö, M. Skoula, M. Kapsokefalou, T. Faresjö (1998). Anti-oxidant effects of herbs in Crete. *Lancet* 352: 1987-1988.

Lockett, C.T., C.C. Calvert, and L.E. Grivetti (2000). Energy and micronutrient composition of dietary and medicinal wild plants consumed during drought. Study of rural Fulani, Northeastern Nigeria. *International Journal of Food Sciences and Nutrition* 51: 195-208.

Lockett, C.T. and L.E. Grivetti (2000). Food-related behaviors during drought: A study of rural Fulani, northeastern Nigeria. *International Journal of Food Sciences and Nutrition* 51: 91-107.

Marshall, F. (2001). Agriculture and use of wild and weedy greens by the *Piik ap Oom* Okiek of Kenya. *Economic Botany* 55: 32-46.

Martinez-Tome, M., A.M. Jimenez, S. Ruggieri, N. Frega, R. Strabbioli, and M.A. Murcia (2001). Antioxidant properties of Mediterranean spices compared with common food additives. *Journal of Food Protection* 64: 1412-1419.

Matalas, A.L., C.E. Franti, and L.E. Grivetti (1999). Comparative studies of diet and disease prevalence in Greek Chians—Part I. Rural and urban residents of Chios. *Ecology of Food and Nutrition* 38: 351-380.

Mertz, O., A.M. Lykke, and A. Reenberg (2001). Importance and seasonality of vegetable consumption and marketing in Burkina Faso. *Economic Botany* 55: 276-289.

Milos, M., J. Mastelic, and I. Jerkovic (2000). Chemical composition and antioxidant effect of glycosidically bound volatile compounds from oregano (*Origanum vulgare* L. ssp. *hirtum*). *Food Chemistry* 71: 79-83.

Moreno-Black, G., W. Akanan, P. Somnasang, S. Thamathawan, and P. Bozvoski (1996). Non-domesticated food resources in the marketplace and marketing system of northeastern Thailand. *Journal of Ethnobiology* 16: 99-117.

Ogle, B.M., H.T.A. Dao, G. Mulokozi, and L. Hambraeus (2001). Micronutrient composition and nutritional importance of gathered vegetables in Vietnam. *International Journal of Food Sciences and Nutrition* 52: 485-499.

Ogle, B.M. and L.E. Grivetti (1985a). Legacy of the chameleon: Edible wild plants in the kingdom of Swaziland, southern Africa. A cultural, ecological, nutritional study. Part I—Introduction, objectives, methods, Swazi culture, landscape and diet. *Ecology of Food and Nutrition* 16: 193-208.

Ogle, B.M. and L.E. Grivetti (1985b). Legacy of the chameleon: Edible wild plants in the kingdom of Swaziland, southern Africa. A cultural, ecological, nutritional study. Part II—Demographics, species, availability and dietary use, analysis by ecological zone. *Ecology of Food and Nutrition* 17: 1-30.

Ogle, B.M. and L.E. Grivetti (1985c). Legacy of the chameleon: Edible wild plants in the kingdom of Swaziland, southern Africa. A cultural, ecological, nutritional study. Part III—Cultural and ecological analysis. *Ecology of Food and Nutrition* 17: 31-40.

Ogle, B.M. and L.E. Grivetti (1985d). Legacy of the chameleon: Edible wild plants in the kingdom of Swaziland, southern Africa. A cultural, ecological, nutritional study. Part IV—Nutritional values and conclusions. *Ecology of Food and Nutrition* 17: 41-64.

Ogle, B.M., P.H. Hung, and T.T. Tuyet (2001). Significance of wild vegetables in micronutrient intakes of women in Vietnam: An analysis of food variety. *Asian Pacific Journal of Clinical Nutrition* 10: 21-30.

Ogle, B.M., M. Johansson, H.T. Tuyet, and L. Johannesson (2001). Evaluation of the significance of dietary folate from wild vegetables in Vietnam. *Asian Pacific Journal of Clinical Nutrition* 10: 216-221.

Ogle, B.M., H.T. Tuyet, H.N. Duyet, and N.N.X. Dung (2003). Food, feed or medicine: The multiple functions of edible wild plants in Vietnam. *Economic Botany* 57: 103-117.

Ogoye-Ndegwa, C. and J. Aagaard-Hansen (2003). Traditional gathering of wild vegetables among the Luo of western Kenya—A nutritional anthropology project. *Ecology of Food and Nutrition* 42: 69-89.

Owen, P.L. and T. Johns (2002). Antioxidants in medicines and spices as cardioprotective agents in Tibetan highlanders. *Pharmaceutical Biology* 40: 346-357.

Paoletti, M.G., A.L. Dreon, and G.G. Lorenzoni (1995). Pistic, traditional food from Western Friuli, N.E. Italy. *Economic Botany* 49: 26-30.

Pemberton, R.W. and N.S. Lee (1996). Wild food plants in South Korea; market presence, new crops, and exports to the United States. *Economic Botany* 50: 57-70.

Perry, N.S.L., P.J. Houghton, J. Sampson, A.E. Theobald, S. Hart, M. Lis-Balchin, J.R. Hoult, P. Evans, P. Jenner, S. Milligan, and E.K. Perry (2001). In-vitro activity of *S. lavandulaefolia* (Spanish sage) relevant to treatment of Alzheimer's disease. *Journal of Pharmacy and Pharmacology* 53: 1347-1356.

Pieroni, A. (1999). Gathered wild food plants in the upper valley of the Serchio river (Garfagnana), central Italy. *Economic Botany* 53: 327-341.

Pieroni, A. (2000). Medicinal plants and food medicines in the folk traditions of the upper Lucca Province, Italy. *Journal of Ethnopharmacology* 70: 235-273.

Pieroni, A. (2003). Wild food plants and Arbëresh women in Lucania, southern Italy. In Howard, P.L. (Ed.), *Women & plants: Case studies on gender relations in biodiversity management and conservation.* New York: Zed Press.

Pieroni, A., V. Janiak, C.M. Dürr, S. Lüdeke, E. Trachsel, and M. Heinrich (2002). In vitro antioxidant activity of non-cultivated vegetables of ethnic Albanians in southern Italy. *Phytotherapy Research* 16: 467-473.

Pieroni, A., S. Nebel, C. Quave, H. Münz, and M. Heinrich (2002). Ethnopharmacology of *liakra:* Traditional weedy vegetables of the Arbëreshë of the Vulture area in southern Italy. *Journal of Ethnopharmacology* 81: 165-185.

Pieroni, A., S. Nebel, R.F. Santoro, and M. Heinrich (2005). Food for two seasons: Culinary uses of non-cultivated local vegetables and mushrooms in a south Italian village. *International Journal of Food Sciences and Nutrition* 56: 245-272.

Pieroni, A. and C.L. Quave (2005). Traditional pharmacopoeias and medicines among Albanians and Italians in southern Italy: A comparison. *Journal of Ethnopharmacology* 101: 258-270.

Pieroni, A., C.L. Quave, and R.F. Santoro (2004). Folk pharmaceutical knowledge in the territory of the Dolomiti Lucane, inland southern Italy. *Journal of Ethnopharmacology* 95: 373-384.

Pignatti, S. (1982). *Flora d'Italia.* Bologna: Edizioni Edagricole.

Prendergast, H.D.V., N.L. Etkin, D.R. Harris, and P.J. Houghton (Eds.) (1998). *Plants for Food and Medicine*. Kew, UK: The Royal Botanical Gardens.

Preuss, A. (1999). Characterisation of function food. *Deutsche Lebensmittel-Rundschau* 95: 468-472.

Price, L. (1997). Wild plant food in agricultural environments: A study of occurrence, management, and gathering rights in Northeast Thailand. *Human Organization* 56: 209-221.

Rommey, A.K. (1989). Quantitative models, science, and cumulative knowledge. *Journal of Quantitative Research* 1: 153-223.

Salminen, P. (1999). *UNESCO Red Book Report on Endangered Languages: Europe*. Available online at www.helsinki.u/~tasalmin/ europe_report.html.

Schackleton, S.E., C.M. Dzerefos, C.M. Shackleton, and R.F. Mathabela (1998). Use of trading of wild edible herbs in the central lowveld savanna region, South Africa. *Economic Botany* 52: 251-259.

Sena, L.P., D.J. Vanderjagt, C. Rivera, A.T.C. Tsin, I. Muhamadu, O. Mahamadou, M. Millson, A. Pastaszyn, and R.H. Glew (1998). Analysis of nutritional components of eight famine foods of the Republic of Niger. *Plants for Human Nutrition* 52: 17-30.

Stepp, J.R. and D.E. Moerman (2001). The importance of weeds in ethnopharmacology. *Journal of Ethnopharmacology* 75: 19-23.

Sundriyal, M. and R.C. Sundriyal (2001). Wild edible plants of the Sikkim Himalaya: Nutritive values of selected species. *Economic Botany* 55: 377-390.

Trichopoulou, A., P. Lagiou, H. Kuper, and D. Trichopoulos (2000). Cancer and Mediterranean dietary traditions. *Cancer Epidemiology Biomarkers and Prevention* 9: 869-873.

Tukan, S.K., H.R. Takruri, and D.M. Al-Eisawi (1998). The use of wild edible plants in the Jordanian diet. *International Journal of Food Sciences and Nutrition* 51: 195-208.

Turner, N.J. (1995). *Food plants of coastal first peoples*. Vancouver, Canada: Royal British Columbia Museum.

Turner, N.J. (1997). *Food plants of interior first peoples*. Vancouver, Canada: Royal British Columbia Museum.

Turner, N.J. (2003). The ethnobotany of edible seaweed (*Porphyra abbottae* and related species; Rhodophyta: Bangiales) and its use by first nations on the Pacific coast of Canada. *Canadian Journal of Botany* 81: 283-293.

Uiso, F. and T. Johns (1995). Risk assessment of the consumption of a pyrrolizidine alkaloid containing indigenous vegetable *Crotalaria brevidens* (Mitoo). *Ecology of Food and Nutrition* 35: 111-119.

Vainio-Mattila, K. (2000). Wild vegetables used by the Sambaa in the Usambarë Mountains, NE Tanzania. *Annales Botanici Fennici* 37: 57-67.

Vierya-Odilon, L. and H. Vibrans (2001). Weeds as crops: The value of maize field weeds in the Valley of Toluca, Mexico. *Economic Botany* 55: 426-443.

Chapter 5

Digestive Beverages As a Medicinal Food in a Cattle-Farming Community in Northern Spain (Campoo, Cantabria)

Manuel Pardo de Santayana
Elia San Miguel
Ramón Morales

INTRODUCTION

When we are hungry we feel that eating is essentially a biological activity. We ingest food for energy and nutrients. Nevertheless, food is a social phenomenon with many biological, agronomic, economic, and social implications. Food habits cannot be reduced to their nutritional, dietetic, or therapeutic values. Coffee, for example, is not just a stimulant beverage that provides caffeine: it is also a tasty beverage used as a relaxant on social occasions. For most cultures, including those in the Mediterranean area, eating is a social activity that expresses social relations such as status, friendship, or kinship (Contreras, 1993).

In every culture, which foods are selected depends not only on their technical or economic availability (Barrau, 1983) but also on individual and social tastes, traditions, beliefs, and taboos that make a specific product acceptable or rejectable. The choice of each product and the way it is cooked, presented, and ingested all have social significance that depends on social class, gender, age, or other social aspects.

Most of the ethnobotanical research carried out in the Iberian Peninsula has been on the medicinal and food plants used by the rural population; the therapeutic potential of food plants and its social implications have scarcely been studied. At the time of this writing a European project on local nutraceuticals was being carried out in the south of Spain (D. Rivera, 2005).

It is almost impossible to draw a clear line separating food from medicine. Etkin (1996) proposed studying "ingestibles" rather than "food" or "medicine." Digestive infusions and spirits are difficult to assign to a sharply defined category of food. These "social foods" are not specifically ingested for their nutritional value, although the caloric contribution of alcohol cannot be ignored. Instead, they are drunk either for their pleasurable taste during convivial conversation, after a meal, in a break from work, or, for health reasons, at breakfast or before going to bed. They are usually offered to visitors, both to ease social relations and because of their medicinal digestive function. Pieroni (2000) and Bonet and Vallès (2002) have also noted the role of homemade spirits as a medicinal food.

We studied the occurrence and social context of the use of digestive beverages in the course of our ethnobotanic research in a small area of northern Spain. Campoo is a mountainous region of 1,012.12 m^2 on the southern slopes of Cordillera Cantábrica, with an average altitude of 800 m but a huge range in altitude: from 670 m at Ebro River near Polientes to 2,200 m at Pico del Cuchillón (see Figure 5.1). The area is on the junction of the Mediterranean and Atlantic ecological regions and the potential vegetation is oak and beech forests. The

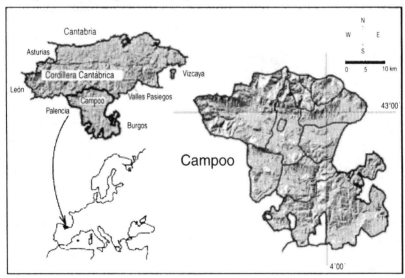

FIGURE 5.1. Geographic location of Campoo (Cantabria, Spain).

population of the area is around 23,000. In recent decades the average age of the population has gone up rapidly because many young people have migrated to urban areas.

The landscape surrounding the villages is dominated by fields of cereals and harvest prairies. Most fields have been abandoned in the past forty years, allowing the grassland and woodland to encroach and become the main elements of the landscape (see Figure 5.2). Farther away from the villages the traditional landscape is grassland for communal grazing and forests that provide wood for multiple purposes and fuel for cooking and heating the houses. Only in the southern regions of Campoo are the fields still cultivated.

In recent decades the economy of Campoo has been mainly based on agriculture, particularly raising livestock. Traditionally, each family kept a few cows and sheep that were managed collectively. The livestock were reared for meat rather than for milk. The economy was fundamentally self-sufficient, with some cash earned from selling animals, handicrafts (wooden shoes, farming implements, tools), and other minor products (milk, butter, eggs). Other income came from working in metal, cement, and glass industries, but salaries were very low and so the workers needed to farm cattle, too. These industries have suffered intense economic decline.

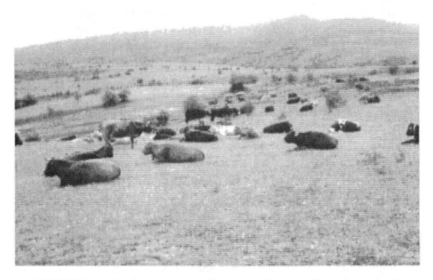

FIGURE 5.2. Cattle grazing at Los Carabeos Campoo (Cantabria, Spain).

In this area, traditional transhumance has survived. It is similar to the transhumance of other cattle-farming systems in the Pyrenees or the *estivage* in the Alps (Gómez Pellón, 1999). In the summer, sheep farmers from Castille or Extremadura also exploited the high-altitude pastures of Campoo, paying rent to the local authority for the privilege.

The extensive cattle-farming system was based on the communal exploitation of high-altitude pastures above the tree line (1,200 m) and below 1,600 m, where the cattle were allowed to roam during the favorable season (i.e., between spring and autumn). The local breed of cattle, *tudanca,* was well adapted to the hostile climate. Their production of litter and milk was low, but they were seldom ill. All the cattle of the community were looked after by cowherds, who were paid in wheat by the other members of the community: each person paid in proportion to the number of cattle contributed to the herd. Some members of the community (usually young men) helped the cowherds according to a rotational system that also depended on the number of cows owned by each family.

In addition to cattle, there were big flocks of sheep or goats in Campoo, comprising all the animals of the neighborhood. These were grazed in the nearby pastures each day, under the supervision of a villager (again, villagers took turns) or of shepherds and their young helpers (male or female). When the average age of the population began to increase it became difficult to find young people willing to herd these animals. These flocks have now disappeared, since people prefer to have cows or horses, which do not roam so much when grazing.

Nowadays people have abandoned aspects of the traditional system and have gradually incorporated the modern market economy. Due to the special incentives for local breeds of livestock, there are a few *tudancas* among the alpine and other breeds of cattle. All the livestock grazing in communal pasture now belong to only a small number of people. The owners visit their animals frequently but there are no longer any shepherds who stay out with the animals all day, looking after them.

The low returns from agriculture (resulting from the difficulties of mechanizing), together with the lack of alternative remunerative employment in industry, resulted in massive rural depopulation during the second part of the twentieth century. Young people moved to cities such as Bilbao, Madrid, Santander, or Barcelona, or to other European and American countries: Germany, France, Argentina, or Mexico. The result has been a social and economic crisis, even leading to entire villages being abandoned and left uninhabited. This phenomenon has also occurred in other mountainous regions of Spain.

Public Rural Development Agencies have played an important role in the recent economic development of the region. Since the 1990s they have attracted European funding through the Leader Program, which was mainly directed toward developing rural tourism. This funding has benefited the local economy and nature conservation, following the ideology of sustainable development.

The information presented in this chapter was gathered during a general ethnobotanic survey based on 117 semistructured interviews with 107 informants, carried out during 1997 and 2000. Local people with traditional knowledge were asked about the medicinal and edible plants they knew; how they were gathered, prepared, or conserved; what kind of illnesses were treated with home remedies; and other aspects of traditional life in which plants played an important role.

CHANGES IN FOOD AND HEALTH HABITS AND CONDITIONS

The recent changes in economic activities have affected the food and medicine habits of the population. Traditionally, the health of the family was essentially cared for using home remedies obtained from the local environment; mainly by mothers and grandmothers. The remedies were intended to heal the most common illnesses: digestive disorders; colds; pneumonia and other respiratory illnesses; and injuries such as burns, wounds or bruises, boils, or other disorders. The consolidation of the free Public Health System pushed aside the traditional use of the home remedies, and chemical pharmacy prevailed.

Traditionally, daily food was based on staple crops cultivated locally: cereals, legumes, potatoes, and other vegetables. The dietary staples were bread, potatoes, and legume soup with pork products. A remarkable variety of legumes (see Table 5.1) was grown in home gardens and fields. Most were cultivated both for people and animals. Other local animal products (milk, butter, eggs, honey) completed the

TABLE 5.1. Legumes cultivated and consumed in Campoo.

Scientific Latin name	Spanish name	English name
Cicer arietinum L.	Garbanzo	Chickpea
Lathyrus sativus L.	Almorta, muela	Chickling vetch
Lens culinaris Medik.	Lenteja	Lentil
Phaseolus vulgaris L.	Alubias	Bean
Pisum sativum L.	Alubias	Garden pea
Vicia ervilia (L.) Willd.	Yero	Bitter vetch
Vicia articulata Hornem	Algarrobas	One-leaved vetch
Vicia faba L.	Habas	Broad bean

diet. Fish, oil, and other foodstuffs had to be bought, and this was not always possible.

Each family had its own home garden, but little time was spent on it because taking care of the livestock and main crops (wheat, barley, hay) was very demanding. Most gardens did not have a water supply, and in the summer it was necessary to carry water in containers from the nearest source (rivers, streams, or springs). The most common vegetables were cabbage, lettuce, onion, and garlic. Cabbage was the only green vegetable available in winter; neither Swiss chard nor spinach were cultivated, and other products were only available to wealthy families who lived on large properties.

The climate (storms, hail, and freezing temperatures late in the season) is not appropriate for most cultivated fruit trees, and in many cold years the fruit cannot be harvested. Rustic trees such as the medlar *(Mespilus germanca)* or the service tree *(Sorbus domestica),* and other wild fruits such as sloes (from the blackthorn *Prunus spinosa),* gooseberries *(Ribes uva-crispa),* wild apples *(Malus sylvestris),* or wild pears *(Pyrus cordata)* are better adapted to the local climate and were gathered instead of commercially available fruits.

Wild food has been gathered in the area since ancient times. Historical evidence suggests that the Cántabros (Iberian tribes who lived in the area before the Roman conquest) used to eat bread made with acorn flour (García Bellido, 1945). They probably gathered other wild berries and products, as did other neighboring tribes such as the Basque tribes called Vascones (Iriarte and Zapata, 1996).

Until recently, wild food was collected regularly. The total contribution of wild plants to the calories of the diet was not large, but there was a great variety of species, especially of berries and other fruits. However, most wild edible plants are no longer gathered. Many people associate modernity with the rejection of all the traditional ideas and habits. They link wild food with manual work and times of scarcity and hunger, which most people would prefer to forget.

Most informants told us that during wars, times were not as hard in Campoo as they were in other rural regions of Spain. A recent study on wild edible plants in Madrid province, a vast and varied territory (about 800 km^2), has revealed that the species gathered have high nutritional value. The consumption of green vegetables such as red campion *(Silene dioica)*, Spanish salsify *(Scolymus hispanicus)*, and docks (*Rumex pulcher* and other species of the genus) is outstanding in this region. It is also common to gather young shoots of asparagus *(Asparagus acutifolius)*, hops *(Humulus lupulus)*, black bryony *(Tamus communis)*, and white bryony *(Bryonia dioica)*, some of which are considered to be toxic plants. The consumption of holm-oak acorns *(Quercus ilex)*, a very common species in the center of Spain, also used to be very important.

Compared to the plant parts consumed in certain Mediterranean areas, including Madrid (see Table 5.2), a high percentage of wild fruits is eaten in Campoo. (Note that in our study we did not consider food plants consumed as spices, used to flavor spirits, or for other infusions or social beverages.) The table shows that in contrast with Campoo, in other Mediterranean areas the percentage of green vegetables is much more important. Reasons for this difference could be that in Campoo the economy is based on cattle farming while in the other areas domesticated plants are more readily available from home gardens, due to the wetter climate. We have already pointed out that one reason wild fruits were so important in Campoo was because cultivated fruit was scarce.

Some current eating behaviors can be interpreted as relics of past times of hunger, especially during the Spanish Civil War (1936-1939) and immediately thereafter (until the 1950s). The generations who lived through these difficult times worked hard and their children are enjoying the present times of abundance. One symptom of the memory of hard times is the custom of not emptying the dish completely, to ensure that nobody will still be hungry after the food is finished.

TABLE 5.2. Wild plants consumed in some Mediterranean areas.

Study area	No. of species	Leaves and shoots	Fruits and seeds	Subterranean part	Flowers
Campoo, Spain (Pardo de Santayana, 2003)	48	14 (29%)	27 (56%)	5 (10%)	5 (10%)
Madrid, Spain (Tardío et al., 2002)	87	49 (56%)	30 (34%)	2 (2%)	8 (9%)
Montseny, Spain (Bonet and Vallès, 2002)	46	28 (61%)	13 (28%)	2 (4%)	4 (9%)
Garfagnana, Italy (Pieroni, 1999)	90	70 (78%)	16 (18%)	6 (7%)	(1%)
Central Anatolia, Turkey (Ertug, 2000)	88	44 (50%)	34 (39%)	7 (8%)	(3%)

Another is the popular saying *"Que no falte de ná "* ("Nothing should be lacking"). Yet another is that in some families the wishes and tastes of each member, including children, are taken into account—to the point that the housewives cook different dishes for each of them. In many families, leftovers are thrown away (González Turmo, 2002).

When locals were asked about the consumption of wild plants, they explained that they used them as snack foods in their childhood. They were consumed on the way to school or to avoid feeling hungry during breaks. Many people consumed these plants and their products more for amusement than food. To avoid having to prepare something to eat between lunch and dinnertime it was also common to send the children to gather wild berries such as blackberries *(Rubus ulmifolius)*, blueberries *(Vaccinium myrtillus)*, or gooseberries *(Ribes uva-crispa);* greens such as sorrel *(Rumex acetosa);* and bulbs such as pig nut *(Conopodium* spp.) or *lezas (Romulea bulbocodium)* as an afternoon snack. People still tell annoying children *"¡Vete a lezas!"* ("Go gather lezas!"). Shepherds and their young helpers also used to eat wild edibles to supplement their meager diet.

The situation is different now. Children prefer sweets and confectionery, and most are not able to recognize wild edible plants or do not like to eat them. As informants said, *"La gente ya no se agacha."*

By comparison with cultivated plants, the contribution of wild plant products to the total food intake was not very important. Nevertheless, the nutritional diversity they provided was important. Wild fruits, for example, provided an important vitamin and sugar intake; beechnuts and hazelnuts provided vegetable fat. Wild greens such as sorrel or watercress are also rich in vitamins and mineral salts, and so are an important source of micronutrients and biochemical substances. None of the wild plants consumed supplied an important quantity of carbohydrates; these were provided essentially by cereals and potatoes. Other very nutritious products, such as vegetable protein, came from legumes. The vegetable fiber intake was quite low, especially in the winter, when for most families the only vegetable eaten was cabbage.

Only a few adult people still consume wild greens such as red campion *(Silene dioica)* or lamb's lettuce *(Valerianella carinata)*. They do so because they like the taste and enjoy the act of gathering plants. Young people who are environmentally inclined also enjoy doing so.

Some people who have migrated to cities yearn for their childhood and the time they lived in the region, so when they stay in the village they like to gather and consume wild edibles and herbs. The familiar flavors remind them of past times.

The only wild edible that is still commonly gathered is watercress (*Rorippa nasturtium-aquaticum*). Mushrooms are also gathered, mostly for home consumption, but the high prices paid by restaurants encourage people to gather and sell them.

Public Rural Development Agencies are trying to promote diversification of economic resources so that people do not rely solely on cattle or rural tourism. They offer courses and other activities with the aim of promoting local quality food products such as cheese, sausages, honey, chocolates, bakery items, or jams made from wild berries.

One interesting fact is that people perceive gathering plants as old-fashioned, unprofitable, and too much hard work. For them, this kind of work is demeaning and a waste of time; they prefer to buy food rather than gather it. However, people do like to work in their home gardens, which is just as uneconomic as gathering wild plants.

The selection of taxa considered to be food is also very interesting. One informant explained that a neighbor from Andalucia in the south of Spain used to eat the young shoots of black bryony. In Cantabria this plant is associated with snakes, as one of its popular names indicates: *comida de culebras* (snake food). No one wishing to be considered a real Cantabrian or *campurriano* (someone who comes from Campoo) would eat such food. Yet this and other species such as Spanish salsify (*Scolymus hispanicus:* the petiole and central nerve of the basal leaves) and white bryony (the young shoots) are widely consumed in other Spanish regions.

Another interesting example of the selection of edible species is the case of fennel (*Foeniculum vulgare* subsp. *piperitum*), which used to be cultivated in home gardens and grows wild in the southwest of the area. This plant is commonly used as a condiment in other regions and countries, but in Campoo only the gypsies gather it; they consume the young leaves as green vegetables cooked with cabbage. This habit, so common elsewhere, is considered in Campoo to be the hallmark of a marginal community. Blanco (1998) indicated a similar perception from Segovia province, which is adjacent to Madrid. In

Madrid, however, it was consumed without this connotation (Tardío et al., 2002).

In Campoo, therefore, most people prefer to buy food or medicines rather than collect them from the wild. At present, though, it is far more common in Campoo to gather medicinal herbs rather than wild foods. A number of locals, both old, traditional people and young people interested in herbal medicine, prefer herbs to synthetic chemicals. For this reason, almost the only wild foods still commonly gathered are those with medicinal properties.

MEDICINAL FOOD: DIGESTIVE BEVERAGES

Medicine and food are concepts that people from Campoo tend to separate, but they still acknowledge the link between them and like to select what kinds of products to eat. Two of the reasons for the high frequency of home garden products in the diet are safety and taste. Nearly everybody considers that in the old days food was tastier and healthier. People are nostalgic for the bread baked by their mothers in home ovens. Then, only local products were consumed, and there were no health problems. People are now afraid of the abuse of fertilizers, pesticides, herbicides, drugs for cattle, and industrial fodder, and prefer to consume their own home-produced products.

Only a few plants are eaten deliberately for health purposes. Watercress is considered an excellent purifier of the blood. Rice, apples, and service tree fruits are consumed for their astringent antidiarrheal qualities. Children used to eat celery against intestinal parasites. Carrots enhance vision and walnuts memory, parsley calcifies the bones; breast-feeding mothers used to drink beer to enhance milk secretion.

Most cultivated food plants are also used as home remedies, but the administration or the part used differs considerably from their food use. For example, onions are heated and used topically to ripen boils; raw garlic is rubbed on the anus, to help expel intestinal worms; a decoction of walnut leaves is used to wash wounds and is considered to be the best disinfectant; figs cooked with wine are one of the best pneumonia or cold remedies, and fig latex is used against warts; an infusion of cinnamon is considered an effective laxative; and a decoction of maize stigmas is drunk as a diuretic.

The medicinal use of some wild species such as elderberry, black-thorn *(Prunus spinosa)*, or hawthorn *(Crataegus monogyna)* also differs widely from their food use. Elderberries *(Sambucus nigra)* are consumed, though some people think that they are not edible. Some people eat them raw, others make them into jams or prepare beverages by boiling the berries with water or squeezing the fresh fruits. Elderberries are also used to make spirits, by leaving the fruits to macerate. As a medicine, the inner bark is used for rheumatism, gout, and as a vulnerary to heal difficult wounds or burns; the decoction of the inflorescence is taken orally against colds and headaches; flowers in steam baths were prescribed for colds and erysipela.

Another kind of food medicine used in Campoo is spirits. Wine and liquors have high alcohol contents (16 percent and 35 to 60 percent, respectively), so when plants are macerated in them, the active compounds dissolve. Wine and liquors were intensely used in popular medicine as extraction agents and as vehicles for the plant extract. Formerly they were prepared mostly as digestive remedies, but now they are consumed for their flavor and as a social beverage (see Figure 5.3).

The new appreciation of natural products has helped to develop new uses for the traditional spirits. It is popular to prepare them at home, and these homemade spirits can be enjoyed in restaurants or pubs as a quality local product. Liquor and anisette are used for macerating herbs and fruits: depending on personal tastes, the two are mixed in different proportions, or only one of them is used. Nowadays people enjoy experimenting with new flavors and they prepare the spirits with new recipes, using acorn, raspberry *(Rubus idaeus)*, wild roses *(Rosa canina* and other species of the genus), and elderberry *(Sambucus nigra)*. Nearly all the edible wild berries are used, together with other kinds of fruits. Herb liquors are prepared solely from *té de los Picos de Europa, té de lastra* (Picos de Europa tea, limestone tea: *Sideritis hyssopifolia*), and anisette *(Scandix australis)*.

In other Spanish regions, different plants are used to prepare spirits. We will discuss only the uses of the species gathered in the Campoo area that are also used in other regions. Sloes (the fruit of the blackthorn, *Prunus spinosa*) are gathered in nearly all the areas in which the species grows, to prepare a special liquor called *pacharán*, a name derived from the Basque name for the plant: *basarana*. In Ma-

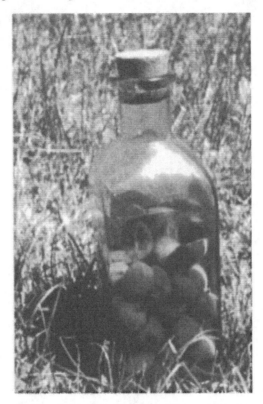

FIGURE 5.3. Wild apple *(Malus sylvestris)* spirit.

drid it is also called *aguardiente de endrinas* (blackthorn liquor). In Campoo and elsewhere in Spain, the fruits are consumed when ripe. This liquor is not only made at home but also industrially, and people from the area have gathered blackthorn fruits to sell to these industries. Usually the beverage is made with anisette and liquor (in proportions depending on personal preferences), blackthorn fruits, cinnamon bark, a few coffee beans, and sugar. Some people like to add chamomile *(Chamaemelum nobile)* flowers, wild apples *(Malus sylvestris),* green walnuts, or raw chickpeas. Other people prefer to make the liquor from European plums *(Prunus insititia)* rather than blackthorns.

Cherries are also macerated in alcohol to make another tonic. In this case it is also common to eat the cherries impregnated in liquor.

An especially interesting liquor called "ratafia" is elaborated in some parts of Catalonia and Aragon. Bonet (2001) studied the composition of many ratafia recipes and found that almost 100 species are used to make this excellent liqueur. It is basically a green walnut liqueur with many plant species added to aromatize it. In half of the recipes studied, seven additional species were found to be essential ingredients: lemon, cinnamon, chamomile, coffee, nutmeg, thyme, lemon balm *(Melissa officinalis)*, and lemon verbena *(Aloysia citrodora = Lyppia triphylla)*. Most of the other brandies are also common in other Spanish areas. Herb spirits are not as common in Campoo as in other areas. In other Cantabrian regions (Liébana) a homemade and home-industrial liquor is prepared from *Sideritis hyssopifolia* and sold as one of the local gastronomic specialties. In Liébana, the excellent tea prepared from this herb is also sold in bars, sometimes with the addition of a dash of brandy. The uncontrolled gathering of this species could endanger its future populations; the area it grows in lies in Picos de Europa National Park, which receives more than one million visitors each year.

Apart from alcohol, the most frequent and readily accessible vehicle for the medicinal properties of plants is water. The most common ways of preparation are heating the water up to boiling point and then adding the plant or boiling the plant in water for several minutes. Another common practice is to macerate the plant in water. Although herbalists usually prescribe an infusion, the most popular preparation is a decoction. Water does not provide as much caloric intake as alcohol does, but the water temperature is very helpful to tone up the body.

Beverages that are ingested both for their flavor and as digestive infusions can also be considered medicinal food. Most of them are made from wild plants that are still commonly gathered. Table 5.3 includes plants called *tés* (teas), which is a generic name denoting plants used to make digestives and tasty infusions. They are given different compound names describing their habitat or their color. Table 5.4 includes the *manzanillas* (chamomiles, see Figure 5.4), which are plants belonging to the Asteraceae family, most of them with tiny yellow flowers in the center enclosed by white ligulated flowers. Only *Helichrysum stoechas* is not ligulate.

None of the infusions prepared in the area are specific to that area. All the chamomiles (see Table 5.4) are used in other Spanish regions.

TABLE 5.3. Tés: Tasty infusions with digestive properties drunk in Cantabria.

Scientific Latin name, local name (English translation)	Mode of use	Applications	Source
Lithospermum officinale té blanco (white tea), té de huerta (garden tea)	Decoction of fruit-bearing plant	Social drink after meals, digestive, colds, heartburn, stomachache, con-stipation	Gardens, wild
Bidens aurea té de huerta (garden tea), té moruno (Moorish tea)	Decoction of leaves	Diarrhea, also for animals (sometimes boiled in milk), di-gestive, sedative	Gardens
Camelia sinensis té (tea)	Decoction of leaves	Social drink after meals	Bought
Jasonia glutinosa té de roca (rock tea)	Decoction of flow-ers	Social drink after meals, digestive, colds, diuretic (cleans kidneys and bladder, helps urina-tion)	Wild
Sideritis hyssopifolia té de lastra (limestone tea), té de peñas (rock tea) té del puerto	Decoction of flow-ers or macerated in liquor	Social drink after meals, digestive	Wild
Thymus pulegioides, T. praecox, T. froelichianus té morado (purple tea)	Decoction of flow-ers	Social drink after meals, digestive, for liver and kidneys	Wild

The most frequent is bitter chamomile *(Chamaemelum nobile)*. It is collected and kept in nearly all homes and consumed regularly. In all cases, the wild plant, gathered and stored, is preferred to the commercial tea bags *(Matricaria chamomilla)*. The use of bitter chamomile is so widespread that, as one informant said, not to have it at home would be a sign of laziness and lack of provision. Remedies of this kind are the only traditional recipes considered more effective than the commercial drugs or herbal remedies bought from pharmacies or herbalists.

Another widely used plant is *Sideritis hyssopifolia,* called "tea" and usually preferred to the tea sold in supermarkets *(Camellia sinensis).* Its use is also common in Asturias and the Pyrenees. In

TABLE 5.4. Plants called "manzanilla" (chamomile) and their medicinal use.

Scientific Latin name	Local name (English translation)	Medicinal and veterinary uses
Achillea millefolium	Manzanilla romana (roman chamomile)	Colic; constipation; diarrhea; menstrual pain; rheumatism; wounds (poultice).
Anthemis arvensis	Manzanilla (chamomile)	Liver; purge for animals.
Chamaemelum nobile	Manzanilla (chamomile)	Digestive: bad digestion, heartburn; constipation (persons or animals); diarrhea (persons or animals); liver; bladder infection; menstrual pain; earache; digestive disorders in cows; eye problems (persons or animals); cleaning placenta after delivery (Moreno and Gutiérrez; 1994). Social drink after meals.
Helichrysum stoechas	Manzanilla de la reina (queen's chamomile), manzanilla de lastra (limestone chamomile)	Digestive (persons or animals); intestinal worms; colds; lungs, kidney.
Matricaria discoidea	Manzanilla silvestre (wild chamomile)	Digestive (animals)

many other areas the American plant *Bidens aurea* is taken as a tea. *Jasonia glutinosa* is an endemic of the Iberian Peninsula and some localities in the south of France and north of Morocco. In the Campoo area, it grows only in the southeast, and here it is consumed. This plant is one of the most important native Spanish wild teas, mainly in the east of Spain, where it is offered in bars and restaurants. It has an excellent aroma and digestive properties. Font Quer (1962) relates how he and other European botanists once ordered tea in San Carlos de la Rápita (Catalonia) and the waiter brought them *Jasonia glutinosa* tea, though they were expecting *Camellia sinensis* tea. They found it strange, so Font Quer asked the waiter what kind of tea it was. He answered that he had served tea, the better tea, *té de roca* (rock tea). *Thymus pulegioides* and other species of *Thymus*, section *Serpyllum*, are also used as digestive teas in Galicia and the Pyrenees.

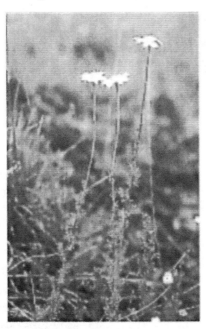

FIGURE 5.4. "Manzanilla" (chamomile, *Chamaemelum nobile*).

Other infusions prepared with species such as mint *(Mentha pulegium)*, lemon verbena *(Aloysia citrodora)*, or wild marjoram *(Origanum vulgare)* could also be considered in this group of medicinal food infusions, because they are consumed daily for their flavor and for their medicinal properties. Mint is also consumed as a digestive infusion, and wild marjoram is especially indicated for respiratory disorders.

These medicinal plants are not the only ones still harvested in Campoo; other plants with vulnerary *(Carduncellus mitissimus, Juglans regia)*, diuretic *(Equisetum arvense, E. telamateia)*, respiratory *(Sambucus nigra, Malva sylvestris, Eucalyptus globulus)*, anti-inflamatory *(Inula montana, I. helenioides, Rosmarinus officinalis)*, or circulatory properties *(Urtica dioica)* are also very common.

A simple analysis of food and medicinal plants of Campoo shows that nearly half of the food plants in a broad sense (including infusions consumed just for their taste, spirits, and spices) have medicinal uses (see Table 5.5). This proportion is not very different from the 60 percent reported by Pieroni (2000) from Lucca Province (Italy).

TABLE 5.5. Comparison between the number of species used as medicine and food.

Use	Number of taxa	% wild taxa	% cultivated taxa
Medicinal	138	61	59
Food	128	46	54
Medicinal food	62	45	55

The total number of edible plants is similar to the number of medicinal plants, but appreciable differences appear in the percentage of wild and domesticated species. The proportion of wild medicinal plants (61 percent) is higher than the proportion of wild edibles (46 percent). The percentage of wild medicinal food species (45 percent) is similar to the percentage of wild food species. This shows that cultivated food plants are used both for medicinal and nutritional purposes, whereas wild plants tend to be solely medicinal. This is reasonable, especially in a settled rural society, because the great cultural significance of cultivated plants has led to many habits, traditions, ideas, and uses regarding them.

Some of the knowledge and practices relating to the use of wild herbs and edibles are not traditional, but have been recently introduced. Our female informant who knew the most different kinds of popular remedies was the only informant who referred to the edible use of lamb's lettuce *(Valerianella carinata)*. She told us that people from other regions had taught her the edible use of this species. Other food species such as dandelion *(Taraxacum officinale)* are mostly gathered by people who were not born in the area or by *veraneantes* (holidaymakers), the term designating people native to the region who have moved to the cities but still own a house in the area and visit regularly.

Most plants are gathered for home consumption, but some minor trading of homemade jams and liqueurs occurs. The new appreciation of natural and quality local products has encouraged the development of new uses, mostly based on traditional ones. A store in Reinosa, the capital of the region, specializes in local food products. These products are also distributed to local craft stores in other tourist cities and villages of Cantabria. The local development office (Agencia de Desarrollo de Campoo) has organized courses on agrofood, in which local producers learn to prepare jams from wild fruits and make other kinds of food. Now elderberry, blackberry, blueberry, or wild berry jams are available, prepared from new and traditional recipes. The medicinal properties of some of them, such as elderberry jam, are well-known; many people in Central Europe use this jam for respiratory disorders, due to its high vitamin C content.

CONCLUSIONS

Big changes have taken place in the rural life of Campoo over the past four decades, as in other European regions. These changes have led to the erosion of traditional knowledge about wild plants and their uses. For example, only 20 percent of the wild food species that used to be eaten in the area are still being consumed. The gathering of wild plants is frequently associated with times of hardship, and only a few people still collect edible and medicinal plants.

The few exceptions to the former are plants used to make infusions that are popular for their flavor and medicinal digestive properties, such as chamomile *(Chamaemelum nobile)* or Picos de Europa tea *(Sideritis hyssopifolia).* Another exception is homemade digestive tonics such as pacharán, which is prepared from sloes *(Prunus spinosa).*

Besides these revitalized uses, new recipes are being incorporated, mostly to make other liqueurs and brandies prepared by macerating wild edible fruits that were not previously used, or to make other kinds of nutraceuticals, such as elderberry jam.

This chapter demonstrates the value of studying changes in the habits of traditional rural societies and the potential of utilizing traditional knowledge for the development and marketing of nutraceuticals.

The average age of the population of Campoo, as in most Spanish rural areas, is very high. This old population has depended on retirement and unemployment pensions and on European and state agrarian subsidies. In order to diversify and revitalize their economy, the people are trying to promote rural tourism and local quality products. To maintain their vitality, rural areas have to rescue traditional valuable practices and knowledge and adopt strategies and information—modern or traditional—from other cultures and regions. This will help them regain some of their attraction and vitality, while maintaining their distinctiveness. The result will be that migration will no longer be the only option for young people, and the European Union objectives of stabilizing the rural population will be successfully achieved.

REFERENCES

Barrau, J. (1983). *Les hommes et leurs aliments. Ësquisse d'une histoire ëcologique et ethnologique de l'alimentation humaine.* París: Temps Actuels.

Blanco, E. (1998). *Diccionario de etnobotánica Segoviana. Pervivencia del conocimiento sobre las plantas.* Segovia: Ayuntamiento de Segovia.

Bonet, M.A. (2001). Estudi etnobotànic del Montseny. Doctoral thesis in biology. Università de Barcelona, España.

Bonet, M.A and J. Vallès (2002). Use of non-crop food vascular plants in Montseny biosphere reserve (Catalonia, Iberian Peninsula). *International Journal of Food Sciences and Nutrition* 53: 225-248.

Contreras, J. (1993). *Antropología de la alimentación.* Madrid: Eudema.

Ertug, F. (2000). An ethnobotanical study in Central Anatolia (Turkey). *Economic Botany* 54(2): 155-182.

Etkin, N.L. (1996). Medicinal cuisines: Diet and ethnopharmacology. *International Journal of Pharmacognosy* 34(5): 313-326.

Font Quer, P. (1962). *Plantas medicinales. El Dioscórides renovado.* Barcelona: Labor.

García Bellido, A. (1945). *España y los Españoles hace dos mil años, según la "geografía" de Strabón.* Madrid: Espasa Calpe.

Gómez Pellón, E. (1999). *Viejas culturas lácteas de Cantabria: Etnografía y patrimonio.* Santander: Universidad de Cantabria.

González Turmo, I. (2002). Comida de pobre, pobre comida. In Gracia Arnaiz (Ed.), *Somos lo que comemos.* Barcelona: Ariel.

Iriarte, M.J. and L. Zapata (1996). *El paisaje vegetal prehistórico en el país Vasco.* Vitoria: Diputación Foral de Álava Departamento de Cultura y Euskera.

Moreno, L.A. and J.A. Gutiérrez (1994). Remedios y creencias de medicina popular en la merindad de Campoo. *Valdeolea* 28: 1-16.

Pardo de Santayana, M. (2003). Las plantas en la cultura tradicional de la Antigua Merindad de Campoo. Doctoral thesis in biology. Universidad Autónoma de Madrid, España.

Pieroni, A. (1999). Gathered wild food plants in the upper valley of the Serchio River (Garfagnana), Central Italy. *Economic Botany* 53(3): 327-341.

Pieroni, A. (2000). Medicinal plants and food medicines in the folk traditions of the upper Lucca Province, Italy. *Journal of Ethnopharmacology* 70(3): 235-273.

Rivera, D., C. Obon, C. Inocencio, M. Heinrich, A. Verde, J. Fajardo, and R. Llorach (2005). The ethnobotanical study of local Mediterranean food plants as medicinal resources in Southern Spain. *Journal of Physiology and Pharmacology* 56: 97-114.

Tardío, J., H. Pascual, and R. Morales (2002). *Alimentos silvestres de Madrid. Guía de plantas y setas de uso alimentario tradicional en la comunidad de Madrid.* Madrid: Real Jardín Botánico, CSIC, La Librería, Instituto Madrileño de Investigación Agraria y Alimentaria.

Chapter 6

"The Forest and the Seaweed": Gitga'at Seaweed, Traditional Ecological Knowledge, and Community Survival

Nancy J. Turner
Helen Clifton

INTRODUCTION

Traditional food systems are an integral part of peoples' cultures and lifeways. Foods provide far more than calories and nutrients; they help define the identity and heritage of a people. Gathering and obtaining food is a primary occupation in land-based societies, and the knowledge required for food procurement is an essential component of peoples' Traditional Ecological Knowledge and Wisdom (TEKW).

We would like to thank all the members of the Gitga'at Nation, Hartley Bay, especially Chief Johnny Clifton, Chief Councillor Pat Sterritt, Belle Eaton, Ernie Hill Jr., Lynne Hill, Cam Hill, Clyde Ridley, Jimmy and Annetta Robinson, Marven Robinson, Art Sterritt, Kayla Wilson, and Mildred Wilson. We are also grateful to Dan Cardinall, Irma Beltgens, Michael Roth, Anne Marshall, Robin June Hood, Sandra Lindstrom, Barbara Wilson (Kii7iljuus), and Judy Thompson (Edosti) for their contributions to this paper. Our research was supported by the Coasts Under Stress Research Project (Rosemary Ommer, PI; http://www.coastsunderstress.ca/home.html, a major collaborative research project between Memorial University of Newfoundland and the University of Victoria and several other universities and partner agencies in Canada and the United States, funded by the Social Sciences and Humanities Research Council of Canada (SSHRC) and the Natural Science and Engineering Research Council of Canada (NSERC) (April 2000-2005). This article was originally published in a volume originating from a workshop (February 2002; Prince Rupert, BC), "Local Knowledge, Natural Resources and Community Survival," organized by Charles Menzies, The University of British Columbia. The volume, edited by Charles Menzies, *Integrating Local Level Ecological Knowledge With Natural Resource Management,* is published by the University of Nebraska Press, Lincoln. We would like to dedicate this paper to the children of the Gitga'at Nation.

As such, this knowledge is embedded in peoples' philosophy and worldview in a vast and complex array of strategies they use to sustain themselves within their territories over many generations, and in the many ways by which they acquire and communicate knowledge to other members of the society and to future generations (Turner et al., 2000) (see Figure 6.1).

For the Gitga'at of Hartley Bay and surrounding territory on the north coast of British Columbia, red laver seaweed *(Porphyra abbottae)*, called *ła'ask,* is a traditional food that represents all of these components of TEKW. The harvesting, processing, and use of this seaweed, undertaken for many centuries by the Gitga'at and their ancestors and still practiced today, is infused within all facets of Gitga'at culture and lifeways, and is vital to their identity, health, and well-being as a people. The continued use of this seaweed by the Gitga'at in the face of economic restructuring and accelerating cultural change since the time of European contact is remarkable. In a sense, the use of the seaweed represents the resiliency of a people. The adaptations that have been made by the Gitga'at to enable and fa-

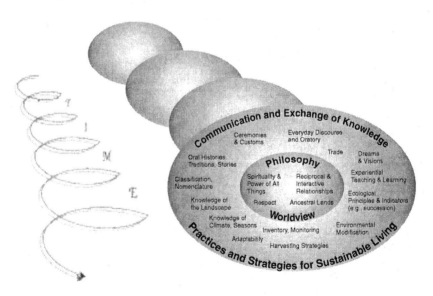

FIGURE 6.1. Components of traditional ecological knowledge and wisdom (TEKW) of Aboriginal peoples of northwestern North America. (*Source:* Turner et al., 2000.)

cilitate its continued harvest and use reflect peoples' abilities to adjust to changing conditions and still retain the essence of their cultures and traditions. In terms of community survival under new and changing economic and cultural regimes, the Gitga'at seaweed harvest represents hope and inspiration for maintaining cultural integrity and provides a model for sustainable resource use based on principles of respect, reciprocity, and cooperation.

In this chapter we present some of the details, particularly the cultural aspects, of the harvesting, processing, and use of this valuable marine alga and describe how they serve to define and strengthen the Gitga'at community and provide continuity and resilience for the Gitga'at people. From a scientific perspective there is still much to be learned about the taxonomy, lifecycles, and ecological aspects of *ła'ask,* but the depth of Gitga'at traditional knowledge about these topics indicates the tremendous value and potential for indigenous knowledge to inform scientists and others about the lifecycles and interrelationships of the natural world. This chapter is called "The Forest and the Seaweed" because in the holistic perspective of the Gitga'at and other first nations, the two are integrally related; a fact we will demonstrate in our discussions here.

Our collaborative research on Gitga'at traditional ecological knowledge relating to plants and the environment is part of this ongoing major research project, Coasts Under Stress. Its goal is to identify the important ways in which changes in society and the environment in coastal British Columbia and coastal Newfoundland and Labrador have affected, or will affect, the health of people, their communities, and the environment over the long run. The Gitga'at community at Hartley Bay, like many other communities of coastal British Columbia, has been subjected to severe economic restructuring, which is the result of the loss of commercial fishing revenues. Their territory has been encroached upon and their resources depleted from logging, commercial fishing, shellfish harvesting, and even tourism. Their efforts to maintain their cultural integrity, community values, health, and well-being in the face of these changes are exemplary. Their continued harvesting and use of traditional resources such as seaweed contributes to these efforts, as we will demonstrate.

SEAWEED USE WORLDWIDE

Seaweeds, or more technically macroscopic marine algae, are used by humans all over the world as sources of food, medicine, and materials. Seaweed accounts for some 10 percent of the diet in countries such as Japan. Japanese seaweed consumption reached an average of 3.5 kg per household in 1973 (Indergaard, 1983). Seaweeds are widely eaten in other regions of the world as well, particularly in China, Korea, parts of Ireland and Scotland, and in Polynesia and Hawaii (Aaronson, 1986; Abbott, 1974; Druehl, 2000; Guiry and Blunden, 1991; Guiry and Hession, 1998; Indergaard, 1983; Kenicer et al., 2000; Madlener, 1977; Milliken and Bridgewater, 2001; Ostraff, 2003). Seaweeds also have many industrial uses, especially in food, cosmetics, and agricultural industries (Guiry, 2004b). Seaweeds are known to be highly nutritious. They are today considered a "health food" in mainstream North American society, although their health and nutritional benefits have long been known and appreciated by the Gitga'at and other Northwest Coast indigenous peoples.

Interest in seaweed products is growing and a few "cottage industries" have developed on the Northwest Coast for harvesting seaweeds for the marketplace, notably at Barkley Sound and in the vicinity of Sooke, both on the west coast of Vancouver Island. A commercial kelp-harvesting plant at Masset, Haida Gwaii (Queen Charlotte Islands), for the purpose of developing industrial kelp and fertilizer products, proved to be economically unviable and existed for only a few years in the 1980s. There are rumored efforts to develop industrial production for red laver on the British Columbia coast as well (Guiry, 2004a), but this has yet to be confirmed. A small red-laver-growing industry has been established in Puget Sound, Washington State (Druehl, 2000), and there are efforts to start cultivating *Porphyra* in the vicinity of Prince Rupert, with Louis Druehl as an advisor to the project.

In contrast, seaweed production in Japan is a multibillion-dollar industry, and many kinds of seaweeds are cultivated, especially for the domestic food market. The most important types are: *nori* (*Porphyra* species), *kombu* (*Laminaria* spp.), and *wakame* (*Undaria* spp.). Today about 350,000 tons of wet nori alone are produced in Japan, with a retail value in excess of U.S. $1 billion. The Japanese nori industry is a highly mechanized, efficient operation that employs some 60,000 people on a part-time basis. Nearly 70,000 hectares of Japanese waters are occupied by *Porphyra*-growing nets (Guiry, 2004a).

Coastal first peoples in British Columbia, especially those of the northern Coast Salish, Kwakwaka'wakw, and peoples of the central and northern coast, all include red laver (*Porphyra abbottae* and other *Porphyra* spp.) in their diets (Turner, 1995, 2003). The Nuu-Chah-Nulth and Ditidaht of the west coast of Vancouver Island evidently did not eat this seaweed themselves, but within the early twentieth century many of these people harvested it for sale to local Asian communities in Victoria and elsewhere (Williams, 1979; Turner et al., 1983). Peoples of the central and northern coast, including the Heiltsuk, Haida, and Coast Tsimshian, have also harvested a variety of seaweeds with herring roe deposited on them, especially the fronds of giant kelp *(Macrocystis integrifolia),* which are eaten not only by these people but are today exported to Japan in large quantities. Traditionally, seaweeds also had many technological and medicinal uses among British Columbia first peoples. For example, bull kelp *(Nereocystis luetkeana)* stipes were cured and used up and down the coast for fishing lines (Turner, 1998). The gelatinous substance from the receptacles of sea wrack (*Fucus* spp.) was, and still is, used as a medicine for burns and sores, to strengthen the limbs, and as an eye medicine.

Seaweeds can be indicators of environmental health. They are dependent on the ocean for their reproduction, growth, and dispersal, may vary in their growth rates, seasonality, and reproductive capacity depending on the ocean currents and tides, temperature, and other factors such as pollution (Druehl, 2000). Humans may also impact the growth and reproduction of seaweeds, including the *ła'ask* of the Gitga'at. In the following section we describe the use of this alga by the Gitga'at, and the multifaceted knowledge system that has supported and continues to support its use.

GITGA'AT SEAWEED USE

The Gitga'at are a Sm'algyax (Tsimshian)-speaking people whose main village is Hartley Bay, situated at the confluence of Greenville and Douglas Channels about 140 km (90 miles) south of Prince

Rupert, where a large number of Gitga'at people also reside (see Figure 6.2). Their territory encompasses a vast number of islands, as well as a substantial portion of the British Columbia mainland. The larger Islands within Tsimshian territory include Gil, Gribble, Campania, and Princess Royal islands.

Like other coastal peoples, the Gitga'at rely on the bounty of the forests and oceans combined to provide them with the foods, materials, and medicines they need for sustenance. They enjoy a diet of plenty of salmon, halibut, and other fish, together with marine mammals such as seal; shellfish such as sea urchins and chitons; land mammals such as deer and bear; gamebirds, including ducks and

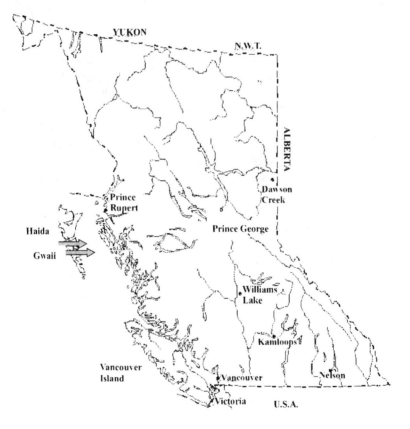

FIGURE 6.2. Map of British Columbia, showing approximate locations of Gitga'at community at Hartley Bay (upper arrow) and the spring seaweed camp at Kiel, Princess Royal Island (lower arrow).

geese, and a variety of plant foods, including berries, root vegetables, green shoots, inner bark of hemlock, and edible seaweed (Port Simpson Curriculum Committee, 1983). Although elders of the Gitga'at community still enjoy many of the traditional foods, many younger people prefer store-bought foods, and some of the traditional foods, especially the wild greens, roots, and inner bark, are scarcely known to them. One elder commented, "The more you eat the [old] foods, the more you like it." This statement reflects a common catch-22 facing those trying to maintain cultural traditions. People like what they are familiar with, and dietary preferences are no different in this regard (Kuhnlein, 1992). Nevertheless, *ła'ask* is one food enjoyed by virtually everyone.

Every year, for most of the month of May, the elders of the community, including Helen and Johnny Clifton, go to the seaweed camp at Kiel *(K'yel)* on Princess Royal Island *(Lax'a'lit'aa Koo)*, to harvest the seaweed, fish for halibut, and other traditional activities[1] (see Figure 6.3). Whenever they are able, the younger adults and school-age children generally come to Kiel during the long weekend in May. Previously, before children were required to be in school at this time, entire families stayed at Kiel while the seaweed harvest and halibut fishing took place. Much has changed in terms of harvesting practices,

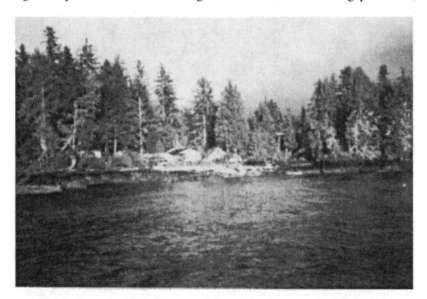

FIGURE 6.3. Kiel, the Gitga'at seaweed camp on Princess Royal Island.

transportation, and living conditions at the seaweed camp, but the seaweed harvest remains a time-honored tradition that brings cohesion to families and communities, provides important opportunities for knowledge acquisition and communication, and promotes health and well-being through providing a nutritious food, requiring a healthy outdoor lifestyle, and promoting cultural values.

Ła'ask: *The Seaweed*

The main species of red laver harvested by the Gitga'at is *Porphyra abbottae* (see Figure 6.4). Other species are known to have been harvested and used by coastal peoples, including *P. torta* and *P. lanceolata* (samples identified by phycologist Sandra Lindstrom). There were likely others as well, since approximately 21 different *Porphyra*

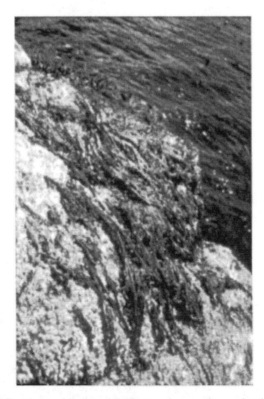

FIGURE 6.4. *Porphyra abbottae, ła'ask,* growing on the rocks, intertidal zone, island at Kiel.

species grow along the Pacific Coast of British Columbia and Alaska, Washington, and Oregon (Lindstrom and Cole, 1991; Turner, 2003), all of which are edible. As noted, *Porphyra* species are eaten in other parts of the world, including Japan, Korea, China, Scotland, and Ireland.

The life history of *Porphyra* is complex. *Porphyra* species, like other algae, reproduce by spores, but also undergo sexual reproduction. They have two main, different mature forms, one with a single complement of chromosomes, the haploid phase, and one with two sets of chromosomes, the diploid phase. This is known as an "alternation of generations" in a life cycle. The best-known, edible phase is haploid.[2] The haploid plants are thin, membranous, and dark greenish purple. Both the haploid and diploid plants produce spores that are released into the water and, depending upon the type of spores and the means of their production, by mitosis or meiosis, they will grow into plants of the same or the alternate generation. This reproductive strategy thus provides various means for the plants to grow, depending on particular environmental conditions. The male and female reproductive parts, or gametes, called spermatia and carpogonia respectively, are produced at the margins of the mature seaweed blades in the case of the spermatia, or inside the margins in the case of carpogonia. The spores produced that result from fertilization are released with the dissolution of the tissues along the margins. These might appear to be "rotting," but in fact are just undergoing another stage in a rather amazing life cycle.

This scientific understanding of the life cycle of *ła'ask* was obviously not known to Gitga'at or other first nations harvesters, as this requires microscopic examination of the seaweed through its life-cycle stages. However, the manifestation of this life cycle, in particular the growth and development of the young haploid phase—the edible seaweed phase—on the intertidal rocks of the shores of the islands where the Gitga'at have ventured to harvest them for generations, was well-known. So, too, was the seaweed's capacity to regenerate itself. The growth rate of the seaweed varies up and down the coast and from site to site, even within Gitga'at territory. On May 18, 2001, Helen explained that people in other communities generally picked seaweed earlier than the Gitga'at: "It's picked earlier than us. We're the last ones to pick seaweed. So, Kitkatla, Metlakatla, Kitasoo way, they will have picked seaweed . . . at Klemtu they picked eighteen sacks of seaweed!" She said that Johnny Clifton, who was born at Kiel, knew all the different places there where the early seaweed grew, as well as the places where the last seaweed was picked, just before they returned home. She said, "So there's places around here, like the island in front of us is one of the first places to pick. . . . There's certain places down here that's the early seaweed . . . Johnny knows, all these years." Helen calls the places where the seaweed grows "seaweed fields" or "seaweed beds," because of the great density of seaweeds grown there (see Figure 6.4). In past decades, people camped out in family groups near the different picking grounds. For example, Johnny's aunt had a place at Fly Bay out at the point; this was the first place they would go and pick—the first seaweed that was mature enough. At other sites, it matured later, even though "It's all the same seaweed. It's just, their growth is slower than the ones at first" (Helen Clifton, May 18, 2001).

The pickers have to learn to differentiate other types of seaweed from the edible type:

> You have seal seaweed that grows in between good seaweed; we call it "seal seaweed." They're wide, and they look like, they've got a rainbow . . . [Iridescent Seaweed, Iridea] but it's very colorful, and so I've learned to pick through that seaweed, if there's good seaweed on that rock.

Helen described how the women traditionally would pick the seaweed systematically:

> They wouldn't spot-pick seaweed. The whole group would go out and clean out one place. . . . And the next time they'd go for seaweed they would start at the place where they stopped the day before, or the tide before. And, so then the island was picked clean, either side—the Campania [Island] side or down here, Princess Royal side. And so you wouldn't have to go searching for seaweed. You knew exactly where the group stopped, and you would start from that point on until you were all finished.

In discussing how sustainable the seaweed harvest is, Helen confirms what many aboriginal harvesters understand about the plants they use routinely:

It's better when it's picked every year. It's just like any plant that has been trimmed; it will grow stronger and better. . . . For seaweed, it's just like any garden: it has to be tended. So if you pick it every year then it grows strong the next year, it keeps coming back. So if it isn't picked for a few years, then it just has rotted away on the rocks there.

One of the concerns Helen has is that people are not picking the seaweed routinely and systematically anymore, and she fears that the seaweed beds and the seaweed produced is deteriorating because they are not being tended. Another major concern of hers is the prospect of climate change, which was manifested for her in the continuous, uncharacteristic rains they experienced through the month of May for four consecutive years (2000-2003). This not only makes predicting the growth of the seaweed problematic, it prevents people from harvesting the seaweed, since one of the important taboos people observe is not to pick seaweed when it's raining. Helen commented: "It's hard to say [about whether they'll be able to pick seaweed] because the weather has changed *so* much, it's hard to say what's happening to the natural growth of whatever. . . . We work with the tides. Whatever we're getting here depends on the tides, and the weather." Another taboo, Helen explained, is that seaweed is not picked when it is floating in the water, but only when it is attached to the rocks, exposed by the low tide. This means that people should not be "greedy" with the seaweed. Limiting the harvest to the time of the lowest tides, when the seaweed is exposed, is both a safety measure—the risk of being washed away by the waves is lessened—and a conservation measure: at least some of the seaweed plants are inevitably left to grow and reproduce when there is such a narrow window for harvesting.

In order to pick the seaweed safely and process it effectively, it is necessary to have the right combination of sunny days and low tides first thing in the morning. As noted, the seaweed can be picked only at low tide from the rocks where it grows, and it can be picked only in dry weather. Picking seaweed in the rain is dangerous because it becomes so slippery, especially on the almost vertical rock faces where some of the best seaweed grows. In any case, seaweed picked in the rain does not taste as good. The seaweed is piled up and packed into large bags, then taken to special locations on sunny rocky headlands to be laid out to dry. It is formed into squares or shapes that conform to the shape and pattern of the rocks and allowed to dry from about eleven o'clock or noon to about three o'clock, when the squares are turned over to dry on the other side, through the late afternoon sun and into the early evening when the rocks start to cool off. Drying occurs both from above and from below, since the rocks themselves are warmed by the sun and they, in turn, help to dry the seaweed on the bottom, while the sun dries it from above. The dried squares are stacked up, about 25 together, and placed into cotton seaweed sheets made by sewing together nine opened-up flour sacks into a large sheet. The seaweed is then packed on people's backs or taken by speedboat to the camp at Kiel to be stored in a dry place, usually in a special "seaweed house," until it can be taken back to people's homes in Hartley Bay for further processing. Instead of the rocky bluffs, some women have used square cedar trays for drying their seaweed. Annetta Robinson, who is originally from Kitkatla, inherited about 100 such trays from her mother; she remembers helping her mother to make them. She kept some of these for drying her own seaweed and gave some of them to her cousins. Helen explained that these trays are used in places where there are no good rocks for drying seaweed, and are especially useful for older women who cannot easily climb around over the rocks to dry their seaweed.

Helen's goal is for her and her family members to pick at least seven large (100-pound) sacks full of the seaweed during the course of their stay at Kiel. This is the minimum amount that she and her family process and use for their personal consumption, trading, and gifts. When this amount is multiplied through all the Gitga'at families (perhaps 10 or more) who harvest seaweed, at least in the past, it translates into about 70 100-pound sacks or more, or perhaps more than 3,000 kg of fresh seaweed.

The seaweed grows quickly. Helen gauges the rate of growth and predicts the stage of readiness of the seaweed by watching the growth of the stinging nettles *(Urtica dioica)* at Kiel; as the stalks of the stinging nettle mature and elongate, so, too, do the seaweed fronds. Helen explained that people could harvest two pickings of seaweed from the same site in the same year, as it regenerates itself quickly. It is pulled off with the fingers, and the small ends remaining attached to the rocks will continue to grow so that, in about a month's time, one can return and pick the next growth. Formerly, the Gitga'at would pick and dry one harvest of seaweed at take it up Douglas Channel to

Kitamaat village to trade with the Haisla people there for oulachen grease, a nutritious fat rendered from a small smelt that comes in large numbers up the rivers to spawn in the spring. They also traded their seaweed with the upriver people for soapberries, *7is*, and other valued products from the Skeena, and with the Nisga'a of the Nass Valley for a different type of oulachen grease. They would then return to Kiel and harvest another crop of seaweed for their own use. The Gitga'at found this second crop preferable because it was said to be more tender and had a finer taste, as noted by Helen:

> I've heard . . . the women from long ago said that they would . . . do the first picking of seaweed and then it would be a month, not even a month, that the second growth would be ready to pick again. And they liked to keep the second growth for themselves because it was a finer seaweed . . . as compared to the first growth.

Helen also noted that the second growth fronds were narrower than the first growth. One Kitkatla man said that the Kitkatla still routinely harvest two crops of seaweed, one at the morning low tide at the beginning of May, and one at the low tides at the end of May.

Obviously, people had to be finely attuned to the tides and the currents, as well as to winds and weather conditions. Any ocean-based activities on the north coast can be treacherous, and this is especially so when people are harvesting from the rocks right at the tide line. They are vulnerable to being swept away by rogue waves or caught by unexpected storms. Helen warned that people have to always be alert and follow the lead of the most knowledgeable ones when it comes to knowing when to stop for rising tides or incoming storms. This type of knowledge comes only with experience and careful attention, and it is one of the concerns of elders that younger people no longer understand these imperatives and may put themselves and others in danger. In the winter of 2000 a young man was drowned, and the reason was in part that he did not understand the power of the currents and tides or the ferocity and bitter cold of the north wind; he tried to swim out to retrieve his boat, which had drifted away from the beach.

Formerly, seaweed harvesting was women's work. The men would venture out to fish for halibut or to hunt or trap, and it was the women who went out in groups in their canoes to get seaweed and bring it home to process. Helen recalled that long ago they used to fix sails to their canoes as well as use paddles. One of the women would steer and guard the canoe, making sure to keep it off the rocks, while the others picked seaweed. She would also watch the tides and weather and warn the others if it was time to stop. Several canoe-loads of women might cross the channel from Princess Royal Island *(Lax'a'lit'aa Koo)* to Campania Island *(Kagaas)* together, to camp out and spend the days picking seaweed. Children usually stayed behind at Kiel or other camps to be cared for by older siblings or young mothers who stayed behind. Older children might be taken along to help look after the canoes or boats. The entire seaweed-picking endeavor was—and still is—one of cooperation and teamwork. Nowadays, men also help out, especially with running the boats and transporting the seaweed. Seaweed harvesting is still very much a family activity.

THE FOREST AND THE SEAWEED

Where does the forest come together with seaweed harvesting? In many ways, the interconnection between forest and seaweed is epitomized in the large dugout canoes made of western red cedar *(Thuja plicata)* that the women used to travel to and from their seaweed grounds. It is also in the location of the seaweed camp itself: nestled at the edge of the towering forest of Sitka spruce *(Picea sitchensis),* western hemlock *(Tsuga heterophylla),* and red cedar, with the cabins intermingled with dense salal *(Gaultheria shallon)* and huckleberry bushes *(Vaccinium parvifolium),* which provide additional food and materials for the Gitga'at people. The trees provide much-needed firewood and construction materials. Helen explained the importance of wood for fuel, some of which is obtained as driftwood: "There's certain little bays and little places where all the driftwood is at. . . . we use a lot of wood; if you don't have the sun, you're using a lot of wood to try to dry your halibut, your fish."

All of the plants around the camp are useful for one purpose or another. Although the salal in the area does not bear fruit at the time the seaweed harvesters are there, the leaves of the salal are important for the later seaweed-curing process. Helen always gathers dozens of large salal leaves or has her granddaughters and the other girls staying at the camp gather them for her. The salal leaves are also made into decorative headbands by these same girls. In fact, over 90 species of plants in Gitga'at territory, most of them from the forests and their associated bogs, marshes, and riverbanks, are named by the Gitga'at and have direct cultural significance.

Another connection between seaweed harvesting and the forest is reflected in one of the Gitga'at taboos associated with picking seaweed: people were warned never to harvest cedarbark (used for clothing, basketry, mats, and even roofing) during the time that people were picking seaweed. Harvesting and working with cedar bark is said to cause rain, and, as already noted, one should not pick seaweed when it is raining. Helen explained that pulling the bark from the cedar tree exposes the wood and can "burn" the tree if it is then exposed to the hot sun. Nature therefore always seems to make a protective blanket for the newly harvested cedar tree by producing a fog, mist, or rain, thus giving the tree time to heal itself and allowing it to continue to live and grow. This is why it inevitably rains when people are harvesting cedarbark, and why these two activities are incompatible. Tradition therefore dictates that women should wait until after the seaweed has been harvested and dried before they go to peel cedarbark.

BACK HOME IN HARTLEY BAY

The squares of seaweed will keep well for several weeks if they are thoroughly dry. Once the people have returned from Kiel, in the fine, sunny days of June, they will undertake the next phase of the seaweed processing. Helen has two bentwood cedar boxes, one of which is probably well over 100 years old, as indicated by the wooden pegs that hold the joined corner ends together and the bottom onto the sides. These are what she uses to shape and cure the seaweed. The square shape of these boxes produces squares of seaweed of a standard, time-honored size that has long served as a form of currency in trading: similar squares of dried soapberries and Saskatoon berries are produced by the Gitxsan, and these squares become an equivalent for exchange. The women moisten the sun-dried squares of dried seaweed, sprinkling them with salt water, then the squares are formed and packed down into the cedar boxes in layers.

Helen explains the whole process:

> You form a square something the way you form an envelope—in
> a triangle. I'm making a square. And so I will put little patches
> of seaweed where it's thin, until I've got the thickness. I would
> make it about, maybe about an inch and a half thick, this square.
> And so I will put it into the box. And . . . I have dish towels and I
> put it on top of that square, and then I'll get somebody that's got
> clean feet and clean socks. And they will step on it and kick—
> it's called kicking—stepping on the seaweed, flattening it out,
> and it's gluing together by the pressure of the foot. And so,
> women that really know how to stamp on the seaweed would
> specifically do the corners . . . after they're finished . . . you take
> the cloth off and you put the salal leaves, face down . . . the light
> side down. And on the seaweed you'd have about nine big leaves
> across the square.
>
> Then . . . you'd lay the cedarbark. . . . And you've got long
> cedarbark [ribbon], let's say you've got about a ten-foot [thin
> strip] piece of cedarbark. (I'm exaggerating a little. I don't think
> it's quite that long.) But you'd lay it diagonally along on top of
> the salal leaves, and then you'd put the next cake of seaweed on.
> Sometimes you have a woman that's pretty strong; she can do
> two cakes at once. And so you would . . . do the same thing, salal
> leaves down, the diagonal cross with the bark, until you get the
> box completely filled. And you would fill it overflowing. And
> so you have a board that fits right on the top of that box. And so
> you put the board on. You put the cloth on top of the seaweed,
> put the board on and then you put big heavy rocks. And so . . . I
> leave that [seaweed] in the box for three days. So, we say, there's
> an expression that it "gets its flavor." It takes three days to ab-
> sorb that . . . salt water [and] . . . to adhere together. So then
> you'd smell real good seaweed.
>
> So then it's time to get the women that come to chop the sea-
> weed. So now we use axes. We use the yew wood block. . . .
> They're sawed-off yew *[Taxus brevifolia]*, a hard wood. They
> put something around it. Sometimes they use cardboard; you
> nail the cardboard around the top of the block [projecting up
> about four inches high]. When they're chopping seaweed on the
> block, [then] it doesn't fall off the block because the cardboard
> outer covering keeps the seaweed in. . . . And so they put that

chopped seaweed in big, big containers and then . . . as soon as the sun shines, that seaweed's going out. And so I'd take a tarp, put a seaweed sheet on there, and sprinkle that seaweed on the seaweed sheet again. . . .

And so you need to dry it in June. This is because of the long daylight hours—hours of sunshine you get in June. Also, you *have* to dry it in June, before the grasses really grow long. If the grasses grow long, then they retain the dew of the evening, you see, and so the evaporation of that dew is coming . . . and you're putting your seaweed close to the ground. So, because right in the village we don't have rocks and things there; we're using boardwalks, and so the top will be the rock. Because the top would warm up the same as a rock. You're putting your white seaweed sheets . . . white . . . retains the heat of the sun. . . . And so then you're sprinkling it in a fine [layer], about half an inch, around all over with seaweed.

So that takes all day to dry. And . . . you're moving that seaweed. About every two hours . . . you'd have a flat stick, like a yardstick. And you would move the seaweed so that it's turning over. It's turning over and drying so that it all dries. . . . After the sun starts to set, the seaweed is cooling off now, and before that dew starts again, you gather the seaweed. You pull up the four corners of the sheets and shake the seaweed down to the center, and pack it inside this way, holding onto the drawn-up corners. . . . You have to let it cool right down, in a dry place. [Helen puts it in her livingroom.] You open up the corners so it doesn't steam or sweat and it dries completely. So overnight you'll let it cool and . . . then you're putting it into tight containers. . . . What we usually do is take a certain amount out of the big containers—just enough seaweed that you're going to eat—and put it into a smaller sealed container; the less you expose the seaweed to the air, the better. Because every time the air hits that seaweed, it changes it. Eventually the seaweed will turn a different color. And it has a different taste. So if you keep the large container closed, and just take out what you're going to eat for that meal . . . it will retain its original flavor from when it was put into there.

Helen explained that some women place green cedar branches instead of salal leaves between the seaweed layers. Women today may also use a length of twine laid diagonally across the seaweed layers instead of a strip of cedarbark.

As in the harvesting of the seaweed, the chopping and drying processes are undertaken with cooperation and reciprocity. Helen described how women all through the village come to help her when it is time to chop the seaweed:

> Somebody will say, "When are you going to chop your seaweed?" And I have to send somebody out: "Well, granny's going to be chopping seaweed on such and such a day." I send word throughout the community and so they drift up. Some people have an hour or so, [but] they'll come out. And so, they all help each other, the women. Some of them have enough daughters or granddaughters to go and help. It works that way in every house, [when] they're chopping seaweed. If you've got an hour to spare, two hours to spare, whatever time you have, you go and help chop seaweed. Especially if you don't have seaweed. You will earn some seaweed; they'll give you some seaweed. You earn it.

Thus, the work of seaweed production is one that brings people—especially women—together to socialize, to learn from one another, and to share the products of their labors. In this way, it is a constructive and healthful activity that contributes to the well-being of the whole community.

Nutritional and Health Contributions

Louis Druehl (2000: 155) wrote that "Nori *(Porphyra)* is probably one of the healthiest foods on our planet. . . . It is rich in carbohydrates, proteins and vitamins." The nutritional constituents of *ɬa'ask* are shown in Table 6.1. Porphyras, like other marine algae, have a high protein content, said to be 25 to 35 percent of dry weight for Japanese *nori* (*Porphyra* spp.). They also contain significant quantities of vitamins and mineral salts, especially iodine. The vitamin C content of the Japanese species is about 1.5 times that of oranges. What is particularly significant is that up to 75 percent of the protein and carbohydrates, at least of the Japanese *nori*, are digestible by humans, which is very high for seaweeds (Guiry, 2004b).

TABLE 6.1. Nutritional constituents of red laver seaweed *(Porphyra abbottae)* and dulse *(Palmaria palmata);* Rhodophyceae (per 100 g fresh weight).

Nutrients	Red laver	Dulse	% of recommended daily requirements
Food energy (kcal)	279	–	2,200 cal/9,204 kj
Water (g)	10	87	–
Protein (g)	24.4	1.8	43
Fat (g)	1.4	–	85
Carbohydrate (g)	58.0	6.1	275
Crude fiber (g)	25.2	–	–
Ash (g)	16.1	3.6	–
Thiamine (mg)	0.37	0.63	.88
Riboflavin (mg)	1.79	0.51	1.1
Niacin (mg)	6.7	0.2	15.8
Vitamin C (mg)	11.6	38.0	45
Vitamin A (RE = retinol equivalents)	263	285	800
Calcium (mg)	230	48	800
Phosphorus (mg)	474	–	–
Sodium (mg)	3,300	–	–
Potassium (mg)	3,140	–	–
Magnesium (mg)	623	60.1	–
Copper (mg)	1.7	0.2	–
Zinc (mg)	1.7	0.8	–
Iron (mg)	10.5	–	13
Manganese (mg)	1.6	0.6	–
Molybdenum (mg)	–	<0.1	–
Chloride (mg)	–	1,306	–

Source: After Morgan et al., 1980; Hooper, 1984; Kuhnlein and Turner, 1991, p. 405; U.S. Department of Agriculture.

Note: The recommended daily intake is based on requirements of a girl aged 13 to 15 weighing 48 kg (Health and Welfare Canada, 1985).

We suspect—although this remains to be demonstrated empirically—that the complex process of drying, rehydrating, curing to "get its flavor," and redrying the seaweed, also helps to break down the complex proteins and carbohydrates and enhances the digestibility of the seaweed. Other peoples along the Northwest Coast also had intricate procedures for curing edible seaweed, including packing them in boxes interspersed with cedarboughs, sometimes even saturating them with juice from chewed rock chitons or clams, presumably to enhance the flavor and/or digestibility of the seaweed (Boas, 1921).

La'ask is also used directly as a medicine. Johnny Clifton explained that eating seaweed will alleviate heartburn and indigestion, just like Tums or Rolaids. It is also used as an antiseptic poultice for a deep cut or swelling; according to Helen, it will take the swelling right down, and will keep a cut from becoming infected.

When eaten as a component of a traditional diet, together with seafood such as halibut and salmon, crabs, game, berries, and wild greens and root vegetables, there is no doubt that seaweed helps to promote good nutrition and health. In addition, the lifestyle associated with the seaweed harvest—being physically active and working outdoors, with safety a prime consideration—would also promote peoples' health and well-being. Culturally and socially, too, the family and community closeness and cooperation, the opportunities for learning and teaching, and the closer understanding of history and traditions of peoples' heritage that comes with harvesting and using traditional foods, promotes emotional and mental health. Environmental health is also a consideration. The seaweed is harvested sustainably, maintaining its capacity for regeneration and renewal. Furthermore, people who are out on the lands and waters on a continuous basis have the opportunity to closely observe any changes or impacts that might be occurring in the environment, including changes in populations and health of other life-forms. Ultimately, this close monitoring can result in adaptive behavior and can enhance a society's resilience and capacity to maintain cultural integrity in the face of change (Berkes and Folke, 1998).

Changes and Adaptations in Seaweed Harvesting and Use

Many changes have occurred over the years relating to the Gitga'at seaweed harvest; some of these have already been mentioned. Fewer people harvest the seaweed today than in the past, at least in part because the younger people have wage jobs and children have to be in school. Thus, they cannot take an entire month to be away from the village. Some Gitga'at people live away from Hartley Bay, in Prince Rupert or Vancouver, and this makes Kiel even less accessible. Men now participate in what was once entirely a women's occupation. Speedboats and skiffs today have replaced the cedarwood dugouts of bygone years. Nylon onion sacks are used in preference to hemp gunnysacks, which had, in turn, replaced original cedarbark containers. The gunnysacks tend to accumulate and hold water instead of allowing it to drain away, thus causing the seaweed kept in sacks to sweat, retain its heat, deteriorate, and rot more quickly. This is why mesh onion bags are preferred today. Fewer of the traditional seaweed beds are used in harvesting and, undoubtedly, less seaweed is picked than in the past—when, according to Helen and Johnny, all the seaweed-producing shorelines of Campania and Princess Royal islands were cleaned off each season. Methods of processing and cooking the seaweed have changed as well. Nowadays, some of the seaweed is dried in thin sheets or left in squares without chopping it; the younger people enjoy just frying these up in lard, like potato chips, and eating them as a snack. Few people have the chance to make halibut-head soup and some of the other dishes that were commonly prepared and traditionally eaten with the seaweed.

People are also concerned about environmental pollution and its impacts on their traditional foods. Seaweeds, for example, can absorb heavy metals (Sirota and Uthe, 1979), but the actual risks of such contamination are little studied or understood.

Changes in the weather have resulted in attempts to adapt by freezing the seaweed so that it could be dried at a later date, when the weather improved. Helen commented:

> For years you could depend on "April showers will bring May flowers." You need that for [predicting] the weather. Worldwide, the weather is so different now, you can't depend on those old sayings. You're lucky if you get one day of sun. And if you're not at the right tide, even if you pick that seaweed for that [day], you might be picking late afternoon, and you can't dry it on those rocks. Some of our people have tried to experiment right now, and tried to put some into the deepfreeze to see [how it does]. And yet, some of our older people will taste it, and

there's a difference. There's a difference to that seaweed that has been frozen. And so they will taste it. Even though we try to save it . . . they'll try many ways because we haven't had the sun that we used to depend so much on.

Helen and Johnny and other Gitga'at elders are concerned that the younger people cannot easily participate in seaweed picking. In part this is also due to the uncertainties of the weather:

And so our young people that can help us—because they're working, they come down here on weekends—and so they get stuck because they're weatherbound.[3] They can't make it down here; they can't help us. They get the wood, they get the water, they do many things for us. We need their help, us elders that live here.

The elders are looked after in other ways, too. Helen noted that there are special seaweed-picking places that are reserved especially for the older women, who are not as nimble and cannot leap from rock to rock or climb down steep rock faces to seek out the best seaweed. The flatter, more even places where the seaweed grows, therefore, are kept for the elders.

Helen also recognizes that the young people are missing out on much of the traditional education that they would have received in the past during stays at Kiel and other places on the land and waters in Gitga'at territory. Because they are not able to experience the effects of tides, currents, and weather first-hand, or how to harvest and process their traditional foods, they may not be able to carry on these traditions or pass them on to the next generations.

The seaweed, too, is affected by the weather. Helen explains:

Sometimes . . . there's a difference of seaweed. With the weather conditions that we've had now—we're having hail, we're having snow—and if the seaweed is just starting to grow on the rocks . . . they're just like any plant: if they've been hit by frost and it's real cold—we did have some really cold north wind in April, it was beautiful weather once the sun came out, but really frosty, icy conditions. So we could tell, all the seaweed, if there was snow, the tide was down, a big snowstorm came in, or hit by hail . . . we'd have to break the ends off of the seaweed there. The seaweed is a beautiful greenish color, and the ends will all start to have curly heads . . . seaweed is smooth, when you feel it. You get to the curly parts [at the ends of the seaweed], they're rotten, they're tough, they're kinky. That seaweed is not good. You learn that with experience.

CONCLUSION

Times are certainly changing, and the Gitga'at, like people of other coastal communities, have had to face the changes and adapt to them. Cultural traditions such as harvesting and eating ɬa'ask are at risk of being lost if a certain threshold of practice and passing on the associated knowledge is not reached. Helen has thought a great deal about these changes, and worries about the future of the young people in her community and about the environmental changes as well:

> I just wonder if [the old people] were alive what they'd say about this weather that we're having now, what they would have to say. They would say somebody did something. . . . [That's] why the weather is the way it is. And of course, we know who that is! But those are some of the things that happened here, that's changed over time. It's the Mickey Mouse [CB Radio], VHS, and TV. Yes, you see kids today, you would find a rare kid that would know whose speedboat that is coming, whose boat that is!

In many ways it is the small details of cultural and environmental knowledge that are the most important, and they are most in danger of slipping away in the societywide rush toward globalization and cultural homogenization. If the details of how to harvest and how to cure seaweed pass out of peoples' knowledge and experience, more than just one food source would disappear. The Gitga'at, and all humanity, would be poorer for this loss. It is thanks to people like the Gitga'at elders, who work hard to keep their cultural traditions alive, that seaweed and other traditional foods are likely to be harvested and enjoyed far into the future.

NOTES

1. Other food people have traditionally gathered from Kiel includes halibut, red snapper, seagull eggs, small and large chitons (China slippers), abalone, and giant mussels ("all the seafood you could get"). However, according to Helen Clifton, the latter were harvested only after the seaweed had been picked and dried; harvesting the mussels is said to cause rain.

2. The life cycle of *Porphyra* is described in full by Michael D. Guiry, phycologist; Web site: http://seaweed.ucg.ie/cultivation.html, from Nelson and colleagues (1999). The haploid plants grow from spores that were produced from the diploid phase through meiosis. The diploid phase, called the Conchocelis phase, was discovered only in 1949 by the British phycologist K. M. Drew-Baker. Before this time, it was not recognized that it was the same plant as the membranous haploid form. The Conchocelis-phase organisms produce two types of spores from the ends of their branchlets. Under some conditions, they produce diploid spores, which will grow into other individuals. However, under other, specific conditions of light quantity, light quality, daylength, and temperature (the permissive conditions differ between species and sometimes between strains of a species), the filaments form swollen branches (called "conchosporangia"), in which the cells, still diploid, develop into branches which protrude from the substrate and eventually release their contents as individual wall-less cells called "conchospores." It is these cells that eventually undergo meiosis—which is a complex process, with secretion of cell walls and splitting of the chromosome pairs. There are usually four haploid cells surviving. Hence, the blades, unlike the plants they are derived from, are haploid. The haploid plants, again under specific conditions of light quality and quantity, daylength and temperature, will eventually produce gametes. Male gametes (called "spermatia") are produced in packets at the blade margins and are released by disintegration of the margin. The female gametes, or "carpogonia," are produced back from the margin. Each carpogonium develops a special receptive surface, to which spermatia attach, allowing fertilization to occur. The fertilized cell, the zygote, now diploid (with a double complement of chromosomes) divides to form a structure called a "carposporangium," which releases diploid spores, or "carpospores," as the blade margin disintegrates. The carpospores germinate to form new diploid Conchocelis-phase filaments which germinate on, and frequently penetrate, a shell substrate. Although the calcium carbonate is not absolutely required for their growth, apparently, it is only within this substrate that the filaments can survive in nature without being browsed by herbivorous snails and other marine grazers.

3. *Note:* On our way down to Kiel with Marven Robinson in May 2001, we had to go to the outside of Campania Island because the waves and currents were too strong on the inside of the island. Marven kept in close radio contact with Johnny, who advised him how the weather was at Kiel.

REFERENCES

Aaronson, S. (1986). A role for algae as human food in antiquity. *Food and Foodways* 1: 311-315.

Abbott, I. (1974). *Limu: An ethnobotanical study of some edible Hawaiian seaweeds.* Lawai, Hawaii: Pacific Tropical Botanical Garden.

Berkes, F. and C. Folke (Eds.) (1998). *Linking social and ecological systems. Management practices and social mechnanisms for building resilience.* Cambridge: Cambridge University Press.

Boas, F. (1921). *Ethnology of the Kwakiutl.* Bureau of American Ethnology, 35th Annual Report, Part 1, 1913-14. Washington, DC: Smithsonian Institution.

Druehl, L. (2000). *Pacific seaweeds. A guide to common seaweeds of the West Coast.* Madiera Park, BC: Harbour Publishing.

Guiry, M.D. (2004a). Nori cultivation. National University of Ireland, Galway. Available online at http://seaweed.ucg.ie/cultivation/NoriCultivation.shtml.

Guiry, M.D. (2004b). The seaweed site. National University of Ireland, Galway. Available online at http://seaweed.ucg.ie/seaweed.html.

Guiry, M.D. and G. Blunden (1991). *Seaweed resources in Europe: Uses and potential.* Chichester, UK: John Wiley & Sons.

Guiry, M.D. and C.C. Hession (1998). The seaweed resources of Ireland. In Critchley, A.T. and M. Ohno (Eds.), *Seaweed resources of the world* (pp. 210-216). Yokosuka, Japan: Japan International Cooperation Agency.

Health and Welfare Canada (1985). *Native foods and nutrition: An illustrated reference resource.* Ottawa, ON: Minister of Supply and Services.

Hooper, H.M. (1984). Nutrient Analysis of twenty southeast Alaska native foods. *Alaska Native News* September: 24-28.

Indergaard, M. (1983). The aquatic resource. I. The wild marine plants: A global bioresource. In Cote, W.A. (Ed.), *Biomass utilization,* NATO Advanced Science Institutes Series. Series A, Life Sciences, Volume 67 (pp. 137-168). New York: Plenum Publishing Corporation.

Kenicer, G., S. Bridgewater, and W. Milliken (2000). The ebb and flow of Scottish seaweed use. *Botanical Journal of Scotland* 52 (2): 119-148.

Kuhnlein, H.V. (1992). Change in the use of traditional foods by the Nuxalk native people of British Columbia. *Ecology of Food and Nutrition* 27: 259-282.

Kuhnlein, H.V. and N.J. Turner (1991). *Traditional plant foods of Canadian indigenous peoples: Nutrition, botany and use.* Philadelphia: Gordon and Breach Science Publishers.

Lindstrom, S.C. and K.M. Cole (1991). A revision of the species of *Porphyra* (Rhodophyta: Bangiales) occurring in British Columbia and adjacent waters. *Canadian Journal of Botany* 70: 2066-2075.

Madlener, J.C. (1977). *The seavegetable book.* New York: Clarkson N. Potter, Inc.

Milliken, W. and S. Bridgewater (2001). Flora Celtica: Sustainable development of Scottish plants. Scottish Executive Central Research Unit and Royal Botanic Garden, Edinburgh. Available online at http://www.scotland.gov.uk/cru/kd01/orange/sdsp-00.asp.

Morgan, K.C., J.L.C. Wright, and F.J. Simpson (1980). Review of chemical constituents of the red alga *Palmaria palmata* (Dulse). *Economic Botany* 34 (1): 27-50.

Nelson, W.A., J. Brodie, and M.D. Guiry (1999). Terminology used to describe reproduction and life history in the genus *Porphyra*. *Journal of Applied Phycology* 11: 407-410.

Ostraff, M. (2003). Contemporary uses of limu (marine algae) in the Vava'u Island Group, kingdom of Tonga: An ethnobotanical study. Doctoral dissertation, School of Environmental Studies and Department of Geography, University of Victoria, Victoria, BC.

Port Simpson Curriculum Committee (1983). *Port Simpson foods: A curriculum development project*. Prince Rupert, British Columbia: The People of Port Simpson and School District No. 52.

Sirota, G.R. and J.F. Uthe (1979). Heavy metal residues in dulse, an edible seaweed. *Aquaculture* 18: 41-44.

Turner, N.J. (1995). *Food plants of coastal first peoples*. Vancouver: Royal British Columbia Museum and University of British Columbia Press.

Turner, N.J. (1998). *Plant technology of British Columbia first peoples*. Vancouver: Royal British Columbia Museum and University of British Columbia Press.

Turner, N.J. (2003). The ethnobotany of "edible seaweed" (*Porphyra abbottae* Krishnamurthy and related species; Rhodophyta: Bangiales) and its use by first nations on the Pacific Coast of Canada. *Canadian Journal of Botany* 81 (2): 283-293.

Turner, N.J., M.B. Ignace, and R. Ignace (2000). Traditional ecological knowledge and wisdom of Aboriginal peoples in British Columbia. *Ecological Applications* 10 (5): 1275-1287.

Turner, N.J., J. Thomas, B.F. Carlson, and R.T. Ogilvie (1983). *Ethnobotany of the Nitinaht Indians of Vancouver Island*. British Columbia Provincial Museum Occasional Paper No. 24. Victoria: British Columbia Provincial Museum.

Williams, M.D. (1979). The harvesting of "slukus" (*Porphyra perforata*) by the Straits Salish Indians of Vancouver Island. *Syesis* 12: 63-68.

Chapter 7

Medicinal Herb Quality in the United States: Bridging Perspectives with Chinese Medical Theory

Craig A. Hassel
Christopher A. Hafner
Renne Soberg
Jeff Adelmann

CONTEXT FROM A BIOMEDICAL PERSPECTIVE

In the United States, medicinal herbs are categorized and regulated as botanical dietary supplements according to the Dietary Supplement and Health Education Act (DSHEA, 1994). The intent of this legislation was to make more nutritional and botanical supplement alternatives available to Americans, in order to improve public health and reduce future health care costs (DSHEA, 1994; Nesheim, 1999). Recently, use of botanical and dietary supplements by the American public has risen by an estimated 380 percent (Eisenberg et al., 1998), to sales exceeding $600 million (Brevoort, 1998). Yet under DSHEA legislation, the quality of plant medicines is ill defined and little guidance is available to growers, processors, distributors, health care providers, or consumers specifically interested in understanding, main-

This work was supported through funding from the following sources: USDA Agricultural Experiment Station Project MIN-54-059; University of Minnesota Extension Service; The Minnesota Institute for Sustainable Agriculture (MISA); the Agriculture Utilization Research Institute (AURI); and the Organic Farmers Research Foundation (OFRF).

taining, or improving the quality of medicinal herbs as tools to improve health (Matthews et al., 1999).

Increasing consumer demand and regulatory ambiguities have led to greater attention toward product quality, understood here as encompassing aspects of both safety and expected health benefits (efficacy). Observers within biomedical science have mapped a broad spectrum of scientific challenges facing the botanical supplement industry "from seed to shelf" (Cardellina, 2002; Costello and Coates, 2001). Growing conditions such as local soil and climate, herbivores, weeds, plant pathogens, time of harvest, and drying/storage conditions are needed research areas that might constitute "good agricultural practices" (GAPs) (Cardellina, 2002). GAP guidelines could address adulteration, contamination, and counterfeiting issues associated with supply of high-quality "raw" or "bulk" herbs, and would require specific research devoted to each herb grown for medicinal purposes. Some 2,048 individual medicinal herbs are delineated in the new reference proposed for use by U.S. regulators (McGuffin et al., 2000). Finding the means to conduct the research needed for creating GAP guidelines for each herb of commerce is unlikely, but presently possible.

A greater obstacle for biomedical scientists is the challenge of determining with assurance that the final product will deliver the maximum health benefits possible to consumers and clinicians. The prevailing approach to medicinal herb quality involves reducing the physiologic effects of an herb to putative active/marker molecular constituents and attempting to create "standardization" with respect to the concentration of the identified constituents (Calixto, 2000; Harkey et al., 2001; He, 2000; Newall et al., 1996; Yan, 1999). In most cases, the bioactive constituents of any given herb are not known with certainty (Cardellina, 2002). This is in part due to the chemical complexity of any naturally occurring plant or food. No medicinal herb to date has been completely characterized with respect to precise chemical composition (Cardellina, 2002). State-of-the-art chemical analyses yield a "fingerprint," or profile of molecular composition, but without positive identification of the individual constituents (Harkey et al., 2001). Thus, scientists may capably differentiate products with respect to chemical profile or pattern, yet in many cases lack the means to confirm the identity of the compounds involved (He, 2000; Yan, 1999). Associating pharmacological effects with specific chemical components is further complicated by the likelihood of interactions among several or many bioactive compounds within the plant material (Chang, 1999). Our best understandings suggest the therapeutic benefits associated with medicinal herbs in many cases come from a complex array of different compound classes within the plant (Lee, 2000; Yan, 1999). Thus, no simple or direct chemical assay or analysis exists that can be used with certainty to predict the "quality" of medicinal herbs with respect to user efficacy or clinical outcome (Cardellina, 2002).

This represents a significant problem because biomedical professionals rely on standards for product quality based upon chemical analysis and pharmacological response (Calixto, 2000; Harkey et al., 2001; Lee, 2000; NCCAM, 2000; Yan et al., 1999). Lacking such basic scientific understandings, current industry quality control measures (good manufacturing processes, GMPs) resort to chemical analysis of identifiable "marker" compounds in an attempt to provide final products with greater homogeneity and product uniformity (Cardellina, 2002; Costello and Coates, 2001). Uniformity and consistency with respect to "marker compounds" are relevant to product identity (does the product contain what the label states?) and to some extent safety, but are not necessarily related to maximizing clinical benefits. In this sense, biomedical efforts to standardize botanical products are concerned with minimizing fraud and possibly adverse effects, but should not be construed with a process of ensuring the best health outcome for patients taking these products.

The pharmacological approach to medicinal herbs has proven useful for creating single-component pharmaceuticals derived from plants, but medicinal herbs themselves are complex systems containing many hundreds of chemical constituents that may act in symphony to produce cumulative physiologic effects (Lee, 2000; Yan, 1999). Efforts to chemically fingerprint each botanical can yield different chemical profiles depending upon where the plant is grown, when it is harvested, how it is processed, and how it is stored (Harkey, 2001; Cardellina, 2002). Significant costs are associated with compositional analysis, and interpreting the pharmacological significance of different fingerprints is ambiguous at best (Harkey, 2001; Chang, 1999). Conclusive understandings of bioactive "cause-and-effect" pharmacology for dose/response and clinical efficacy comparisons requires expensive randomized controlled trial (RCT) design. The cost for one well-executed RCT can range from under $1 million to many millions, depending upon the size and duration of the protocol. RCT costs are a significant part of the escalating costs associated with pharmaceutical products (patent protection is used to recover these formidable investments). Medicinal herbs lie beyond patent protection, so it is unrealistic to expect such costs to be recovered from the marketplace. Cardellina (2002) suggests that if simple, cost-effective bioassays could be established and linked to performance in RCTs, the challenge of defining standards of quality from a biomedical perspective become more viable. Given the magnitude of the challenges, one might question whether developing scientifically sound and reliable bioassays can be accomplished without adding significant cost to final products. DSHEA legislation was enacted to provide consumers with alternatives to reduce health care costs (DSHEA, 1994; Nesheim, 1999), not to raise them further. However, perhaps it may be possible to create cost-effective bioassays by looking at other, well-established knowledge systems already in place.

CONTEXT FROM A CHINESE
MEDICAL THEORY PERSPECTIVE

Biomedical-based standards of medicinal herb quality offers Chinese medicine (CM) practitioners little help with quality assurance on one hand and a series of significant obstacles to providing patients with the best possible health outcomes on the other (Chevallier, 1996; Chiu, 1997; Hassel et al., 2002; Yang, 2002). Aside from the challenges previously posed, practitioners of CM use different language, systems of logic, and criteria for understanding health and diagnosing illness (Chevallier, 1996; Leslie and Young, 1992). The fundamental ideas upon which Chinese medical theory rests do not fit well within a biomedical model and are often discounted or ignored (Leslie and Young, 1992). Consequently, ideas of medicinal herb quality as understood and used within CM (Bensky and Gamble, 1993; Chiu, 1997; Hsu et al., 1986; Yang, 2002) are not well recognized by established biomedical scientific and regulatory organizations. Yet CM practitioners face the prospect of mounting restrictions, increased costs, and continued disregard by U.S. regulations oriented exclusively toward biomedical understandings (Hassel et al., 2002).

Overview of Chinese Medical Theory

In order to offer the reader a fuller appreciation of these dilemmas, we introduce a few fundamental concepts of CM considered general knowledge among its students, practitioners, and scholars. This overview, written by Christopher Hafner, is largely excerpted from a prior work (with kind permission of Kluwer Academic Publishers) and serves to illustrate how the CM system of knowledge can serve as an independent foundation for determining and guiding appropriate, safe, and effective use of medicinal herbs (Hassel et al., 2002).

CM has existed for over 2,500 years (Kaptchuk, 2000; Maciocia, 1989) and is one of many societal systems of ancient medical practice devoted to understanding and diagnosing illness and using plants to restore and maintain health (Balick and Cox, 1997; Chevallier, 1996). The theory of yin and yang is integral to CM and defines its most fundamental principle (Kaptchuk, 2000; Maciocia, 1989). Yin/yang theory addresses the dual nature of perceivable reality. Based upon a principle of relativity, the theory explains the interaction between opposite forces and qualities that make up the known universe. Yin and yang are interdependent—each defines the other. Originally, the Chinese characters for yin and yang depicted the interplay of sunlight and shadow upon a hillside. Yin represents the side of the hill that is cast in shadow while yang represents the side of the hill that is bathed in light. By extension, yin represents all that is relatively dark, cool, moist, receding, passive, quiet, heavy, and descending, while yang represents all that is relatively bright, warm, dry, advancing, active, restless, light, and ascending. Yin is potential, yang is kinetic. Yin is form, and yang is function.

Inherent in the relationship between yin and yang is the potential for both harmony and disharmony (Kaptchuk, 2000; Maciocia, 1989). When harmony exists between yin and yang, an appropriate balance between the opposite forces and qualities at play (whether it is an ecosystem, a community or society of human beings, or the anatomy and physiology of an individual human being), there is peace, contentment, health, and sustainability. When disharmony exists between yin and yang, then there is conflict and discord, illness, disease, suffering, and disintegration.

CM applies this understanding of the dynamics of yin and yang to human health and wellness. Specifically, Chinese medical practice guides the careful cultivation and preservation of harmony between yin and yang (and thus safeguard health, prevent disease, and promote well-being), and seeks to treat the illnesses and suffering that are created from identified disharmonies. Disharmonies between yin and yang occur in four ways: yin excess, yin deficient, yang excess, and yang deficient. These patterns of disharmony frequently occur in combination and can engender subsequent patterns of disharmony that can increase exponentially, giving rise to all the different disease states known to humans. In all cases, the general treatment strategy for resolving disharmony between yin and yang is to remove that which is in excess and to supplement that which is deficient.

Based on the fundamental theory of yin and yang, there are two general categories of CM (Kaptchuk, 2000; Maciocia, 1989). The first category includes everything dedicated to understanding, diagnosing, and developing strategies to resolve patterns of disharmony. The second category includes that body of knowledge dedicated to identifying, understanding, and classifying *qualities* and forces in nature in terms of yin and yang, and the effects these qualities and forces have upon the relationship between yin and yang in human beings. Combining the knowledge gained in these two categories provides the practitioner of CM with the rationale and information necessary to manipulate the forces in nature and thereby promote good health and prevent or treat illness through harmonization of yin and yang in the patient (Maciocia, 1989).

CM does not rely upon the chemical composition of food or herbs as a basis for understanding medicinal efficacy, safety, or quality. In Chinese dietary and herbal therapies the yin/yang qualities that are inherent in foods and medicinal herbs are identified and classified through the sensory attributes that naturally occur in these substances. These sensory attributes are called "property" and "flavor" (Bensky and Gamble, 1993; Hsu et al., 1986; Yang, 2002). Property (*si xing*, literally "four natures") refers to the attribute of a food or medicinal substance that, once ingested or applied externally, is experienced by the individual as one of the "four natures": cold, cool, warm, or hot. This effect is on the subjective experience of an individual's body temperature and is independent of (but not necessarily exclusive of) the objective assessment of body temperature by outside means, such as by palpating the skin or by a thermometer reading. Foods or medicinal substances are referred to as being "cooling" or "warming" or as having a "cold," "cool," "warm," or "hot" property (Bensky and Gamble, 1993; Hsu et al., 1986; Yang, 2002). Mint, for example, is said to be cooling, as is watermelon, cucumber, and tofu. Ginger is said to be warming, as is cayenne pepper, cinnamon, and lamb. The property of a food or medicinal substance is assessed independently of the temperature at which that food or substance is consumed or applied, although various methods of cooking and preparation can occasionally be used to augment or mitigate a property.

Flavor *(wei)* refers to the sensory attribute that occurs with the sensation of "taste" when a substance is placed in the mouth (Bensky and Gamble, 1993; Chiu, 1997; Hsu et al., 1986; Yang, 2002). CM identifies five primary flavors: sweet, pungent, salty, sour, and bitter. According to Chinese medical theory, flavor is considered to be a manifestation of the *Qi* that is inherent in a substance. *Qi* is usually translated as "energy" or "vital energy," although there is no one word in English that adequately captures the full meaning of the word as it is used in Chinese, and particularly as it is used in CM. *Qi* is the manifestation of the interaction of yin and yang and therefore refers simultaneously to both form and function and to both potential and kinetic energies. Different flavors embody different qualities of *Qi* and manifest the particular interactions of yin and yang.

Each flavor, as a manifestation of *Qi,* has a unique effect on the *Qi* of a human being (Bensky and Gamble, 1993; Hsu et al., 1986). The sweet flavor is said to engender *Qi* and nourish fluids in the body, promote structure and form in the body, strengthen and protect the digestion, relieve pain, and harmonize the effects of the other flavors. The pungent flavor disperses *Qi* in the body, promotes movement and function, and can have a drying effect. The salty flavor softens hardness and purges accumulations of *Qi*. The sour flavor consolidates, gathers, and binds *Qi* in the body and stabilizes secretions and discharges. The bitter flavor clears heat from the body and dries dampness.

The sensory attributes of property and flavor inherent in a particular food or medicinal substance can be used to create an energetic profile of that substance (Bensky and Gamble, 1993, Hsu et al., 1986). This energetic profile can then be used by the CM practitioner to guide the appropriate use of that food or substance to safely and effectively manipulate *Qi* and promote harmony between yin and yang in a patient (Bensky and Gamble, 1993; Chiu, 1997; Hsu et al., 1986; Yang, 2002).

For example, a patient suffering from an excess of cold with acute symptoms of strong chills and body aches but an absence of thirst or sweating (symptoms of excess heat) might be advised to consume substances that have a pungent flavor (to disperse the excess) and a warming property (to counter the effect of cold). A strong broth made from ginger, scallions, and cayenne pepper, all of which are considered to be both pungent and warming, would remove the excess of yin responsible for the disharmony and subsequently help the patient to feel better. A patient suffering from a deficiency of warmth with chronic symptoms of chilliness, weakness, and fatigue, may be advised to consume substances that are classified as sweet (to engender *Qi*, and therefore tonifying to the body) and warming (again, to counter the chilliness). A diet that regularly included chicken, lamb, trout, and venison (all of which are considered in CM to be sweet and warming) perhaps cooked with ginger, garlic, and onions (for their warming property), would be warming and tonifying and would supplement the deficiency of yang that is responsible for the disharmony in this situation. Gradually, the patient would feel stronger and less chronically chilly.

Quality Discrimination Using CM

In this way, CM offers a system that recognizes and discriminates characteristics of all food and medicinal substances in terms of sensory attributes. Some 5,700 different plant-, mineral-, and animal-derived substances are used medically and characterized and categorized according to "property" and "flavor" attributes within the *Zhong Yao Da Ci Dian* (Encyclopedia of traditional Chinese medicinal substances), representing classification during the past 2,500 years (Bensky and Gamble, 1993; Hsu et al., 1986; Yang, 2002). As with biomedicine, CM recognizes that altering soil, growing, harvest, processing, and storage conditions can change the qualities of any given food or herb. Unlike biomedicine, CM recognizes physiologic manifestations of medicinal herb qualities that are subjectively experienced by the senses. Discriminating CM practitioners and pharmacists can independently assess quality of medicinal herbs through careful assessment of sensory qualities by recognizing the "property" and "flavor" attributes found in the plant material (Bensky and Gamble, 1993; Yang, 2002). This process is akin to recognizing the quality of a fine meal by discrimination of sensory qualities associated with each food. Indeed, CM does not make distinctions between food and medicinal herbs in terms of quality assessment. CM thus offers an alternative system through which to understand, determine, and guide appropriate use of medicinal herbs for treating patterns of disharmony and to restore and maintain health.

CM practitioners have expressed frustration over the lack of serious attention by most biomedical research to medicinal herb quality as understood by CM or other knowledge systems (Hassel, 2002). Biomedical approaches may improve product uniformity, but could represent a lateral or even backward step in terms of end-use efficacy, as the standardization process does not take into account the characteristics of medicinal herbs as understood by CM (Cheviallier, 1996; Hassel et al., 2002). Regulations to ensure public safety offer another case in point. In a clinical study in Europe of a weight-loss product comprised of Chinese herbs, a number of patients developed severe nephrotoxicity after *Aristolochia fangchi* had been inappropriately substituted for the expected *Stephania tetranda* (Vanherweghem, 1999). This unfortunate mistake was probably the result of confusion with Chinese names for the two plants (*Guang fang ji* and *Han fang ji,* respectively) by clinicians lacking sufficient training in CM. The subsequent adverse effects were linked to aristolochic acid, a constituent of *Aristolochia.* The U.S. Food and Drug Administration (FDA) responded by issuing warnings and a recall of all supplements containing aristolochic acid. The FDA recall was very broad, including approximately 600 species of plants, many of which contain little or no detectable aristolochic acid (Cardellina, 2002). The broad recall includes many plants that have been safely and effectively used in CM for millenia, compromising the practice of knowledgeable CM practitioners and the health benefits of patients across the United States. The FDA cannot be faulted for acting quickly to protect public safety, but overattachment to a pharmaceutical approach, combined with underappreciation for the coherence of CM as a knowledge base for determining appropriate use, has led to a regulatory response that further erodes the practice of CM. Regulator focus on chemical identification and pharmacology as the exclusive means to determine appropriate use of medicinal herbs furthers disregard for the fundamental principles and logical coherence of CM. If biomedical models continue to form the exclusive basis for regulation, medicinal herbs available to practitioners would likely become unavailable or more expensive while quality, as understood from a CM perspective, could actually decrease.

DILEMMA OF "INTEGRATING" TWO DIVERGENT EPISTEMOLOGIES

Historically, CM represents a heterogeneous array of ideas and practices developed over the past 3,000 years (Unschuld, 1985). Over the past century, CM has been exposed to increasing influence from outside forces, such as Marxism and Western science (Unschuld, 1992). Given the advancement and hegemony of biomedical science, many indigenous medical systems, including CM, have suffered disintegration and dismantling of their philosophical underpinnings (Aldrete, 1996; Fruehauf, 1999; Semali and Kincheloe, 1999; Smith, 1999). This disintegration is a result of biomedical inquiry into the tools of practice employed by the systems under investigation (Fruehauf, 1999; Leslie and Young, 1992).

From a biomedical perspective, CM presents itself as a series of potentially useful and exploitable technologies (tangible artifacts or practices such as medicinal herbs or acupuncture), each to be evaluated through well-conducted RCT methodology. The purpose of such inspection is to expand the realm of biomedical practice by including specific herbs or practices proven efficacious or safe through controlled scientific experiment (or as illustrated in the case described earlier, to exclude by regulation specific herbs proclaimed as unsafe). Left behind are the underlying theories and epistemologies (such as *Qi* and yin/yang theory) that do not fit with the biomedical model (Fruehauf, 1999; Leslie and Young, 1992). From the perspective of CM practitioners, the safety and efficacy of CM lie not only with the toolbox of specific herbs or practices used but also with underlying concepts that determine and govern their appropriate use (Unschuld, 1987). However, to biomedical researchers, these ideas are discounted, dismissed, or ignored (Leslie and Young, 1992). Biomedical inspection of the herbs and procedures of CM propagates expansion and globalization of the biomedical paradigm at the expense of the underlying integrity of the CM perspective (Fruehauf, 1999). Significant concerns have been raised about the viability of the fundamental essence of CM in the face of ongoing attempts to "integrate" diversity through biomedical expansion (Farquhar, 1987; Fruehauf, 1999; Scheid, 1999). The outcome of such "integration" is unclear, but could result in further disintegration or destruction of CM as an independent medical tradition (Scheid, 1999).

FOUNDING A MEDICINAL HERB NETWORK

Against this background context, the Medicinal Herb Network was formed several years ago to establish a marketing, communication, and programmatic relationship between health care practitioners seeking quality medicinal herb products and farmers looking for opportunities to diversify operations and increase profitability (Hassel et al., 2002). The purpose of the network was to bring together expertise among medicinal herb growers and health care practitioners in the upper midwestern United States to explore opportunities in the production, processing, marketing, and use of botanicals. An extensive Web search for similar endeavors begun elsewhere revealed several organizations comprised of either medicinal herb growers or herbalist health care practitioners, but none that deliberately included both within the same network. A participatory, community-based action research approach (Greenwood and Levin, 1998) was employed where participants defined issues and research questions, developed agendas, and conducted research based upon areas of opportunity identified by ongoing discussion.

Network members quickly came to the understanding that disconnections between medicinal herb producers and end-user practitioners kept both groups from realizing the significant benefits and opportunities that might exist for domestically grown herbal medicines. Local herb growers expressed their readiness to grow a variety of medicinal herbs, but had concerns related to profitability and sustainability. Price volatility observed over the course of the growing season heightened a sense of uncertainty of the demand and potential for profit generated by their products. They reported receiving mixed messages from distributors concerning future prices for given herbs and premium pricing for "higher quality" products. They indicated poor definition, understanding, and communication regarding the concept of "high quality" within the marketplace. When growers engaged in contract negotiations, processors/distributors were often unclear about the desired qualities of the medicinal herbs to be produced.

CM practitioners indicated that they relied significantly upon products imported from Asia, South America, and Europe, but were suspicious of dubious quality, including concerns of contamination and/or adulteration. Because of DSHEA regulations and poor oversight of imported products, they had no way of certifying authenticity or the conditions under which the product was produced or processed. Practitioners suggested that locally grown herbs produced with specific attention to generating a high-quality product would provide added value to their practice. As one practitioner indicated, "my diagnosis can be flawless, yet if the herbs I prescribe are of substandard quality, the patient will not see the best results" (Hassel et al., 2002).

Network Initiatives

Practitioners expressed confidence that higher quality medicinal herbs would translate into better health care for patients. The network produced a survey that was distributed to CM practitioners in the upper Midwest to gather data on specific medicinal herb product use and sought insights regarding quality concerns with available products (Cooperative Development Services, 2000). The survey was part of a larger, broad-based market research study of medicinal herbs conducted by the Minnesota Grown Opportunities (MGO) Project. Practitioners stated their willingness to pay a premium price for assurance of quality as recognized within the system of CM practice (Cooperative Development Services, 2000).

Another initiative resulted in the development of the Organic Herb Producers Cooperative to focus specifically on producing and marketing high-quality medicinal herbs. The cooperative brings together organic herb growers with a wide range of backgrounds and expertise throughout the upper Midwest to deal with issues regarding growing; harvesting; postharvest processing, including dry-cut/sift and essential oil production; and marketing. Some 80 different medicinal herbs used in CM were propogated and field tested by Cooperative members. Growers are especially interested in a means to assess quality throughout the production and processing cycle without having to rely upon the time and expense associated with chemical analysis procedures.

A third activity directly addresses the issues of medicinal quality described previously. Indications from the practitioner survey suggest standards of quality would enhance market opportunities for domestic growers by making their products more attractive to CM practitioners. A product certified under a system that could verify growing, harvest, processing, and storage conditions would give producers a market advantage by providing practitioners with medicinal herbs assured to meet certain criteria for quality. Quality benchmarks would include certification of organic production, botanical authenticity, and postharvest processing methods and practice. Most important, quality recommendations would include a means of assessment that would employ the fundamental principles of CM as a basis for clinical efficacy and safety.

Quality As Determined Using CM

Practitioners suggested that quality assessment using CM principles already in place may offer an alternative perspective to chemical analysis and standardization efforts that predominate in the pharmaceutical industry (Bensky and Gamble, 1993; Hsu et al., 1986; Yang, 2002). As described previously, CM recognizes and discriminates characteristics of medicinal herbs—and indeed categorizes them—in terms of their property *(si xing)* and flavor *(wei)* attributes as accessed by the senses. CM practitioners with expertise in classical principles of CM have the capacity to evaluate the quality and potential for clinical efficacy of a given herb by its smell and/or taste characteristics (Chiu, 1997; Hsu et al., 1986; Yang, 2002). The Medicinal Herb Network has developed a project to take advantage of both CM knowledge and descriptive sensory analysis, a subdiscipline within food science where panelists are trained to detect specific sensory characteristics ("attributes" or "notes") present in food (Gacula, 1997).

This project includes the expertise of CM practitioners with experience in the evaluation of medicinal herbs and graduate food scientists trained in the procedures of descriptive sensory analysis. Its purpose is to establish a means of communicating the concepts of quality as understood by CM practitioners using a vocabulary of terms developed by descriptive sensory analysis procedures. A given herb is selected for analysis and a wide variety of samples (both imported and domestic) are procured from the marketplace. Expert CM practitioners are then asked to evaluate the overall quality of the herb samples with regard to their *si xing* and *wei* characteristics and to offer a cursory description of its taste/smell characteristics. The graduate-food-scientist panelists are then employed to more fully elucidate and identify the sensory attributes or "notes" inherent within the spectrum of samples for a given species of medicinal herb. Once the attributes are discriminated, identified, described, and labeled, intensity scores for each attribute in each sample can be assessed. In this way, different sources of the same herb species can be compared and evaluated with respect to the presence and intensity of sensory attributes. The assessment of quality by CM practitioners can then be correlated with the presence and intensity of attributes as determined by the panelists using descriptive sensory analysis. By evaluating several different species of medicinal herbs, a dictionary of attributes could be compiled that might be used to convey information about medicinal herb characteristics and qualities. CM practitioners envision that as more species are analyzed the redundancy of attributes would increase, so that a fairly complete dictionary of attributes could be derived from several species of medicinal herbs. Such a dictionary of attributes would form a lexicon (vocabulary) that could be used to communicate a sense of quality, as understood from the CM knowledge system, to others less familiar with CM. The lexicon would not replace chemical analysis, but could offer a different and perhaps more cost-effective means to perceive and distinguish medicinal herb quality, using the lens of CM theory. Once learned by medicinal herb growers, processors, health care practitioners, and other professionals, the lexicon could be used to create a common understanding of quality that would not depend solely upon more expensive and exhaustive chemical analysis methodologies. In addition, growers could potentially use sensory assessment as a means to add value to their products, making them more attractive to CM practitioners seeking quality products.

The Medicinal Herb Network has begun working on a pilot study to test the feasibility of these ideas, using a cross-section of eight to ten samples of two different herbs (of both imported and locally grown origin) of varying quality. Briefly, a critical mass of local and knowledgeable CM practitioners was assembled to offer an initial quality assessment of each herb sample. Practitioners were asked to judge overall quality for clinical use and then to briefly describe sensory characteristics for each sample. Descriptive analysis sensory panels were organized using graduate students trained at the Sensory Center in the Department of Food Science & Nutrition at the University of Minnesota. Student panelists were trained using individual descriptor-element reference "attribute" standards, deciphered from the herb samples. During these sessions, students developed their ability to discern and rate the intensity of the individual attributes for a given sample. Based upon the practice sessions, students were able to discern some thirty individual notes or descriptor characteristics found among all herb samples. Intensity scores for each attribute were aggregated into mean data for each individual herb sample. Attributes rated by students in samples are statistically correlated with medicinal herb quality as assessed by qualified practitioners. Thus, establishment of a lexicon of quality attributes based upon descriptive sensory analysis appears feasible. Additional studies and analysis of several other medicinal herb species will yield a lexicon that could be incorporated into clinical trials that include the CM system of diagnosis and treatment as part of the randomization protocol. If successful in such trials, a lexicon could potentially offer medicinal herb growers a means through which to target growing and processing protocols, thereby adding value and quality to locally grown products sought by practitioners of CM.

REFERENCES

Aldrete, E.W. (1996). The formulation of a health research agenda by and for indigenous peoples: Contesting the Western scientific paradigm. *The Journal of Alternative and Complementary Medicine* 2(3): 377-385.

Balick, M.J. and P.A. Cox (1997). *Plants, people and culture: The science of ethnobotany.* Scientific American Library Series, Number 60. New York: W.H. Freeman & Co.

Bensky, D. and A. Gamble (1993). *Chinese medicine materia medica,* Revised edition. Seattle: Eastland Press.

Brevoort, P. (1998). The booming U.S. botanical market; a new overview. *Herbalgram* 44: 33-48.

Calixto, J.B. (2000). Efficacy, safety, quality control, marketing and regulatory guidelines for herbal medicines (phytotherapeutic agents). *Brazilian Journal of Medical & Biological Research* 33(2): 179-189.

Cardellina, J.H. (2002). Challenges and opportunities confronting the botanical dietary supplement industry. *Journal of Natural Products* 65: 1073-1084.

Chang J. (1999). Scientific evaluation of traditional Chinese medicine under DSHEA: A conundrum. Dietary Supplement Health and Education Act. *Journal of Alternative and Complementary Medicine* 5(2): 181-189.

Chevallier, A. (1996). *The encyclopedia of medicinal plants.* London: Dorling Kindersley Ltd.

Chiu, D.C. (1997). Traditional Chinese herbal therapies. In Gao, D. (Ed.), *Chinese medicine* (pp. 54-85). New York: Thunder Mouth Press.

Cooperative Development Services (2000). *Medicinal herbs market research.* St. Paul, MN: The Minnesota Grown Opportunities Project.

Costello, R.B. and P. Coates (2001). In the midst of confusion lies opportunity: Fostering quality science in dietary supplement research. *Journal of the American College of Nutrition* 20(1): 21-25.

Dietary Supplement Health and Education Act (DSHEA) of 1994, Public Law 103-417 (1994) (codified at 42 USC 287C-11). Available online at http://www .fda.gov/opacom/laws/dshea.html.

Eisenberg, D.M., R.B. Davis, S.L. Ettner, S. Appel, S. Wilkey, M. Van Rompay, and R.C. Kessler (1998). Trends in alternative medicine use in the United States, 1990-1997. *JAMA* 280(18): 1569-1575.

Farquhar, J. (1987). Problems of knowledge in contemporary Chinese medical discourse. *Social Science & Medicine* 24(12): 1013-1021.

Farquhar, J. (1994). *Knowing practice: The clinical encounter of Chinese medicine.* Boulder, CO: Westview Press, Inc.

Fruehauf, H. (1999). Chinese medicine in crisis. Science, politics and the making of "TCM." *Journal of Chinese Medicine* 61: 6-14.

Gacula, M.C. Jr. (1997). Descriptive sensory analysis methods. In Gacula, M.C., Jr. (Ed.), *Descriptive sensory analysis in practice* (pp. 5-15). Trumbull, CN: Food & Nutrition Press.

Greenwood, D.J. and M. Levin (1998). *Introduction to action research.* Thousand Oaks, CA: Sage Publications.

Harkey, M.R., G.L. Henderson, M.E. Gershwin, J.S. Stern, and R.M. Hackman (2001). Variability in commercial ginseng products: An analysis of 25 preparations. *American Journal of Clinical Nutrition* 73(6): 1101-1106.

Hassel, C.A., C. Hafner, R. Soberg, J. Adelmann, and R. Haywood (2002). Using Chinese medicine to understand medicinal herb quality: An alternative to biomedical approaches? *Agriculture & Human Values* 19: 337-347.

He, X.G. (2000). On-line identification of phytochemical constituents in botanical extracts by combined high-performance liquid chromatographic-diode array detection-mass spectrometric techniques. *Journal of Chromatography* 880(1-2): 203-232.

Hsu, H.Y., Y.P. Chen, S.J. Shen, C.S. Hsu, C.C. Chen, and H.C. Chang (1986). *Oriental materia medica: A concise guide.* Long Beach, CA: Oriental Healing Arts Institute.

Kaptchuk, T.J. (2000). *The web that has no weaver: Understanding Chinese medicine.* Chicago: Contemporary Publishing.

Lee, K.H. (2000). Research and future trends in the pharmaceutical development of medicinal herbs from Chinese medicine. *Public Health Nutrition* 3(4A): 515-522.

Leslie, C. and A. Young (1992). *Paths to Asian medical knowledge.* Berkeley, CA: University of California Press.

Maciocia, G. (1989). *The foundations of Chinese medicine: A comprehensive text for acupuncturists and herbalists.* New York: Churchill Livingstone.

Matthews, H.B., G.W. Lucier, and K.D. Fisher (1999). Medicinal herbs in the United States: Research needs. *Environmental Health Perspectives* 107(10): 773-778.

McGuffin, M., J. Kartesz, A. Leung, and A. Tucker (Eds.) (2000). *Herbs of commerce,* Second edition. Silver Spring, MD: American Herbal Products Association. Available online at http://www.ahpa.org/update_03HOCRule.htm.

National Center for Complementary and Alternative Medicine (NCCAM) (2000). *Expanding horizons of health care. Five year strategic plan, 2001-2005.* Available online at http://nccam.nih.gov/about/plans/fiveyear/index.htm.

Nesheim, M.C. (1999). What is the research base for the use of dietary supplements? *Public Health Nutrition* 2(1): 35-38.

Newall, C.A., L.A. Anderson, and J.D. Phillipson (1996). *Herbal medicines: A guide for health-care professionals.* London: The Pharmaceutical Press.

Scheid, V. (1999). The globalisation of Chinese medicine. *Lancet* 354(9196 Suppl. 1): 10.

Semali, L. and J. Kincheloe (1999). What is indigenous knowledge and why should we study it? In Semali, L. and J. Kincheloe (Eds.), *What is indigenous knowledge? Voices from the academy* (pp. 3-57). New York: Falmer Press.

Smith, L.T. (1999). *Decolonizing methodologies: Research and indigenous peoples.* New York: Zed Books Ltd.

Unschuld, P. (1985). *Medicine in China: A history of ideas.* Berkeley, CA: University of California Press.

Unschuld, P. (1987). Traditional Chinese medicine: Some historical and epistemological reflections. *Social Science & Medicine* 24(12): 1023-1029.

Unschuld, P. (1992). Epistemological issues and changing legitimation: Traditional Chinese medicine in the twentieth century. In Leslie, C. and A. Young (Eds.), *Paths to Asian medical knowledge* (pp. 44-61). Berkeley: University of California Press.

Vanherweghem, J.L. (1999). Misuse of herbal remedies: The case of an outbreak of terminal renal failure in Belgium (Chinese herbs nephropathy). *Journal of Alternative and Complementary Medicine* 4: 9-13.

Yan, X., J. Zhou, and G. Xie (1999). *Traditional Chinese medicines: Molecular structures, natural sources, and applications.* Brookfield, VT: Ashgate.

Yang, Y. (2002). *Chinese herbal medicines. Comparisons and characteristics.* New York: Churchill Livingstone.

Chapter 8

Balancing the System:
Humoral Medicine and Food
in the Commonwealth of Dominica

Marsha B. Quinlan
Robert J. Quinlan

INTRODUCTION

People in many societies—Western cultures included—believe that a well-balanced lifestyle yields a healthy mind and body. People strive for a "balanced" diet and some harmony between work and play, sitting and exercise, and so forth. Humoral medicine is a similar concept, in which wellness is maintained or restored by balancing opposite forces (or humors) such as heat and cold or dryness and wetness. In the Commonwealth of Dominica, villagers assert that much illness is the result of hot or cold humors that enter a person's body and disrupt the balance of his or her "system." Disruptive humoral forces may enter a person's body in a number of ways. For example, a wound might allow a hot or cold element to contaminate a person, the body might become deeply chilled in cool weather, or a person might become overheated by hard work in the tropical sun. Most commonly, however, disruptive hot or cold forces are thought to enter the body by eating. People are expected to become unhealthy by eating

We thank Mark V. Flinn for introduction and project support in the study site. We thankfully acknowledge Dominica's Ministry of Health for sponsoring this research. We are most grateful to villagers of the study community, especially Edith Coipel, Juranie Durand, and the Warrington family. Research in this chapter was funded in part by the Earthwatch Institute (1998 Grant for "Dominica Family Environment and Child Health Project" to M. Flinn, R. Quinlan, and M. Quinlan) and by the National Science Foundation (Grants BNS 8920569 and SBR 9205373 to M. Flinn).

an unbalanced diet or by neglecting to adjust their diet to their lifestyle. Logically, when people feel that they are suffering from a diet-
related disorder, they adjust their diet. The reader should find this sce-
nario familiar. The idea that ill health results from an unbalanced diet
is not unique to Dominica; in fact it may be a human universal.

The hot/cold humoral system has been documented throughout the
New World, particularly in Latin America (for an overview, see Foster, 1994). Foster claims, in fact, that "humoral medicine in the Americas is the most completely described of all ethnomedical systems"
(1994, p. 2). In the hot/cold humoral system, people group mental and
physical states, plants, and animals into "hot" and "cold" categories.
Here, "cold" or "hot" may refer to the temperature of air or bathing
water; however, "hot" and "cold" often refer to culturally ascribed
symbolic values having nothing to do with thermal state. North
Americans similarly refer to chili peppers as "hot" regardless of the
temperature at which they are served. Some mental states also carry
hot or cold labels. The North American view of anger as hot-headed-
ness and indifference as coldness reveals a glimpse of similar
symbolic use of heat and cold.

In addition to associating temperatures and emotions with heat and
cold, the humoral approach associates heat and cold with all living
things. Every plant or animal (therefore everything one eats) has an
assumed inherent humoral temperature.

People who live by the hot/cold humoral system believe that the
human body functions best at a warm state that is in-between the hot
and cold extremes that exist in other species of the plant and animal
kingdoms.

Heat and cold are reckoned as transferable; not only can temperatures of water and air in the physical environment be absorbed or
transferred to the internal and external body, but one can also transfer
the humoral quality of something one ingests to one's own body. Just
as people must avoid overexposure to hot or cold temperatures, they
must also avoid overexposure to hot or cold humoral states. They
must therefore balance the hot or cold humoral qualities of the foods
they eat.

The Dominican version of the balanced diet presents an example
of the internal logic of one hot/cold humoral belief system. In Dominica, much illness is blamed on eating too much humorally hot or
humorally cold food, thereby changing the body's optimal warm state

to a hot or cold one. The remedy to a hot or cold condition is to ingest a food which has cooling or heating properties to counteract the perceived causes of illness. Health maintenance through balancing humorally hot and cold properties in the diet is a fundamental component of "bush medicine," the folk medical system of Dominica and much of the Caribbean.

SETTING

The Commonwealth of Dominica is a small island nation located between the French Departments of Guadeloupe to the North and Martinique to the South (15°N, 61°W). The island is mountainous, relatively undeveloped, and supports little agriculture or tourist industry compared to other Caribbean islands. Dominica's population (approximately 68,000) is composed of people from a mixed African, European (French and English), and Native American (Island-Carib) descent. Most Dominicans are bilingual in Creole English and French-Patois.

This research took place in an east (windward) coast village nestled at the crux of two mountain ridges (see Quinlan, 2004). The mountains trap rain blown in from the ocean, so the village's annual rainfall is between 100 and 150 inches per year, making for lush vegetation. The site is primarily a subsistence agricultural community. Almost everyone gardens. In addition to subsistence gardens at the village periphery, most land within the village is cultivated with fruit trees and other plantings. Many families also maintain small house gardens for condiments and herbs for cooking and medicine.

Remote even by Dominican standards, the site is located about a 40-minute drive from the main road at the dead-end of a narrow, mountainous, sometimes washed-out lane. There are approximately 650 full- and part-time residents. Relative isolation reduces residents' economic opportunities. Average annual income is approximately 5,000 East Caribbean dollars (U.S. $1,850). Villagers earn their living through subsistence gardening, fishing, bay oil production, and banana production, and a few residents engage in wage labor.

The village's location also limits residents' access to outside (Western) health care. There is a local health center that offers inoculations and a small supply of common medications (e.g., ibuprofen) and first-aid materials. The nearest pharmacy is a two-hour drive away. A doctor is available at the government health center, approximately a 45-minute drive from the village. No villager owns a private automobile, however, and rides are expensive and sometimes difficult to arrange. Hence, all villagers rely heavily on home remedies—locally called bush medicine. Villagers assert over and over that everyone in the village is his or her own bush doctor. Diet is a fundamental component of bush medicine.

METHODS

Fieldwork for this project was conducted during five trips to the study site between 1993 and 1998. Ethnographic data on bush medicine were collected using informal key-informant interviews, a village health survey, semistructured key-informant interviews with bush-medicine experts, and free-list tasks with 160 village residents (90 percent of adults).

Informal Interviews

The informal interviews were conversational and involved asking a representative sample of village adults about their own experiences with and responses to illness events. Informal interviewing was also conducted during the course of participant observation, such as working with people in their gardens, cooking meals with them, and so forth.

Health Surveys

The health survey involved asking every village mother a series of questions regarding the health of family members. Women were asked about the general health history and condition of all household residents. They were asked to recall any illness or injuries their family members had suffered in the past week, past month, and past year. Each time a woman mentioned an illness event she was asked how the family member became sick, in order to probe for the perceived etiology of the illness. Women were next asked what, if anything, anyone did to treat the sick person. If someone at home treated the sick person (which was usually the case), the woman was asked to describe the treatment. Mothers were also asked who they sought out for bush medical advice and which villagers knew the most about bush medicine.

Key-Informant Interviews

From the survey of mothers, five village residents stood out as particularly sought after for their bush medical advice. These five experts became key informants, or project consultants. They included three women, ages 39, 55, and 68, and two men, ages 25 and 49.

Each consultant was interviewed three times. The first interview was a long, general interview on the medical system, including the kinds of health practitioners villagers use under certain circumstances, local notions of ethnophysiology, and which illnesses the expert treated with bush medicines. During the second interview the experts were asked which bush remedies they used for each sickness they listed during the previous interview. Next, the informant was asked about the use(s) of each bush medicine that he or she had listed. Finally, the consultants helped to gather samples of every remedy they had mentioned during the previous two interviews (the majority of the remedies were plants, for which voucher specimens were collected; however, there were also many nonherbal treatments, including foraged animal and mineral ingredients and purchased products).

Free-List Interviews

Interviews eliciting the health problems that villagers treat with bush medicine were conducted with 30 residents to identify salient illnesses in the community.[1] Next, free-list interviews for remedies were conducted with every willing adult villager ($N = 160$, about 90 percent) in residence during the summer of 1998. Villagers were asked to list all bush medicines (many foods are considered bush medicine as well as nourishment) used to treat each of the salient illnesses.

RESULTS AND DISCUSSION

Rural Dominicans emphasize the importance of maintaining a balanced body "system." Balance is necessary regarding how much blood one has; how often one eats, drinks, and eliminates waste; the size of one's intestinal parasite load; and the hot/cold humoral state of one's body. The balance of hot and cold, however, is the primary concern expressed in many rural Dominican conversations about illness.

Dominican Daily Diet

There is a lot of variation in what, when, and how much Dominican villagers eat. However, three general dietary rules predominate. First, every villager starts his or her day with "tea." Second, everyone eats lunch, the main meal of the day, between noon and 2:00. Finally, everyone's food and drink intake attempts to follow the basic guidelines of local hot/cold humoral theory.

The hot/cold humoral qualities inherent in things people eat correspond to the local models of nutrition. Human bodies are reckoned to contain the same elements present in animals; therefore, animal products (meat, milk, and eggs), like the healthy human body, are seen as neither too hot nor too cold, or humorally neutral. Dominicans regard animal foods as essential, at least in small amounts. They state that the body can easily transform animal products into human fluids and tissue. Staples such as legumes and boiled tubers or starchy fruits are also neutral and eaten together. Processed starch foods (i.e., kinds of flour) are "hot" (and cause constipation) while fruits and greens are "cool" (and alleviate constipation). These notions make sense in terms of two opposing Dominican food preoccupations: keeping the belly full and keeping the belly and bowels (or intestines) blockage-free.

In addition to water, Dominicans drink three kinds of beverages: juice, "tea," and alcohol. Dominicans make most fruit juices by grating, squeezing, or blending fruit and adding water and some raw sugar. Dominicans include unripe coconuts *(Cocos nucifera)*, or "jellies" as a kind of juice, though a good portion of it is actually eaten. One "has a jelly" by opening a hole in a green coconut with a machete, drinking the liquid endosperm, then splitting the drained coconut open and scooping out the unripe coconut meat (which has a gelatinous, or jelly-like consistency). All juice is reckoned humorally cold, though coconut, pineapple *(Ananas comosus),* and papaya *(Carica papaya)* are especially cold. Drinking plenty of juice (two to three servings a day) is thought to provide refreshment, keep one's digestive tract moving as it should, keep one's skin blemish-free, and protect against heat exhaustion.

Dominicans use the word *tea* to refer to any hot, nonmeat beverage. It is rarely store-bought green tea (i.e., cured leaves of Asian tea shrubs *[Camellia sinensis]*—green, orange pekoe, black oolong, or otherwise). Rather, people drink some kind of plant-based infusion from materials that they harvest themselves. These "teas" include coffee, "cocoa tea" (hot chocolate), or "bush tea" (any herbal tea, such as mint and orange-leaf tea). People drink morning "tea" every day to "ease off" two bodily accumulations that occur during sleep in the cool air: (1) the gas that accumulates in the belly overnight and (2) the cold that builds in the body overnight (i.e., "tea" loosens up mucus and joints). Most people drink at least one more cup of "tea" in the late afternoon, though some men skip their afternoon tea in favor of alcoholic beverages.

Alcohol, especially cask rum, has a large, visible presence in Dominican village life. With the exceptions of a few strict Seventh-Day Adventists, all villagers, from teenagers through the elderly, drink on occasion. Middle-aged and older men drink the most, and some adult males are routinely publicly inebriated. Alcohol doubtless comprises a large proportion of the calories that these men consume. Beer, ginger wine, brandy, and bottled rum are usually available at village shops, but the typical (and most economical) drink is a "shoot" (shot) of cask rum followed by a chaser of water. Villagers reckon alcohol and alcohol-related illnesses as humorally "hot." Drinkers try to balance their humoral intake by eating "cold" fruits.

Lunch, the main meal, is "food" complimented with "peas" (any kind of bean) and usually meat or bouillon-based gravy. Rural Dominicans use the word "food" only to refer to the starchy provisions that form the base of their diet. Dominicans especially refer to their principal subsistence crop, dasheen (taro, *Colocasia esculenta*) as "food." However, plantains (*Musa* × *paradisiaca*), breadfruit *(Artocarpus altilis),* sweet and Irish potatoes (*Ipomoea batatas* and *Solanum tuberosum*), and yams (*Dioscorea* spp.) are also "food." Processed starches including manioc flour *(Manihot esculenta),* arrowroot starch *(Maranta arundinacea),* rice *(Oryza sativa),* cornmeal

(Zea mays), and anything made with wheat *(Triticum aestivum)* flour (e.g., bread, pasta, dumplings) is "like food" but is not "real food." "Food" "fills your belly" and "stays with you" without causing constipation. Edibles "like food" fill the belly, but only for a short time. Further, these processed starches are humorally hot. Eaten alone they cause "inflammation," which swells up the inner body, causing constipation by blocking the bowels. Dominicans occasionally eat "hot things" (e.g., dumplings) as a "food" replacement. They must then accompany "hot" starches with fruit juice, greens, cucumber, or another humorally "cold" item to "keep the system free of blockage."

"Food" and things "like food" are not said to "build" the body. Rather, they provide simple sustenance—give energy and fill hungry bellies. Fruits and vegetables build the body, especially digesting into components of body fluids (blood, breastmilk, and semen). Meat, milk, eggs, and (to a lesser extent) legumes digest directly into body components, such as muscles and blood. People discuss these edibles as the essence for strength, growth, and wound healing.

Humoral Quality of Food

How do cultures ascribe certain foods with hot or cold humoral values? The enthnography points to factors that some groups use to assign "hot" versus "cold" values. For example, Nahuatl Indians in the Valley of Mexico make humoral distinctions between certain foods in their raw versus cooked state (Madsen, 1955). This is not the case in Dominica where, for example, a humorally "hot" "bush tea" remains "hot," even if it cools completely. Likewise, "cold" food remains "cold" (such as papaya in goat stew), even if it is hot or cooked. In some populations (e.g., Guatemala [Logan, 1973]) color is an ascription factor, but not in Dominica. The Central American Quichés' humoral definition of meat is tied to the animal's wild or domestic status (Neuenswander and Souder, 1977). Meat is neutral in Dominica, so a distinction contrasting natural to human-altered food is not an issue. However, Dominicans do make one similar type of distinction: processed versus unprocessed staples. Dominicans view processed starches (e.g., wheat flour, manioc flour *[farín]*, and cornmeal) as hot foods. Whole carbohydrate foods that—other than peeling or cooking—do not require processing (plantain, dasheen [taro], potatoes, yams, and breadfruit) are neutral staples.

Food's perceived sensory effect is another factor for assigning hot or cold humoral quality. How does the food or seasoning feel to the skin or mouth? Does exposure to it burn one's skin, as with the bay leaf that Dominicans distill as a fragrance and eat as a seasoning, or does it feel cool and soothing like the flesh of banana fruit *(Musa ×️ paradisiaca)*? After one ingests the plant, does it feel refreshing (i.e., "cool") or piquant (i.e., "hot") on one's mouth/throat? Organoleptic qualities such as taste, appearance, and odor may be passed down as explanations of plants that work, yet it is doubtful that Dominicans assign hot, cold, or neutral values to foods based *solely* on sensory, or organoleptic properties.

Messer (1981) and Brown (1976) found that people in their re-search areas (Oaxaca, Mexico, and Highland Ecuador, respectively) classified some foods according to their sensory qualities (e.g., spicy foods are "warming"). However, both studies found that the per-ceived physiological effect on people was more important in assign-ing a hot or cold value than the immediate organoleptic sensation a food/herb produced. People in both populations reasoned that, ulti-mately, their experience and observations of what the substance did was the main issue in determining humoral quality.

Organoleptic indicators are present in a small minority of foods and medicine. However, when present, they function as mnemonic aids in Dominica as elsewhere (Leonti et al., 2002). After seeing a fire-roasted banana, one will not likely forget its use as a laxative (and, as laxatives are always viewed as cold in Dominica, one is un-likely to forget the banana's humoral property). Papaya fruit remains protected from the sun's heat because the tree's large leaves shade the fruit and the fruit's skin protects the flesh from the heat. Hence fresh, moist papaya fruit might seem cool to Dominicans. Papaya is indeed regarded as a cold food in Dominica. Rum produces a burning sensa-tion when swallowed and is regarded as a hot drink, yet other sub-stances that produce burning oral effects, such as curry, seasoning peppers, and ginger are regarded as neutral. Further, burning sensa-tion from acid in lime *(Citrus aurantifolia)*, pineapple, and tomato *(Lycopersicon esculentum)*, though potentially hot to the senses, does not effect the Dominican classification of these fruits as humorally cold.

One might argue that, for most people, tradition provides the basic guidelines for knowing whether a food is hot or cold. Children know the humoral qualities of many foods through traditional learning. Through casual observation and conversation, children memorize the names, medicinal uses, and humoral qualities of many foods that their families and neighbors eat, as well as the "bush teas" that they drink. In some societies, hot/cold assignment of plant humoral quality appears to be entirely memorized, in that it has nothing to do with a human's physiological reaction to the plant. For example, New York Puerto Ricans classify lima beans and white beans as "cold" and kidney beans as "hot," though they all offer very similar benefits and effects on the body (Harwood, 1971).

However, in Dominica, as in Ecuador and Mexico (Brown, 1976; Messer, 1981), a plant's humoral value comes from the effects the plant produces when people ingest or apply it. The most important factor that Dominicans use to determine a substance's humoral value is the effect that the substance has on the human body. Though people may memorize the hot or cold status of foods as children, adults usually discuss a food or medicine's use (and ascribe a hot/cold/neutral quality) in terms of the internal logic of the ethnomedical system. For example, in Dominica, a rash is a hot condition. Dominicans would thus refer to a plant that soothes rashes as a cold plant (whether eaten, drunk, or applied topically) because it counteracts a hot condition. The Dominican ethnomedical system is one in which the assumed humoral state of human maladies takes precedence in determining the humoral value of a food or herb. In fact, people do not seem to have the humoral qualities of plants committed to memory as well as they have the humors of illnesses. Thus, when asked if a plant had a hot or cold value, informants generally had to reason out a response. For example, one might say that a food makes one feel "refreshed" or helps "clean your bowels," and that is why it is "cooling."

In many respects, the Dominican humoral system conforms to the general pattern of humoral theory found across cultures. It differs, however, from most New World hot/cold humoral systems in one important aspect. In most New World cultures, humans are viewed as the only living thing (or one of a few) that is humorally neutral (or warm—in-between hot and cold). All other animals and plants (therefore all edibles) are regarded as either colder or hotter than humans (Foster, 1994). Dominicans regard only *certain* foods and diseases as hot or cold, while others—approximately one-third of illnesses—are neither hot nor cold, but rather humorally neutral

(Quinlan, 2004). People treat a cold illness by ingesting something humorally hot and likewise ingest cold things for a hot illness, but treatments for neutral illnesses are not typically regarded as hot or cold. In these cases, they target areas of pollution or imbalance that residents associate with the particular humorally neutral health problem.

Humoral Illness in Dominica

The foundation of rural Dominican humoral theory is that humans are made of meat. Locals compare the behavior of human flesh and fluids to that of the meat and gravy in their daily stewpot, which becomes thin or supple when warm and thick or hard when cool. Thus, if temperature, food/drink, or emotions create too much cold inside a person's body, his bodily fluids and tissues presumably thicken or harden. Hard tissues or thick body fluids are the perceived etiology of a cold illness. Conversely, when temperature, food/drink, or emotions result in too much bodily heat, a person's insides soften and thin, or (in extreme cases) cook. Cold and heat are thought to affect all body tissues and the viscosity of bodily fluids, but especially blood and mucus.

The body can regulate its own temperature to some degree. If a person needs to cool down, his or her pores will allow some heat to escape from his or her body and the person will perspire. The body is particularly good at heating itself up. When one has a cold illness, the body often heats up on its own to "melt out" the cold. Sometimes, "melting out" a tenacious "cold" overheats the body. In the Dominican view, a fever (a hot condition) comes from overheating in response to a cold illness. Self-cooling during the daytime is difficult, Dominicans say, because the air temperature is hot. Sweating and open pores do not cool the body well when it is hot out. Usually, cooling requires external forces such as shade, breeze, bathing, and ingestion of humorally cool foods and fluids.

In Dominican ethnomedicine, humoral states can have an important influence on illnesses relating to blood and the circulatory system. Dominicans describe the heart as a muscular pump that receives blood from two blood entrance tubes. Informants explain that the bottom tube receives clean, new blood from the kidneys and liver, while the top one takes in old blood from the body for recirculation. The heart pumps, squeezing the blood from the entrance veins into one big exit vein (presumably the aorta) that divides three ways. The left vein division fuels the left side of the body with blood, the middle division goes up to the head, and the right division delivers blood to the right side of the body. The quality of the blood pumping through one's veins, Dominicans allege, is a primary cause and indicator of health or illness. Dominicans judge the quality of one's blood by three basic criteria: viscosity, quantity, and purity.

Blood viscosity, in particular, is thought to vary with temperature or humoral status. Blood congeals when it is cool and thins when it is hot. Warm blood is too thin. It does not scab quickly and flows through cuts or menstruating women too fast. The ambient temperature, humoral "heat" in food or "teas," or overexertion can cause warm blood. Warm blood usually goes away on its own as the body cools and rests. Prolonged warm, thin blood leads to weakness or may make some "anemic." Villagers say that "anemic" people are thin, always tired, have poor color, and tired eyes. According to locals, anemics have thin, weak, pale blood. Folk diagnosis involves checking the color and texture of the veins on the underside of a person's arms. Rest and eating "plenty peas" (beans), especially wild "pigeon peas," or *pwa angol (Cajanus cajan)*, are prescribed for people who seem anemic. Anemics also need to eat "plenty meat," especially wild *manikou* (opossum) and agouti, but goat or beef is also good.

Cold blood is thick. It clots too easily, potentially causing a "mass" that blocks circulation. If a mass blocks circulation to the "brains" or heart, a person could drop dead suddenly. Otherwise, cold blood might just slow a person down. It also might cause one's mucus to thicken and one's joints to stiffen. Respiratory illnesses (such as asthma and the common cold) and arthritis are thus cold. A person's blood can become "cold" through exposure to cold temperatures (locals describe air below about 68°F as "cold"), which is a relatively rare experience for Dominicans. Dominicans have occasion to feel cold during tropical depressions, at higher elevations, and when wet in the rain, out at sea, or swimming in cold water for extended times. Shock or fear, humorally cold emotions, can also lead to cold illnesses, including respiratory illnesses and a folk illness called "fright" (similar to post-traumatic stress syndrome), in which one's blood is thought to chill. Although the Dominican humoral system recognizes food and herbs that are cold enough to cause vomiting or diarrhea, no food or herb has a humoral quality so cold that it can cause cold, thick blood, or mucus. There are, however, foods to treat cold blood. They are all seasoning or condiment foods, including wild basil *(Ocimum basilicum)*, bay leaf, garlic *(Allium sativum)*, Cuban oregano *(Plectranthus amboinicus)*, cinnamon *(Cinnamomum zeylanicum)*, "male garlic," or *ajo sacha (Mansoa alliacea,* syn *M. hymenaeamanilkara)*, lemon grass *(Cymbopogon citratus)*, and goatweed *(Capraria biflora)*.

There is a folk blood condition that Dominicans refer to as "pressure." "Pressure" is *not* the same as "high blood pressure," or hypertension. "Pressure" is a hot condition in the blood and the veins that can be caused by diet, digestion, or stress. The body of someone suffering from "pressure" is internally hot and inflamed. Inflammation causes the veins to swell, making the tubes for blood circulation narrower. A large gas build-up can also push against veins, restricting the amount of blood that can pass through them. A person with "pressure" also has hot blood. Hot blood generally becomes thin and weak. However, hot blood under "pressure" goes one step further and actually begins to cook, as if boiling off the water in the blood. This makes the blood too concentrated or too "rich." Because this blood is extra rich and thick, the body has a hard time pushing it through the already compromised veins. Hence, pressure builds up in the veins.

"Pressure" can result from the stress of worrying, studying too hard, and having strained relationships. These stressors cause the mind to work overtime, which is said to generate heat in the blood. Dietary "pressure" can result from eating too many processed starches, the "hottest" foods. Drinking too much rum (also very hot) exacerbates the possibility of developing "pressure." Digestion is involved with "pressure" because some people with otherwise healthy diets are said to digest too efficiently, leading to "pressure." If people are particularly good digesters, or have a diet particularly rich in foods that "build the blood" (meat), their blood will be too thick and rich. The local ethnophysiology of the digestive and circulation systems provides for "building" blood, but not for thinning blood or taking blood away. Females with "pressure" rid some supposed extra blood or extra blood richness with menstruation, but this might be temporary, so the blood becomes too rich again.

The typical reaction to "pressure" is to exclude all hot (flour-based) foods from the diet, eliminate or limit animal products from the diet, and eat a cold (high-fiber) diet that is heavy in fruits and vegetables. Favored foods for "pressure" are papaya, christophine or *chayote (Sechium edule)*, and passion fruit *(Passiflora laurifolia)*. If a change in diet does not sufficiently relieve the "pressure," a Dominican thought to have too much blood (or blood richness) in the veins may resort to cutting (bleeding) himself or herself to relieve the vein pressure.

Dominicans theorize that blood may become polluted by dirt that gets inside the body. As dirty blood flows through the body, it is imagined to irritate and abrade body tissues. The result is what Dominicans call "inflammation" (internal humoral heat and occasional swelling). "Inflammation" can be in a specific body part, but more often it is generalized. General inflammation eventually moves outward, to the limbs and the head, and finally to, or through, the skin. Dirt enters the body via an open wound, air pollution, or on food. Dominicans claim that cuts—especially cuts on feet—and bites—especially dog and witch bites—are wounds that put people most at risk for dirty blood. Dirt can also enter the body system by breathing it in. Smoke is said to carry dirt in it, and smoke is all around the village. Villagers use fire to cook, clear gardens, distill bay oil, and burn rubbish. People also breathe in dirt in dusty air. The study site is on the wet, eastern side of the island, so dust is uncommon, although one can breathe in dust and ashes while cleaning out a hearth or planting in a newly cleared garden on a dry day. If one goes to Roseau, the capital, he or she will certainly breathe in some dust. Roseau is on the island's drier side, and the relative bustle of its 15,000 inhabitants results in airborne dust. Villagers always complain about feeling dirty and run down after a trip to town.

Any dirt that enters the body with food (or on food) may be pushed through the walls of the "worm bag,"[2] stomach, and intestines into the "belly," and through the "belly" walls, where it pollutes the outer body and blood as it circulates through the body. People wash their food thoroughly to avoid eating dirt. However, if they suspect that there is dirt inside the body already (evidenced by pimples and rashes on the skin where the dirt is trying to "force" itself out) Dominicans follow a few steps. First, they drink extra water to help "wash" the dirt through the body's pores. Second, they eat "plenty" of cold (high-fiber) fruits and vegetables (the same as those mentioned for "pressure"). Finally, they take a "washout" (laxative or emetic treatment) with castor oil or various herbal infusions (see Quinlan, 2000).

CONCLUSION

Illnesses in rural Dominica tend to have associated explanatory models and treatments consistent with the internal logic of their ethnomedical system. The purely cold illnesses are associated with respiratory problems or are stress induced. Hot remedies for cold illnesses relax a sufferer and/or ease breathing. They are typically administered in the form of herbal "teas" (infusions), as seasonings in the daily stew, or as a tincture in an alcoholic drink. Hot illnesses in the Dominican system have to do with (thermal) heat, redness, and/or swelling usually thought to stem from dirt or feces in the body. Hot illnesses are treated with cold foods and "teas," which often have laxative properties. Conditions that do not have respiratory, stress, constipation, or inflammation symptoms are typically "neither hot nor cold."

In sum, for rural Dominicans, health is largely maintained through balance. One important issue is the balance between hot and cold humors. Balance is maintained on a daily basis by ingesting humorally hot or cold food or drink in accordance with the body's present state. In case of illness, health can often be regained by ingesting foods with certain humoral qualities that compensate for the humoral imbalance associated with the particular illness.

NOTES

1. The sample was stratified by age, sex, and village location (see Quinlan, 2004).

2. Worms in the worm bag (see Quinlan et al., 2002) function in the digestive process to refine chewed food, turning it into rich blood, much the way that earthworms convert compost to rich soil. The rich blood that the worms expel passes through the walls of the worm bag and into the belly. From the worm bag, semidigested solids, waste, blood, and nutrients travel into the intestines or "tripe."

REFERENCES

Brown, M. (1976). Patterns of variability in two folk systems of classification. *Michigan Discussions in Anthropology* 2: 76-90.

Foster, G.M. (1994). *Hippocrates' Latin American legacy: Humoral medicine in the New World.* Langhorne, PA: Gordon & Breach Science Publications.

Harwood, A. (1971). The hot-cold theory of disease: Implications for treatment of Puerto Rican patients. *Journal of the American Medical Association* 216: 1153-1158.

Leonti, M., O. Sticher, and M. Heinrich (2002). Medicinal plants of the Popoluca, México: Organoleptic properties as indigenous selection criteria. *Journal of Ethnopharmacology* 81(3): 307-316.

Logan, M.H. (1973). Humoral medicine in Guatemala and peasant acceptance of modern medicine. *Human Organization* 32: 385-395.

Madsen, W. (1955). Hot and cold in the universe of San Francisco Tecospa, Valley of Mexico. *Journal of American Folklore* 68: 123-139.

Messer, E. (1981). Hot-cold classification: Theoretical and practical implications of a Mexican study. *Social Science and Medicine* 15B: 133-145.

Neuenswander, H.L. and S.D. Souder (1977). El sidrome calient-frio, humedo-seco entre los Quiches de Joyabaj: Dos modelos cognitivos. In Neuenswander, H.L. and D.E. Arnold (Eds.), *Estudios Cognitivos del Sur de Mesoamerica* (pp. 92-121). Dallas: SIL Museum of Anthropology.

Quinlan, M.B. (2000). Bush medicine in Bwa Mawego: Ethnomedicine and medical botany of common illnesses in a Dominican village. PhD dissertation, University of Missouri–Columbia.

Quinlan, M.B. (2004). *From the Bush: The front line of health care in a Caribbean Village.* Belmont, CA: Wadsworth Press.

Quinlan, M.B., R.J. Quinlan, and J.M. Nolan (2002). Ethnophysiology and herbal treatments of intestinal worms in Dominica, West Indies. *Journal of Ethnopharmacology* 80: 75-83.

Chapter 9

Medicinal Foods in Cuba:
Promoting Health in the Household

Gabriele Volpato
Daimy Godínez

INTRODUCTION

Food and beverages play a vital role in the lives of men and women, as they reflect people's ethnic, historical, and cultural heritage. They represent a link between the material and spiritual: on the one hand satisfying hunger, thirst, and basic health necessities and on the other contributing to human social relations by generating traditions and customs. In certain circumstances, foods and beverages are consumed for medicinal purposes. Although foods and medicines are often approached as two separate fields of study, the nutritional and pharmacological properties of plants are often not easily distinguishable (Johns, 1990, 1996; Johns and Chapman, 1995). Thus, many plants generally considered as foods have important therapeutic roles and are used in different contexts (Etkin and Ross, 1982), according to socioeconomic and cultural factors.

Since colonial times, due to the complex links between the original ethnic components of the main expressions of Cuban material and spiritual culture have been connected to the historic process of settlement (Rivero de la Calle, 1992). Cuban people rely for food and medicine on a mixed culture that draws upon wisdom originating mainly from indigenous Cuban, African, Spanish, and Antillean ethnic groups (Guanche, 1983; Esquivel and Hammer, 1992a; Rivero de la Calle, 1992; Núñez and González, 1999; Sarmiento, 2001b). This multiethnic legacy has resulted in a rich pharmacopoeia, food knowledge, and food traditions. Due to the economic crisis following the collapse of trading relations with the socialist bloc and the tightening of the U.S. blockade of the country during the twentieth century, these are presently being revalorized (Deere, 1992; Garfield and Santana, 1997). The general population has moved toward greater reliance on urban communal garden production, home-grown and wild food (Chaplowe, 1998; Wezel and Bender, 2003), local folk medicine (Acosta de la Luz, 2001), and hence also on medicinal food lore and practices.

The knowledge of medicinal foods lies primarily within family traditions, particularly in the mothers' and grandmothers' experiences with dietary items employed medicinally in the fabrication of inexpensive and simple remedies. The medicinal uses of these remedies in primary health care are common knowledge, passed down through generations via traditions, and do not require the specialized and trained *curanderos,* traditional Cuban healers.

Through open-ended interviews (Levy and Hollan, 1998), mostly with elderly women in the provinces of La Habana, Santiago de Cuba, and Camagüey, an attempt has been made to investigate the local perception and use of medicinal foods as components of health maintenance and disease prevention. In this chapter we report on the findings and also highlight the role of medicinal foods and related knowledge in the Cuban historic process and present economic crisis.

RESULTS AND DISCUSSION

Table 9.1 lists the medicinal food plants most used in Cuba, with their scientific and popular names, used part(s), traditional gastronomic use, and medicinal properties as reported by the informants. Seventy-one species belonging to 60 genera and 37 families were recorded. These figures include most of the major food crops used in Cuba since colonial and precolonial times.

About 80 percent of the plants are cultivated in traditional Cuban home gardens or *conucos* (Hammer et al., 1992). Among the plants collected from the wild, most live as weeds and synanthropic species around cultivated fields and human habitations (e.g., *Amaranthus viridis, Cleome gynandra*), while a few of them are primary or secondary forest species (e.g., *Guazuma ulmifolia, Smilax domingensis*). Only one species endemic to Cuba was reported by the informants *(Gastrococos crispa).* Thus, managed and disturbed landscapes are

TABLE 9.1. Medicinal food plants used in Cuba.

Botanical taxon	Botanical family	Cuban phytonym	Part(s) used	Traditional gastronomic use(s)	Medicinal use(s)
Abelmoschus esculentus (L.) Moench	Malvaceae	Quimbombó	fr	C boiled (*calalú*)	Depurative, refreshing, nourishing
Acrocomia aculeata (Jacq.) Lodd. ex Mart.	Arecaceae	Corojo	fr	R; C toasted	Diuretic, refreshing
Amaranthus viridis L.	Amaranthaceae	Bledo	le	C boiled	Depurative
Anacardium occidentale L.	Anacardiaceae	Marañón	fr	R	Astringent
Ananas comosus (L.) Merr.	Bromeliaceae	Piña	fr	R juice	Stomachic
			fr	R juice with *Annona muricata*	For asthma and colds
Annona cherimolia Mill.	Annonaceae	Chirimoya	fr	R *champola*	Antianemic
Annona muricata L.	Annonaceae	Guanábana	fr	R *champola*	Antihypertensive
			fr	R juice with *A. comosus*	For asthma and colds
Annona squamosa L.	Annonaceae	Anón	fr	R juice	Digestive
Artocarpus communis J.R. et J.G. Forster	Moraceae	Mapén	fr	C boiled	Stomachic
Averrhoa carambola L.	Oxalidaceae	Carambola or Pera China	fr	R	Astringent
Beta vulgaris L. var. *vulgaris*	Chenopodiaceae	Remolacha	le	R juice with orange juice	Nourishing for children

TABLE 9.1. *(continued)*

Botanical taxon	Botanical family	Cuban phytonym	Part(s) used	Traditional gastronomic use(s)	Medicinal use(s)
Bromelia pinguin L.	Bromeliaceae	Piña de ratón	fr	R	Antihelmintic
Cajanus cajan (L.) Huth	Fabaceae	Frijol Gandul	fr	C boiled	Nourishing
Canavalia gladiata (Jacq.) DC.	Fabaceae	Frijol de Machete	se	C coffee substitute	Digestive
Canella winterana (L.) Gaertn.	Canellaceae	Canela	ba	C infusion	Tonic, antinausea, hypertensive
Capsicum frutescens L. var. *frutescens*	Solanaceae	Ají guaguao	fr	R juice with *Petroselinum crispum*	Antianemic
Carica papaya L.	Caricaceae	Frutabomba, Papaya	fr	R juice	Refresh the stomach, antihypertensive, diphtheria
			se	R with milk of the green fruit	Antihelmintic
			yf	C chopped and boiled with milk	Digestive, against colics in children
			yf	C decoction	Antidiarrheic, against gastrointestinal infections
Cassia fistula L.	Fabaceae	Cañafistola	fr	R before breakfast	Antihelmintic
			fr	R snack/ with milk and sugar	Antianemic, mild laxative
Cassia grandis L.	Fabaceae	Cañandonga	fr	R snack/ with milk and sugar	Antianemic, mild laxative

Species	Family	Common name	Part	Preparation	Uses
Chenopodium ambrosioides L.	Chenopodiaceae	Apasote	yl	R salads	Antihelmintic
Citrus aurantium L.	Rutaceae	Naranja Agria	fr	R juice	Astringent, antihypertensive
Citrus limon (L.) Burm. f.	Rutaceae	Limón	fr	R juice	Astringent, digestive, antihypertensive
Citrus medica L.	Rutaceae	Cidra	fr	R juice	Antihypertensive
Citrus sinensis (L.) Osbeck	Rutaceae	Naranja Dulce	fr	R juice	Astringent, antihypertensive
			fr	R eaten with salt	Stomachic
			fr	R juice with oil of *R. communis*	To treat *empacho*
Cleome gynandra L.	Capparaceae	Uña de Gato, Volantín	yl	R salads	Diuretic
Cocos nucifera L.	Arecaceae	Coco	fr	R "water"	Diuretic, antihypertensive
			fr	C "milk"	Laxative, antihelmintic
			fr	C *manteca*	Antihelmintic
Colocasia esculenta (L.) Schott et Endl.	Araceae	Malanga Isleña	rh	C boiled	Nourishing, stomachic
Corchorus siliquosus L.	Tiliaceae	Malva tè	yl	C boiled	Depurative, nourishing
Cucurbita maxima Duch.	Cucurbitaceae	Calabaza	fr	C boiled	Nourishing
Cymbopogon citratus (DC.) Stapf.	Poaceae	Caña Santa	le	C infusion	Carminative, tonic

TABLE 9.1. *(continued)*

Botanical taxon	Botanical family	Cuban phytonym	Part(s) used	Traditional gastronomic use(s)	Medicinal use(s)
Daucus carota L. ssp. *sativa* (Hoffm.) Schuebl. et Mart.	Apiaceae	Zanahoria	fr	R with orange juice	Good for the blood
Dioscorea alata L.	Dioscoreaceae	Ñame	rh	C boiled	Nourishing
Dioscorea bulbifera L.	Dioscoreaceae	Ñame Volador	rh	C boiled	Stomachic
Foeniculum vulgare Mill.	Apiaceae	Hinojo	le	R with orange juice	Diuretic, stomachic
Gastrococos crispa (H.B.K.) H. E. Moore	Arecaceae	Corojo	fr	R	Diuretic, refreshing
			fr, se	C toasted/oil	Internal anti-inflammatory
Gouania polygama (Jacq.) Urban	Rhamnaceae	Bejuco de Indio	ba	C *pru* component	Hypotensive *(pru)*
Guazuma ulmifolia Lam	Sterculiaceae	Guásima	fr	R	Antianemic, antihelmintic
Ipomoea batatas L.	Convolvulaceae	Boniato	ro	C boiled	Nourishing
Lepidium virginicum L.	Brassicaceae	Mastuerzo	yl	R salads	Diuretic
Lycopersicum esculentum (L.) Karsten	Solanaceae	Tomate	fr	R juice with orange juice	Good for the blood
Mammea americana L.	Clusiaceae	Mamey de Santo Domingo	fr	R juice	Antianemic
Mangifera indica L.	Anacardiaceae	Mango	fr	R juice	Digestive, laxative, stomachic
Manilkara zapota (L.) P. Royen	Sapotaceae	Níspero	fr	R juice	Stomachic

218

Species	Family	Common name	Part	Preparation	Property/Use
Maranta arundinacea L.	Marantaceae	Sagú, Yuquilla	rh	D with milk	Digestive, antidiarrheic
Melicocca bijuga L.	Sapindaceae	Mamoncillo	fr	R	Antihypertensive
Momordica charantia L.	Cucurbitaceae	Cundeamor	fr	C salads/condiment	Antihelmintic
Musa × paradisiaca L.	Musaceae	Plátano	fr, le	C infusion	Antihelmintic
			fr	C boiled with sugar, jam	Refreshing, good for the blood
			fr	C boiled, *fufú*	Nourishing for children, antidiarrheic, antihelmintic
			fr	D with milk, *bananina*	Nourishing for children, antidiarrheic, antihelmintic
Nasturtium officinale L.	Brassicaceae	Berro	le	R juice with orange juice	Nourishing for children
Persea americana Mill.	Lauraceae	Aguacate	fr	R salads	Digestive
Petroselinum crispum (Mill.) Nym.	Apiaceae	Perejil	le	R juice with mashed *C. frutescens*	Antianemic
Phaseolus lunatus L.	Fabaceae	Frijol Caballero	fr	C boiled	Nourishing for children
Phyllantus acidus (L.) Skeds	Euphorbiaceae	Grosella	fr	R	Stomachic
Pimenta dioica (L.) Merr.	Myrtaceae	Pimienta dulce	le	C *pru* component	
Portulaca oleracea L.	Portulacaceae	Verdolaga	yl	R salads	Astringent, for stomach ulcers
Pouteria campechiana (Kunth) Baehni	Sapotaceae	Canistel	fr	R	Antianemic

TABLE 9.1. (continued)

Botanical taxon	Botanical family	Cuban phytonym	Part(s) used	Traditional gastronomic use(s)	Medicinal use(s)
Pouteria sapota (Jacq.) H.E. Moore et Stearn	Sapotaceae	Mamey Colorado	fr	R	Antihelmintic
Psidium guajava L.	Myrtaceae	Guayaba	fr	R juice/in syrup	Antianemic, antidiarrheic
Ricinus communis L.	Euphorbiaceae	Higuereta	fr	C oil with orange juice	To treat *empacho*
Roystonea regia (H.B.K.) O.F. Cook	Arecaceae	Palma Real	yl	R salads (*palmitos*)	Nourishing
Sechium edule (Jacq.) Sw.	Cucurbitaceae	Chayote	fr	R, C snacks	Diuretic
			le	R salads	Antihypertensive
Senna obtusifolia (L.) Irwin et Barneby	Fabaceae	Guanina	se	C coffee substitute	Digestive, antianemic, against migraine and stomach spasms
Senna occidentalis (L.) Link.	Fabaceae	Guanina	se	C coffee substitute	Digestive, antianemic, against migraine and stomach spasms
Sesamum orientale L.	Pedaliaceae	Ajonjoli	se	C toasted/oil	Nourishing, antiasthmatic, anti-inflammatory
Smilax domingensis Willd.	Smilacaceae	Raíz de China	rh	C *pru* component	
Smilax havanensis Jacq.	Smilacaceae	Alambrillo	rh	C boiled	Stomachic

Solanum americanum Mill.	Solanaceae	Yerba Mora	yl	R salads, condiment	To treat stomach ulcers, depurative, aperitive, stomachic
Spondias mombin L.	Anacardiaceae	Jobo	fr	R	Stomachic
Spondias purpurea L.	Anacardiaceae	Ciruela	fr	R	Laxative, stomachic
Tamarindus indica L.	Fabaceae	Tamarindo	se	R juice	Antianemic, antihypertensive, mild laxative, febrifuge
Xanthosoma sagittifolium (L.) Schott	Araceae	Malanga	bu, rh	C boiled	Nourishing for children
			rh	C mashed with milk	Stomachic, against gastritis and stomach ulcer
			rh	C with plantain	Antidiarrheic
Zingiber officinale Rosc.	Zingiberaceae	Jengibre	rh	C infusion	Antispasmodic, digestive, carminative, tonic

Part(s) used: ba, bark; bu, buds; fr, fruits; le, leaves; rh, rhizome; ro, root/ tuber; se, seeds; yf, young fruit; yl, young leaves.

Traditional gastronomic use(s): C, cooked; D, dried; R, raw.

the most important foraging places for wild food and medicinal plants, as has been found for many native peoples of America and worldwide (e.g., Alcorn, 1981; Frei et al., 2000).

The interviews defined three main categories of medicinal foods. These will now be discussed in the following sections.

Functional Viandas: *Starchy Root and Tuber Crops from Africa*

African influence can be considered the strongest in the Caribbean (Laguerre, 1987); this also holds for Cuba (López, 1985; Esquivel et al., 1992). Afro-Cuban foodstuffs and meals, for human consumption and sometimes for religious practices, have shaped popular Cuban food systems. The plant composition of these dishes and drinks varied according to the available species that the African slaves were faced with, although several species originating from Africa were used as well. About 15 percent of the plants reported in Table 9.1 are of African origin; they include important crops such as *Dioscorea* species, *Abelmoschus esculentus* and *Cajanus cajan*. At present, foods from the era of slavery still represent the staple foods of Cuban rural populations, and starch-rich tubers, vegetables, and legumes have come to be of paramount importance to people's health. Species such as *malanga* (*Xanthosoma sagittifolium* and *Colocasia esculenta*), *calabaza* (*Cucurbita maxima*), *platano* (*Musa paradisiaca*), *boniato* (*Ipomoea batatas*), *ñame* (*Dioscorea* spp.), and many species of beans (i.e., *frijol gandúl: Cajanus cajan; frijol caballero: Phaseolus lunatus*) are cultivated in home gardens throughout Cuba (Hammer et al., 1992; Wezel and Bender, 2003). These food items, popularly called *viandas,* are boiled in water and eaten as mashed vegetables *(fufú)* or in soups and regarded as nourishing foods to be given to children, "to let them grow strong," and to the ill.

All of these *viandas* have been cultivated in home gardens since the sixteenth century. They were the food of the slaves, who had to rely on an energy- and pharmacologically rich diet in order to be able to cope with the harsh workload of cutting and milling sugarcane. Staple foods such as *Xanthosoma* spp., *Dioscorea* spp., *Musa paradisiaca,* and *Abelmoschus esculentus* were brought to Cuba from Africa soon after the conquest or with the slave shipments (Esquivel et al., 1992), and often retained their African names. Words such as *ñame, malanga,* and *calalú* are subsaharianisms that have become part of the Cuban vernacular (Valdés, 1987). *Malanga* means aquatic plant in the Quicongo language (Valdés, 1987), and the word *ñame* has a possible Bantú origin, as it means "eat" in several Bantú languages (Mendoza, 1948). *Abelmoschus esculentus* is the main ingredient of the *calalú,* a soup of wild and cultivated vegetables of African origin sparsely distributed throughout America (Ortiz, 1956; Núñez and González, 1995, 1999). It is often prepared with *bledo (Amaranthus viridis)* and is regarded as a depurative and refreshing food "good for the health of the children and whatever person feeling ill or tired." *Quimbombó* (the Cuban folk name for *A. esculentus*) derives from the African *quim'-gombo* (Ortiz, 1956), and variants of this term are widespread throughout American countries with populations of African origin (Valdés, 1987).

Having to rely on a few food items for their general health, in the past people sought ways further to exploit the available resources. Plant varieties and congenerics (i.e., different species of *Dioscorea* and *Xanthosoma*) with different maturation periods were cultivated, wild relatives such as wild yam (*ñame cimarrón: Smilax* spp.; *ñame volador: Dioscorea bulbifera*) were used as famine foods (Roig, 1965), and less-important starchy foods such as *Artocarpus communis* were cultivated. These may have been used also as medicinal resources, particularly for gastrointestinal disorders. The *vianda* regarded as the favorite and most nourishing by Afro-Cuban people is probably *Xanthosoma* spp.; the rhizome and buds are widely regarded as children's food (Núñez, 1999). The *fufú* with milk is used as a stomachic, against gastritis and stomach ulcer. Cut into pieces and mashed with plantain, it is given to children as a healthy and antidiarrheic food. The plantain is a main component of the Cuban diet: it is consumed as a strengthening food, particularly for breakfast in the morning; its *fufú* and *bananina* (plantains cut into pieces, dried, mashed, and added to the milk given to children) are two traditional dishes used to make children grow strong and to treat intestinal parasites and diarrhea. As well, the jam made from mature plantain is considered to be "refreshing" and "good for the blood." *Maranta arundinacea* is cultivated on a small scale mainly in the Eastern Provinces of Cuba (Esquivel and Hammer, 1992b). Its rhizome, grated, sun dried and given to children with milk, is considered a digestive and antidiarrheic.

Among medicinal foods used by Cuban people, palms play an important role in spiritual, religious, and material terms (Fuentes, 1992). They were among the first plants to attract the attention of Colon when he landed in Cuba (Esquivel and Hammer, 1992b; Jiménez, 1999), and the Arecaceae family is one of the most important food resources to Native Americans (Henderson et al., 1995; Leiva, 2001). The young leaves of the *palma real (Roystonea regia),* locally called *palmitos,* are eaten raw in salads and regarded as highly nutritious; they were also one of the main staples of the *mambises* during the Cuban secession war against Spain (Sarmiento, 2001b). The coconut, *Cocos nucifera,* was brought to Cuba soon after the conquest (Whitehead, 1984) and is now a major local resource. The "water" inside the young fruits is drunk as a diuretic and an antihypertensive, while the "milk" (grated endosperm) is reported to be laxative and antihelmintic. The *manteca* (butter), made by toasting the "milk," is said to be good against intestinal parasites, and is often used as a frying oil in Cuban households. Two more species of spiny palms called *corojo* are similarly used, often as coconut substitutes in more restricted geographical areas (e.g., Sierra de Cubitas in the province of Camagüey). *Acrocomia aculeata,* distributed throughout tropical America, and *Gastrococos crispa,* endemic to Cuba, are appreciated for the food and medicinal properties of their fruits (Leiva, 2001). The inner part of the fruits of both species *(masa)* is eaten and considered refreshing, and it is also used for its diuretic properties. The fruits are also toasted to make cooking oil, and because the economic crisis has led to shortages of cooking oil throughout Cuba, wild populations of these species are being exploited.

Fufú and soups of African origin are often accompanied with vegetables cultivated in home gardens or present in Cuban plantations as weeds (Gutte, 1994). As examples, the young leaves of *Lepidium virginicum* and *Cleome gynandra* are eaten in salads and considered diuretic, while those of *Chenopodium ambrosioides* are considered antihelmintic (Kliks, 1985). *Portulaca oleracea* and *Solanum americanum* are collected from the wild to be eaten in salads. They are both considered good to treat stomach ulcers, while *P. oleracea* is also used as an astringent against diarrhea and *S. americanum* as a depurative, aperitive, and stomachic.

Many of the ritual dishes of African origin include depurative and nourishing species (e.g., *Corchorus olitorius, Portulaca oleracea,*

Amaranthus spp., *Gastrococos crispa*) which can be regarded as secondary and famine foods within Afro-Cuban populations, transmitted through generations via ritual and religious offerings (cf. Esquivel et al., 1992; Valdés, 1987). As stated by Johns (1994), and Huss-Ashmore and Johnston (1994), some edible wild plants consumed on an infrequent and opportunistic basis or as minor components in complex dishes appear in the intergenerational transmission of knowledge using myths and rituals as vehicles. Similarly, Afro-Cuban ritual dishes could have played a role to offset food shortages during the 1990s in Cuba, following a resurgence of forgotten religious practices and reinforcement of ethnic identity. A large number of plants used in Afro-Cuban religions are also used as foods and medicines (Aguilar and Herrera, 1995; Cabrera, 1954; Fuentes, 1992), which highlights the link between the spiritual and material activities of these people in the selection of plants to be used.

Fruits: A Widespread Medicinal Food Resource

Fruits are important secondary and medicinal food resources worldwide (e.g., Fleuret, 1986). They are used as simple remedies, mainly for gastrointestinal afflictions, and their therapeutic properties are orally transmitted as common social knowledge across generations.

According to historical and archeological records, the selection of fruits consumed by Cuban aboriginal peoples was restricted (Wilson, 1999; Liogier, 1992; Hernández and Navarrete, 1999) and included species such as *Spondias mombin, Annona* spp., and *Pouteria sapota,* which were probably not grown as crops. Many species of fruits were later introduced by the Spanish from the Mediterranean and Asiatic areas (e.g., *Citrus* spp., *Mangifera indica*), Africa (i.e., *Tamarindus indica*), and other areas of America (i.e., *Persea americana*) (cf. Esquivel et al., 1992). Fruits are at present a main resource to local people and represent more than half of the medicinal foods reported in Table 9.1. Species such as *Anacardium occidentale, Carica papaya, Psidium guajava, Mangifera indica, Spondias purpurea, Phyllantus acidus,* and *Tamarindus indica,* among others, are widely grown in traditional home gardens (Hammer et al., 1992; Wezel and Bender, 2003). These fruits may be prepared in syrup, juice, or *batido* (milkshake) and also used in old, traditional preparations such as the *aliñao* (fruits fermented under the ground in rum). Fruits are mainly used to help the digestive process (e.g., *C. papaya*, *M. indica*), as vermifuge (e.g., *C. papaya*), against diarrhea (e.g., green *P. guayava*), or as a laxative (e.g., *Spondias purpurea*), and the medicinal food use of available fruits is perceived by people as a simple, cheap, and effective remedy for many common ailments, especially gastrointestinal disorders. During the food shortages and deterioration of the general health of the population in the 1990s (Garfield and Santana, 1997; Rodríguez-Ojea et al., 2002), fruits represented a primary food for people; they were consumed as snacks in the field or bought at markets and in the streets (e.g., the fruits of *Melicocca bijuga* are sold in the streets as snacks or to be sucked as an antihypertensive). Fruits were a major source of vitamins and minerals, and the lore of their use as medicinal food came to be of paramount importance to maintain health within the households. As examples, the green fruit of *C. papaya* is chopped and boiled with milk to prevent bad digestion and colic in children, and its decoction is used to treat diarrhea and gastrointestinal infections. *C. sinensis* is cut in half and eaten with salt to clean the gastrointestinal tract after bad digestion, and its juice is mixed with a tablespoon of oil of *Ricinus communis* and used to treat *empacho*, a kind of stomach congestion described by an informant as "something like a ball *[bola]* of undigested food that develops within the stomach."

Although most common fruits are eaten in a food rather than in a medicinal context, others are more often sought for specific medicinal purposes. For example, this is highlighted in the fruits of *Guazuma ulmifolia* and *Bromelia pinguin*, which are regarded as antihelmintic and eaten sometimes as snacks in the field. Other food species specifically sought as a treatment for intestinal parasites include *Pouteria sapota* and *Momordica charantia*, eaten before breakfast. In Cuba, fruits of the latter species are mainly grown as vegetables by people of Asiatic origin (Hammer and Esquivel, 1992; Pérez et al., 1994), and they are sometimes used as fresh snacks, especially by children. The habit of consuming antihelmintic foods or teas before or during breakfast is particularly common among Cubans of Haitian origin. The continuous ingestion of the low doses of allelochemicals in these species may be an effective means of preventing massive parasite infestations, especially in children.

Medicinal foods in Cuba are widely used for the treatment of anemia and hypertension, two major health problems that may be alleviated by the high iron and vitamin B content of some fruits and green leafy vegetables and the high potassium and vitamin C content of others (Roberts et al., 2001). As examples, the fruit of *G. ulmifolia, Pouteria campechiana,* the green fruit of *Mammea americana,* and the seeds of *T. indica* are ingested (or sucked) as antianemics. In spite of the Cuban government's policies of promoting the equity of vulnerable groups and giving them priority, since the early 1990s protein intake has dropped by 36 percent, dietary fats by 65 percent, and nutritional deficiencies have led to major health imbalances among the population and to the outbreak of new diseases (Gay et al., 1995; Tucker and Hedges, 1993). In this context, fruits and vegetables have played an important role as suppliers of iron and vitamins, and traditional antianemics and vitamin-rich formulas based on local biodiversity have been revalorized. Juices and *batidos* (milkshakes made from juice and sugar) of various fruits are commonly prepared as refreshments and for specific medicinal purposes. *Batidos* of the fruits of *Annona* spp. (e.g., *A. cherimolia*) are called *champolas* and regarded as useful to treat conditions of anemia. The term *champola* probably derives from the Congo *sámpula* (to shake rapidly), an allusion to how this drink is prepared (Ortiz, 1956). Fruit juices are often mixed with vegetable juices to prepare refreshing drinks that are also used within Cuban households as home remedies with high nutritional and antianemic value. Orange juice is mixed with the juice of the leaves of *Nasturtium officinale* and *Beta vulgaris* as a functional food for children, with *Lycopersicum esculentum* and *Daucus carota* "for the blood," and with *Foeniculum vulgare* as a diuretic and stomachic. In the same way, the fruits of *Capsicum frutescens* var. *frutescens* are mashed and eaten with the juice of *Petroselinum crispum* as an antianemic.

Medicinal Drinks and Coffee Substitutes

Beverages play a special role that overlaps both food and medicine. Infusions or teas are often the preferred way of consuming medicine, but herbal teas also form part of the routinely dietary food items, and the distinction between teas consumed as a refreshing drink and teas used as medicine is unclear (Johns, 1990).

Pru is a traditional refreshing drink produced from the decoction and fermentation with sugar of the following main components: stems of *Gouania polygama,* the rhizome of *Smilax domingensis,* and the leaves of *Pimenta dioica.* It is purported to have depurative and diuretic properties; it is taken as a medicinal drink by people with chronic high blood pressure, to help digestive process, and to heal *empacho* "by cleaning stomach walls" (Volpato and Godínez, 2004; Hernández and Volpato, 2004). *Pru* has long been confined to a number of traditional villages in eastern Cuba, and its origin may be traced back to the ethnobotanical knowledge of French-Haitian people who migrated to Cuba from the end of the 1700s. During the 1990s, *pru* spread almost throughout the island, and its prevalent consumption shifted from being a medicine to a food; at present it is sold in almost every Cuban city as a refreshment. In the historical development of food and medical systems, the original consumption of herbal preparations as medicines can shift to a food context and vice versa. With the commercial exploitation of *pru,* its consumption may have become associated with food habits, just like coffee (also a former medicinal tea; Johns, 1990) or soft drinks, with little regard to its purported health benefits.

Beverages containing caffeine and other stimulants may also have been more important in the past as medicines, and teas originally taken with therapeutic aims could have culturally shifted to a prevalent consumption as food. Indeed, as well as retaining their original medicinal properties, teas may make important nutritional contributions of vitamins and minerals (Johns, 1990). The habit of drinking coffee for breakfast is widespread throughout Cuban cities and countryside, although coffee is sometimes not available to Cuban farmers. They thus substitute it with the seeds or sometimes the leaves of other more easily available species collected from the wild and from the gardens, such as *guanina* (*Senna obtusifolia* and *Senna occidentalis*) and *frijol de machete* (*Canavalia gladiata*). Seeds of these species are roasted and ground and have the food and medicinal (mainly digestive) role of coffee. The habit of drinking "coffee" made from the seeds of *guanina* is widespread throughout Africa and America (Correa and Bernal, 1990; Roig, 1974), and it was probably brought to Cuba with the African slaves or by Antillean immigrants of African origin. This infusion is also drunk as a diuretic and to treat bad digestion, stomach spasms, migraine, and anemia. As one informant explained, "*guanina* coffee when drunk in the morning is the best for the blood, but care must be taken to prepare it light and not to drink it much, because it makes too much blood and be harmful." The seeds of the species have been found to be rich in proteins (Flores et al., 1988) and antraquinonic glycosides (Lal and Gupta, 1973, 1974), though no toxicity to humans has been reported yet to confirm Cuban ethnomedical lore.

As emphasized in other works (Johns, 1990; Leonti et al., 2002), the palatability and the taste of plants used in traditional medicine are related to their perceived and expected medicinal properties. Bitter foods and teas are often used as marginal food sources but regarded as "strong" (*fuerte*) medicinal foods (e.g., as antihelmintic). People perceive that the common characteristic of these coffee substitutes is their bitter taste, which is often related to the allelochemicals present in the species. *Momordica charantia (cundeamor)* is a common medicinal plant almost worldwide, and in Cuba the infusion of the leaves is taken as febrifuge, vermifuge, to treat colitis, renal calculus, and liver afflictions, and to regulate menstruation (Fuentes, 1988; Roig, 1974; Seoane, 1984). Its bitterness and medicinal properties are mainly related to the presence of cucurbitacins (Ng and Yeung, 1984; Raman and Lau, 1996; Rathi et al., 2002), and the bitter taste is perceived by people as imparting health properties to the resulting drink. An old woman reported: "In my childhood, my mother gave me to drink every morning a little cup of an infusion of a few leaves of *cundeamor*. We used to drink it without sugar, in spite of its bitterness, first thing in the morning before breakfast, as a coffee. The infusion cleans the blood and prevents *lombrices* [stomach and intestinal parasites] moving upward looking for sweet food. If in fact someone having parasites drinks or eats something with sugar first, parasites move, causing stomach pains and even coming out from mouth and nostrils. We used to take it every morning."

Many systems of traditional medicine emphasize proper diet as a requirement for health, along with prophylactic uses of herbal medicines (Johns, 1990). Using herbal teas such as that of *M. charantia* as preventive medicine could represent an evolutionary step toward their consumption in a medicinal food context in specific cultural and social situations (e.g., when coffee is not available and substitutes are needed).

Cuban medicinal food habits draw upon the hot-cold *(frío-caliente)* dichotomy (Fuentes, 1984; Núñez, 1999), widespread in Latin American and Afro-Caribbean medical cultures (Harwood, 1971; Wiese, 1976; Laguerre, 1987; Foster, 1994). It is believed that the balance of the hot and cold in the body should be maintained by adding to the diet equal amounts of foods with hot and cold qualities; disrupting this can result in illness. The classification of many food items in terms of their hot and cold properties, and the empirical relation between the consumption of these items and the state of health of a person, make these items important as medicinal and preventive foods. Thus, eating "cold" food such as *Ananas comosus, Persea americana,* and *Annona muricata* while one is warm or hot (e.g., after one has been engaging in physical activity such as collecting coffee or cutting sugarcane) could lead to "cold" illnesses such as asthma and colds. *A. muricata* is considered a cold fruit, not to be given to young children or to people with *resfriado* (cold). However, hot items such as honey and teas made from "hot" plants such as *cañasanta (Cymbopogon citratus),* locally called *calientura,* are regarded as useful in such cases. The infusion of the leaves of this plant is reported as either a medicinal or an everyday tea, depending on the informant: that is, it can be taken as a medicine or as a hot tea for breakfast. Infusions of *Zingiber officinale* and *Canella winterana* are sometimes used as everyday "hot" tonics "like coffee," while the former is also regarded as an antispasmodic, digestive, and carminative, and the latter as an antinausea and hypertensive. Moreover, they are both used as spices in traditional dishes and cakes. Spices are used worldwide to increase the palatability and the variety of foods, but also to give dishes some medicinal properties due to the allelochemicals contained in these species (Johns, 1990). The contemporary use of these plants in Cuba as teas, spices, foods, and medicines highlights the overlap that exists within traditional systems between "what is food" and "what is medicine," and the multiple ways to exploit the nutritional and therapeutic properties of plant species.

CONCLUSIONS

The food habits of a population are the result of cultural and social changes determined by historical developments. Cuban "ethnoalimentation" has been shaped by the interaction of the different ethnic actors in the history of the island, each bringing its own knowledge of foods and drinks for health and medicinal purposes.

Within Cuban households, staple and secondary foods are regarded as the main way to preserve good health and treat minor ailments. Most starch-rich tubers and *viandas* of African origin are regarded as nourishing foods, as they were used and cultivated by slaves faced with hard work on the sugarcane plantations. Fruits and, to a lesser extent, vegetables, are used mainly as depuratives ("good for the blood") and in the treatment of gastrointestinal afflictions.

Medicinal foods are among the more available home remedies for treating certain common ailments. The economic crisis that affected Cuba in the 1990s brought shortages of food and medicine and led to a revalorization of traditional lore on local plant resources. Medicinal foods and related knowledge of restricted ethnic and/or geographic origin diffused and their traditional forms of consumption changed. Ritual dishes and emergency foods have been included in the diet, and teas formerly used therapeutically have become dietary drinks as coffee substitutes. The medicinal and food uses of plants overlap and are continuously changing, highlighting the multiple ways with which people deal with plants and the local environment.

REFERENCES

Acosta de la Luz, L. (2001). Producción de plantas medicinales a pequeña escala: Una necesidad de la comunidad. *Revista Cubana de Plantas Medicinales* 2:63-66.

Aguilar, A. and P.P. Herrera (1995). El significado sociocultural de las plantas alimenticias, en las religiones afrocubanas. *Fontqueria* 47:279-287.

Alcorn, J.B. (1981). Huastec noncrop resource management: Implications for the prehistoric rain forest management. *Human Ecology* 9:395-417.

Cabrera, L. (1954). *El Monte*. Havana: Ediciones Letras Cubanas.

Chaplowe, S.G. (1998). Havana's popular gardens: Sustainable prospects for urban agriculture. *The Environmentalist* 18:47-57.

Correa, J.E. and H.Y. Bernal (1990). *Especies vegetales promisorias de los países del convenio Andrés Bello*. Tomo III. Bogotá: Talleres de Editora Guadalupe.

Deere, C.D. (1992). *Socialism on one island? Cuba's national food program and its prospects for food security*. The Hague: Institute of Social Studies, Working Paper Series No. 124.

Esquivel, M., V. Fuentes, C. Martínez, J. Martínez, and K. Hammer (1992). The African influence from an ethnobotanical point of view. In Hammer, K., M. Esquivel, and H. Knüpffer (Eds.), *". . . Y tienen faxones y fabas muy diversos de los nuestros . . ."* Origin, evolution and diversity of Cuban plant genetic resources, Vol. 1. Gatersleben, Germany: Institut für Pflanzengenetik und Kulturpflanzenforschung.

Esquivel, M. and K. Hammer (1992a). The Cuban homegarden "conuco": A perspective environment for evolution and in situ conservation of plant genetic resources. *Genetic Resources and Crop Evolution* 39:9-22.

Esquivel, M. and K. Hammer (1992b). Native food plants and the American influence in Cuban agriculture. In Hammer, K., M. Esquivel, and H. Knüpffer (Eds.), *". . . Y tienen faxones y fabas muy diversos de los nuestros . . ." Origin, evolution and diversity of Cuban plant genetic resources,* Vol. 1. Gatersleben, Germany: Institut für Pflanzengenetik und Kulturpflanzenforschung.

Etkin, N.L. and P.J. Ross (1982). Food as medicine and medicine as food: An adaptive framework for the interpretation of plant utilisation among the Hausa of northern Nigeria. *Social Science and Medicine* 16:1559-1573.

Fleuret, A. (1986). Dietary and therapeutic uses of fruit in three Taita communities. In Etkin, N.L. (Ed.), *Plants in indigenous medicine and diet.* New York: Redgrave Publishing Company.

Flores, J.S., C.A. Martínez, M.A. Olivera, R. Galván, and C. Chávez (1988). Potencial de algunas leguminosas de la flora yucatense como alimento humano o animal. *Turrialba* 38:159-162.

Foster, G.M. (1994). *Hippocrates' Latin American legacy: Humoral medicine in the New World.* Langhorne, PA: Gordon and Breach Science Publisher.

Frei, B., O. Sticher, and M. Heinrich (2000). Zapotec and Mixe use of tropical habitats for securing medicinal plants in Mexico. *Economic Botany* 54:73-81.

Fuentes, V. (1984). Sobre la medicina tradicional en Cuba. *Boletín de Reseñas: Plantas Medicinales* 10:1-39.

Fuentes, V. (1988). Plantas medicinales de uso popular referidas como tóxicas. *Boletín de Reseñas: Plantas Medicinales* 19:1-37.

Fuentes, V. (1992). Plants in Afro-Cuban religions. In Hammer, K., M. Esquivel, and H. Knüpffer (Eds.), *". . . Y tienen faxones y fabas muy diversos de los nuestros. . ." Origin, evolution and diversity of Cuban plant genetic resources,* Vol. 1. Gatersleben, Germany: Institut für Pflanzengenetik und Kulturpflanzenforschung.

Garfield, R. and S. Santana (1997). The impact of the economic crisis and the U.S. embargo on health in Cuba. *American Journal of Public Health* 87:15-20.

Gay, J., M. Padrón, and M. Amador (1995). Prevención y control de la anemia y la deficiencia de hierro en Cuba. *Revista Cubana de Alimentación y Nutrición* 9:52-61.

Guanche, J. (1983). *Procesos etnoculturales en Cuba.* Havana: Editorial Letras Cubanas.

Gutte, P. (1994). Weeds in the fields and plantations. In Hammer, K., M. Esquivel, and H. Knüpffer (Eds.), *". . . Y tienen faxones y fabas muy diversos de los nuestros . . ." Origin, evolution and diversity of Cuban plant genetic resources,*

Vol. 3. Gatersleben, Germany: Institut für Pflanzengenetik und Kulturpflanzen-forschung.

Hammer, K. and M. Esquivel (1992). The role of ethnic minorities—the East Asiatic case. In Hammer, K., M. Esquivel, and H. Knüpffer (Eds.), ". . . *Y tienen faxones y fabas muy diversos de los nuestros . . ." Origin, evolution and diversity of Cuban plant genetic resources*, Vol. 1. Gatersleben, Germany: Institut für Pflanzengenetik und Kulturpflanzenforschung.

Hammer, K., M. Esquivel, and H. Knüpffer (1992). Inventory of the cultivated plants. In Hammer, K., M. Esquivel, and H. Knüpffer (Eds.), ". . . *Y tienen faxones y fabas muy diversos de los nuestros . . ." Origin, evolution and diversity of Cuban plant genetic resources*, Vol. 2. Gatersleben, Germany: Institut für Pflanzengenetik und Kulturpflanzenforschung.

Harwood, A. (1971). The hot–cold theory of disease: Implications for treatment of Puerto Ricans. *Journal of the American Medical Association* 216:1153-1158.

Henderson, A., G. Galeano, and R. Bernal (1995). *Field guide to the palms of Americas*. Princeton: Princeton University Press.

Hernández, J. and R. Navarrete (1999). Semillas carbonizadas del residuario protoarcaico La Batea, Santiago de Cuba. Presunciones Etnobotánicas. *El Caribe Arqueológico* 3:70-73.

Hernández, J. and G. Volpato (2004). Herbal mixtures in the traditional medicine of Eastern Cuba. *Journal of Ethnopharmacology* 90:293-316.

Huss-Ashmore, R. and S.L. Johnston (1994). Wild plants as cultural adaptations to food stress. In Etkin, N.L. (Ed.), *Eating on the wild side: The pharmacologic, ecologic, and social implications of using noncultigens*. Tucson: The University of Arizona Press.

Jiménez, J. (1999). Cristobal Colón. Primeras referencias sobre la biodiversidad de Cuba. *Biodiversidad de Cuba Oriental* 3:31-40.

Johns, T. (1990). *The origins of human diet and medicine: Chemical ecology*. Tucson, Arizona: The University of Arizona Press.

Johns, T. (1994). Ambivalence to the palatability factors in wild food plants. In Etkin, N.L. (Ed.), *Eating on the wild side: The pharmacologic, ecologic, and social implications of using noncultigens*. Tucson: The University of Arizona Press.

Johns, T. (1996). Phytochemicals as evolutionary mediators of human nutritional physiology. *International Journal of Pharmacognosy* 34:327-334.

Johns, T. and L. Chapman (1995). Phytochemicals ingested in traditional diets and medicines as modulators of energy metabolism. In Arnason, T. (Ed.), *Phytochemistry of medicinal plants*. New York: Plenum Press.

Kliks, M.M. (1985). Studies on the traditional herbal anthelmintic *Chenopodium ambrosiodes* L.: Ethnopharmacological evaluation and clinical field trials. *Social Science Medicine* 21:879-886.

Laguerre, M. (1987). *Afro-Caribbean folk medicine*. South Hadley, MA: Bergin and Garvey Publishers.

Lal, J. and P.C. Gupta (1973). Anthraquinone glycoside from the seeds of *Cassia occidentalis*. *Experientia* 29:141-142.

Lal, J. and P.C. Gupta (1974). Two new anthraquinones from the seeds of *Cassia occidentalis*. *Experientia* 30:850-851.

Leiva, Á. (2001). *Cuba y sus palmas*. Havana: Editorial Gente Nueva.

Leonti, M., O. Sticher, and M. Heinrich (2002). Medicinal plants of the Populuca, México: Organoleptic properties as indigenous selection criteria. *Journal of Ethnopharmacology* 81:307-315.

Levy, R.I. and D.W. Hollan (1998). Person-centered interviewing and observation. In Bernard, H.R. (Ed.), *Handbook of methods in cultural anthropology*. Walnut Creek, CA: Altamira Press.

Liogier, A.H. (1992). Preface. In Hammer, K., M. Esquivel, and H. Knüpffer (Eds.), *". . . Y tienen faxones y fabas muy diversos de los nuestros . . ." Origin, evolution and diversity of Cuban plant genetic resources*, Vol. 1. Gatersleben, Germany: Institut für Pflanzengenetik und Kulturpflanzenforschung.

López, R.L. (1985). *Componentes Africanos en el etnos Cubano*. Havana: Editorial de Ciencias Sociales.

Mendoza, R. (1948). *A influencia Africana no Portugués du Brasil*. Rio de Janeiro: Porto Ediciones.

Ng, T. and H. Yeung (1984). Bioactive constituents of Cucurbitaceae plants with special emphasis on *Momordica charantia* and *Tricosanthes kirilowii*. Proceedings of the 5th Symposium on Medicinal Plants and Spices, Seoul, Korea.

Núñez, N. (1999). Algunas concepciones alimentarias de los cubanos. *Revista Cubana de Alimentación y Nutrición* 13:46-50.

Núñez, N. and E. González (1995). Diferencias regionales en las comidas tradicionales de la población rural de Cuba. *Revista Cubana de Alimentación y Nutrición* 9:79-83.

Núñez, N. and E. González (1999). Antecedentes etnohistóricos de la alimentación tradicional en Cuba. *Revista Cubana de Alimentación y Nutrición* 13:145-150.

Ortiz, F. (1956). *La cocina Arocubana*. Havana: Imprenta Oscar García S.A.

Pérez, E., N. Enríquez, and N. Sarduy (1994). Plantas alimenticias silvestres y cultivadas para el consumo humano en la provincia de Camagüey. *Acta Botánica Cubana* 104:1-20.

Raman, A. and C. Lau (1996). Anti-diabetic properties and phytochemistry of *Momordica charantia* L. *Phytomedicine* 2:349-362.

Rathi, S.S., J.K. Grover, and V. Vats (2002). The effect of *Momordica charantia* and *Mucuna pruriens* in experimental diabetes and their effect on key metabolic enzymes involved in carbohydrate metabolism. *Phytotherapy Research* 16:236-243.

Rivero de la Calle, M. (1992). Cuba: A mosaic of races and cultures. In Hammer, K., M. Esquivel, and H. Knüpffer (Eds.), *". . . Y tienen faxones y fabas muy diversos de los nuestros . . ." Origin, evolution and diversity of Cuban plant genetic re-*

sources, Vol. 1. Gatersleben, Germany: Institut für Pflanzengenetik und Kultur-pflanzenforschung.

Roberts, A.J., M.E. O'Brien, and G. Subak-Sharpe (Eds.) (2001). *Nutraceuticals: The complete encyclopedia of supplements, herbs, vitamins, and healing foods.* New York: The Berkeley Publishing Group.

Rodríguez-Ojea, A., S. Jiménez, A. Berdasco, and M. Esquivel (2002). The nutritional transition in Cuba in the nineties: An overview. *Public Health Nutrition* 5:129-133.

Roig, J.T. (1965). *Diccionario botanico de nombres vulgares Cubanos.* Havana: Editora del Consejo Nacional de Universidades.

Roig, J.T. (1974). *Plantas medicinales, aromáticas o venenosas de Cuba.* Havana: Ciencia y Técnica, Instituto del Libro.

Sarmiento, I. (2001). Raíces de la cultura alimentaria cubana. *Del Caribe* 36:80-94.

Seoane, J. (1984). *El folclor médico de Cuba.* Havana: Editorial de Ciencias Sociales.

Tucker, K. and T.R. Hedges (1993). Food shortages and an epidemic of optic and peripheral neuropathy in Cuba. *Nutrition Review* 51:349-357.

Valdés, S. (1987). *Las lenguas del África subsaharana y el Español de Cuba.* Havana: Editorial Academia.

Volpato, G. and D. Godínez (2004). Ethnobotany of *pru*, a traditional Cuban refreshment. *Economic Botany* 58:381-395.

Wezel, A. and S. Bender (2003). Plant species diversity of homegardens of Cuba and its significance for household food supply. *Agroforestry Systems* 57:39-49.

Whitehead, R.A. (1984). Coconut. *Cocos nucifera* (Palmae). In Simmonds, N.W. (Ed.), *Evolution of crop plants.* New York: Longman.

Wiese, J.H. (1976). Maternal nutrition and traditional food behavior in Haiti. *Human Organization* 35:193-200.

Wilson, S.M. (Ed.) (1999). *The indigenous people of the Caribbean.* Gainesville: University Press of Florida.

Chapter 10

Healthy Fish: Medicinal and Recommended Species in the Amazon and the Atlantic Forest Coast (Brazil)

Alpina Begossi
Natalia Hanazaki
Rossano M. Ramos

INTRODUCTION

Food as medicine, recommended in diets for ill individuals, includes certain specific species that are eaten or mixed with other foods. These medicinal foods may be roasted, boiled, or made into beverages. Such use of specific foods to cure illness goes back a long way in human history. As pointed out by Etkin and Johns (1998, p. 3), a key organizing principle of this practice is that all foods contain a single element that when digested repairs the body and provides energy, thereby mediating disease.

The practices of the Hippocratic school included curing by providing a beneficial environment for the patient and a regimen of suitable diet and exercise (Porter, 1997, p. 20). The spiciness of Indian cuisine is well-known, and its ingredients may have the role of maintaining health or preventing illness. According to Handa (1998, p. 57), the In-

We are grateful to FAPESP (Brazil) grants for the fieldwork along the Araguaia and the Negro rivers, and to the MacArthur Foundation for the fieldwork along the Juruá River. FAPESP has also supported fieldwork on the Atlantic Forest coast since 1992. One of the authors (A.B.) thanks CNPq (Brazil) for a productivity scholarship (1B) and for a research grant in 1992. We thank M. Quinlan, Ball State University, IN, USA, for the valuable review of and suggestions for a draft of this paper. An interim report of this study was presented at the XV ICAES 2K3, Florence, Italy, July 5th-12th, 2003 (travel funded by FAPESP).

dian diet has components to balance the body's equilibrium in order to prevent illnesses, and diet is considered the most important component of health (Handa, 1998). Prohibitions of plants and animals during illness, menstruation, and puerperium have historical roots and are widespread around the world, as exemplified by food taboos on fish, animals, and vegetables (Begossi, 1998, pp. 41-43; Begossi et al., 2002). Other food may be recommended to treat illnesses or included in diets prepared to alleviate illnesses or their related symptoms.

In many cases, the interface between a recommended food and a medicine includes a threshold that is difficult to define. Beverages used in treatments often include plants, but in many cases they also contain animal parts. Mystic or supernatural factors may be associated with treatments. In many different parts of rural Brazil, among coastal populations, or in riverine environments, the association of supernatural factors with diseases is fairly common. Maués (1990) found different categories of diseases in a fishing community in the northern part of Brazil, where some illnesses were associated with natural (biological) causes and others were associated with supernatural causes. In rural Brazil there are specialists such as the *curandeiro,* who gives recipes and beverages to the ill, the *rezador,* who prays and uses magical practices to induce cures, and the *raizeiro,* who prepares and gives recipes on radish leaves and essences to be used in cures (Araújo, 1979; Campos, 1967, pp. 32-33).

Most medicinal recipes and practices are usually based on the vegetal world, as exemplified in the medicine found in the colonial Brazil of the sixteenth to eighteenth centuries (Beltrão Marques, 1999; Ribeiro, 1971) or by the relative abundance of publications on the use of plants by peoples such as the Caiçaras in the Atlantic Forest and the Caboclos of the Amazon (Begossi et al., 1993; Begossi et al., 2000; Begossi et al., 2002; Hanazaki et al., 2000; and Rossato et al., 1999).

The animal world, even as a secondary source of medical treatments, is also used in medicinal practices in other parts of Brazil, such as the northeast. Fish are also used. In particular, the oils of some fish species are used in treatments to cure illnesses such as leishmaniosis, rheumatism, cystitis, and earache (Begossi, 1992; Begossi and Braga, 1992; Seixas and Begossi, 2001). Other fish are used not strictly as a medical treatment, but as part of a diet to be given to ill persons. These species are the main focus of this chapter, and they straddle the threshold between the realms of food and medicine.

METHODS

The results shown in this chapter are from research projects carried out in the Amazon since 1987, and in the Atlantic Forest coast since 1985. The methods included interviews with adult couples of riverine fishers (Caboclos) and coastal Atlantic fishers (Caiçaras), based on questionnaires. Along the Araguaia, Juruá, and Negro Rivers in the Brazilian Amazon, the sampling effort varied from 25 percent (Juruá River) to 50 percent (Araguaia). Along the Negro River, we sampled about 50 percent of the residences at the mouth of tributaries between Ponta Negra (Manaus) and the Unini River. The data obtained in the Atlantic Forest coast area came from two communities from Juréia, on the southern coast of São Paulo state; eight communities, including two islands (Búzios and Vitória) from the northern coast of São Paulo; and one island (Gipóia), from the southern coast of Rio de Janeiro state (see Figure 10.1). For details of the methods used in the specific sites, see Begossi (1992), Begossi and colleagues (1999, 2000), and Hanazaki and Begossi (2000). The freshwater fish were identified by J. Zuanon of the National Institute of Amazonian Research (INPA, Manaus), and by O. Oyakawa of the Zoology Museum of the University of São Paulo. Marine fish were identified by J. L. Figueiredo of the Zoology Museum of the University of São Paulo, and with the help of identification keys (Figueiredo, 1977; Figueiredo and Menezes, 1980, 2000; Menezes and Figueiredo, 1980, 1985). Other sources of identification were Begossi and Garavello (1990), Ferreira and colleagues (1998), Santos and colleagues (1984), and Silvano and colleagues (2001). The English names have been taken from Begossi (1989), Begossi and Figueiredo (1995), and the database of www.fishbase.org.

RESULTS AND DISCUSSION

The Caiçaras and Caboclos are people of mixed Amerindian, Portuguese, and other descent. The Caiçaras are rural inhabitants of

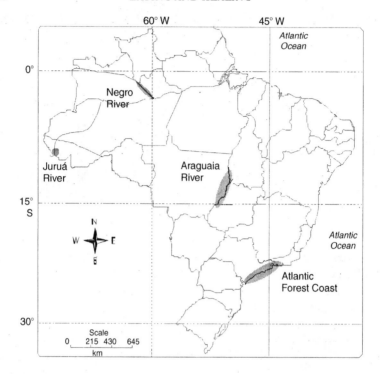

60° W   45° W

Atlantic
Ocean

0°

Negro
River

Juruá
River

Araguaia
River

15°
S

N

W   E

S

Atlantic
Ocean

Atlantic
Forest Coast

30°

Scale
0   215   430   645
km

Research areas

FIGURE 10.1. Map of the research areas.

coastal sites of the Brazilian Atlantic Forest, and the Caboclos are rural inhabitants of the Amazon (in this study, riverine Caboclos). Their livelihood depends on aquatic resources and forest resources, along with shifting cultivation, in which cassava is the staple crop.

The Caiçaras include coastal artisanal fishers. Most riverine Caboclos in the Amazon area are also engaged in artisanal fishing. Fish is an important part of their daily intake of animal protein, and both peoples include certain fish species in the recommended diet prescribed to invalids.

In both fieldwork areas, the list of recommended fish is much longer than the list of specifically medicinal fish. In the Amazon, the interviews yielded the names of 49 fish recommended for specific diets, compared with 28 names of medicinal fish. The comparable figures for the Atlantic Forest coast were 64 and 16 fish names. Because of the great diversity and dispersion in the data from the interviews, here we have included only those fish species mentioned by at least ten interviewees in any community studied.

Recommended Fish for Ill Persons and Puerperal or Menstruating Women

In the Amazon fieldwork area, the fish mentioned as recommended during illness in the three research areas (Araguaia, Juruá, and Negro rivers) were pacu (*Mylossoma* sp., *Myleus* sp., *Metynnis* sp.), anchovy or sardine (*Triportheus* sp., Clupeidae, Engraulidae), and *traíra (Hoplias malabaricus)*. In specific areas it seems to be very important to eat certain species during illness. Area-specific examples are pacu, piranha (Serrasalmus), and sardines along the Araguaia River, *bode* (Loricariidae) and sardines along the Juruá River, and *acará* (Cichlidae) and pacu along the Negro River (Figure 10.1). The differences in uses found between the rivers may be due to regional differences in the abundance of fish species, since Loricariidae are easily available at the research site along the upper Juruá River and are also very important in the diet of the riverine Caboclos (Begossi et al., 1999).

On the Atlantic Forest coast, the Caiçaras in all the study sites mentioned eating *corvina (Micropogonias furnieri* and *Umbrina coroides)* and bluefish *(Pomatomus saltatrix)* during periods of illness and during puerperium and menstruation. The relative importance of the fish recommended per study area fluctuated. Grouper (*Epinephelus* spp.), spottail pinfish *(Diplodus argenteus),* and yellow chub (*Kyphosus* spp.) were mentioned especially often on Búzios and Vitória Islands; tomtate (*Haemulon* spp., *Orthopristes ruber*) and weakfish *(Cynoscion, Nebris, Macrodon)* were mentioned on Gipóia Island; the cichlid *(Geophagus brasiliensis), caratinga (Diapterus* spp.) and snook (*Centropomus* spp.) were mentioned in the Juréia communities of Barra do Una and Praia do Una; and grouper, spottail pinfish, weakfish, and especially the southern kingfish *(Menticirrhus americanus)* were mentioned by the Caiçaras of the six communities studied in Ubatuba district (Table 10.2 and Figure 10.1). Piso (1658), a Dutch physician who came to Brazil in 1637 and organized a scientific expedition, recorded the names of some fish recommended in invalid diets. They included a fish called *caraúna,* which Freire (1939, p. 120) gives as *G. brasiliensis* (the *acará* found in Table 10.2) and a freshwater fish called *amoré-guaçú,* which Freire (1939, p. 503) gives as *Chronophorus taiacica,* a Gobiidae. Such references show that some of these feeding behaviors have an earlier historical origin, predating the arrival of Portuguese colonists in Brazil. Most fish recommended to be eaten during illness eat invertebrates, or they are detritivorous or even omnivorous (data in Ferreira et al., 1998; Santos et al., 1984; Silvano et al., 2001, 2002). In the Amazonian case, these are *acará, aracu, aruanã (Osteoglossum bicirrhosum), bode, caranha (Colossoma brachypomum), corvina (Plagioscion, Pachyurus), jaraquí (Semaprochilodus* spp.), *mandí (Pimelodina, Pimelodella,* among others), *matrinchã (Brycon), mocinha (Potamorhina altamazonica),* pacu, *piau* (Anostomidae), *saburú (Steindachnerina* spp.), and sardine (see Table 10.1). Some fish may occasionally eat other fish species such as *acará, corvina,* and *mandí.* A few exceptions, such as piranha, *traíra,* and *tucunaré (Cichla* spp.) are usually piscivorous. On the Atlantic Forest coast, with the exception of king mackerel *(Scomberomorus cavalla),* bluefish, and *traíra,* the fish recommended are not piscivorous, but instead are invertebrate eaters, omnivorous, or detritivorous. Therefore, *acará,* round scad *(Decapterus punctatus), carapeba (Diapterus* spp.), *carapicú (Eucinostomus* spp.), *caratinga,* tomtate, *corvina,* grouper, *goete (Cynoscion, Larimus),* southern kingfish, spottail pinfish, white mullet *(Mugil curema),* weakfish, *piragica, robalo,* and mullet *(Mugil platanus)* are in these categories (see Table 10.2). Some of them, such as *corcoroca* and *garoupa,* may sometimes eat fish.

The importance of recommending nonpiscivorous fish for ill people is especially relevant, given that most fish species prohibited from the diets of puerperal or menstruating women or invalids, are piscivorous (Begossi, 1992; Begossi and Braga, 1992; Begossi et al., 2004). One reason for recommending a diet based on nonpiscivorous prey is that fish from low trophic levels are probably very digestible, as at higher trophic levels there is an increasing probability of accumulating toxins. The accumulation of toxins at upper trophic levels is referred to as biological magnification, and it is widely known for substances such as DDT and mercury (Kormondy and Brown, 1998).

TABLE 10.1. Fish recommended to be eaten during illness, puerperium, or menstruation by riverine fishers of the Amazonian rivers Araguaia, Juruá, and Negro, and by fishers from 18 coastal communities of the Atlantic Forest coast. Data on fish cited by at least ten interviewees at one of the study sites.

Local name	English name	Species, genera, or family	Number of citations per study area		
			Araguaia	Juruá	Negro
Acará	Cichlid	Cichlidae	4	8	37
Aracu	Leporinus	Anostomidae	–	–	12
Aruanã	Arawana	*Osteoglossum bicirrhosum*	–	–	–
Bode		Loricariidae	–	70	–
Caranha		*Colossoma brachypomum*	12	–	–
Corvina	Croaker	*Plagioscion, Pachyurus* sp.	13	1	–
Jaraquí		*Semaprochilodus* spp.	10	–	19
Mandí	Catfish	*Pimelodina, Pimelodella, Pimelodus,* among others	9	18	–
Matrinchã		*Brycon*	17	–	–
Mocinha		*Potamorhina altamazonica*	–	13	–
Pacu	Pacu	*Mylossoma duriventre, Myleus* spp., *Metynnis* spp.	45	1	40
Piau	Leporinus	Anostomidae	16	17	–
Piranha	Piranha	*Serrasalmus* spp.	21	1	–
Saburú		*Steindachne rina* spp.	–	13	–
Sardinha	Anchovy, Hatchetfish	*Triportheus* spp., Clupeidae Engraulidae	24	50	12
Traíra	Trahira	*Hoplias malabaricus*	19	18	18
Tucunaré	Peacock cichlid, Speckled pavon	*Cichla* spp.	–	–	–
Total Number			113	120	64

Note: Amazonian fish (freshwater) $N = 297$.

TABLE 10.2. Fish recommended to be eaten during illness, puerperium, or menstruation by riverine fishers from five areas of Atlantic Forest coast, including nine fishing communities. Data on fish cited by at least ten interviewees at one of the study sites.

Local name	English name	Species, genera, or family	Number of citations per study				
			Búzios	Gipóia	Juréia	Ubatuba	Vitória
Acará	Cichlid	Geophagus rasiliensis	–	–	22	7	–
			–	–	–	–	–
Cacao	Small shark	Carcharhinidae	9	–	–	22	1
Carapau	Round scad	Decapterus punctatu	–	7	–	13	–
Carapeba	Mojarra	Diapterus spp.	–	–	1	11	–
Carapicú	Mojarra	Eucinostomus spp.	–	–	–	23	–
Caratinga	Mojarra	Diapterus spp.	–	–	28	7	–
Cavala	King mackerel	Scomberomus cavalla	–	7	–	13	–
Corcoroca	Tomtate, Grunt	Haemulon spp. Haemulon spp.r.	4	10	–	2	–
Corvina	Croaker, Sand drum	Microponias furnieri Umbrina coroides	1	7	6	23	1
Enchova	Bluefish	Pomatomus saltarix	1	3	1	25	4
Garoupa	Grouper	Epinephelus spp.	25	6	–	34	7
Goete	Weakfish	Cynoscion, Larimus	–	1	–	15	–
Imbetara	Southern kingfish	Menticirrhus americanus	–	2	12	93	–
Marimba	Spottail pinfish	Diplodus argenteus	27	–	–	30	4

Pampo	Pompano	*Trachinous* spp.	–	–	2	10	–
Parati	White mullet	*Mugil curema*	–	–	13	3	–
Pescada	Weakfish	*Cynoscion, Nebris, Macrodon*	–	10	9	37	–
Piragica	Yellow chub	*Kyphosus* spp.	21	1	–	9	5
Robalo	Snook	*Centropomus* spp.	–	–	31	26	–
Tainha	Mullet	*Mugil platanus*	–	–	7	29	–
Traira	Trahira	*Hoplias malabaricus*	–	–	10	–	–
Total number			113	120	64	–	–

Note: Atlantic Forest coast (estuarine or marine species) $N = 374$.

Prey that feed at lower trophic levels are expected to contain less toxins; thus herbivorous preys should be very acceptable.

Medicinal Fish

Some fish are used as medicine or used to treat certain diseases when prepared in a certain way. Rays are medicinal in both the Amazon and the Atlantic Forest areas. In the 297 interviews from the Araguaia, Juruá, and Negro river areas, the fish mentioned most often as having medicinal uses were rays (different species: 45 mentions), *poraquê* (*Electrophorus electricus:* 21 mentions), *traíra* (*H. malabaricus:* 19 mentions), and *pirarara* (*Phratocephalus hemiliopterus:* 17 mentions). The oil from these fish is used to treat asthma and bronchitis (rays); rheumatism (*poraquê*, also *pirara*), skin burns, cough, and wounds; and, in particular, asthma *(pirarara);* and earache *(traíra)*. The fish oil is usually drunk, but in the case of rheumatism it is rubbed on the body. The liver of rays may also be used, toasted and drunk as an infusion (locally referred to as "tea") for bronchitis and flu.

In the Atlantic Forest coast area, none of the medicinal fish were mentioned by more than 10 interviewees from each community. The "ray egg," mentioned at Búzios Island and Ubatuba in less than five interviews, is used against hemorrhages by puerperal women. It is often toasted and drunk as an infusion, also locally referred to as "tea." At Ubatuba, the "ray egg" is mentioned to cure bronchitis as well. The most-mentioned medicinal fish is sea horse *(Hippocampus reidi)*, with a total of 29 mentions on the Atlantic Forest coast. It is used toasted in a beverage (as an infusion or as a tincture in *pinga*, a Brazilian rum) to treat bronchitis and puerperal hemorrhages. An aquatic animal mentioned on the coast is a turtle *(Chelonia mydas);* it is used to treat asthma, bronchitis, and rheumatism (29 mentions). On the coastal islands of Jaguanum and Itacuruçá (Rio de Janeiro), *peixe porco* (filefish; *Aluterus monoceros, Stephanolepis hispidus*) was mentioned in 100 interviews as a medicinal fish to treat bronchitis. The filefish's skin is toasted and drunk or mixed with food. Three interviews on Gipóia Island and at Ubatuba also mentioned the medicinal properties of filefish. In communities on Grande Island, on the southern coast of Rio de Janeiro, *H. reidi* (sea horse), *M. furnieri* (croaker), and *Balistes capriscus* (other filefish) were mentioned to treat bronchitis. The skin of *H. reidi* or the skin of *B. capriscus* are toasted, ground, and drunk as an infusion or eaten during meals, and the otolith of *M. furnieri,* also toasted and ground, is drunk as an infusion (Seixas and Begossi, 2001).

In other Brazilian fishing communities, such as Siribinha Beach in the state of Bahia (northeastern Brazil), black prochilodus, marine electric fish, marine catfish, shark, and *traíra* are also used as medicinal fish (Costa-Neto and Marques, 2000). In fishing communities in northeastern Brazil, such as Várzea de Marituba, some fishermen recognize medicinal uses for the oil of fishes, such as *Tarpon atlanticus, Parauchenipterus galeatus, Erythinus* cf. *erythrinus, Schizodon kneery,* and *Leporinus* sp. *(piau), Serrasalmus brandtii,* as well as *Hoplias* aff. *malabaricus (traíra)* (Marques, 2001).

CONCLUSIONS

The riverine Caboclos of the Amazon differ slightly from the coastal Caiçaras of the Atlantic Forest, Brazil, in modifications to the diet that involve particular fish species and are a response to a particular condition of the consumer (e.g., fish recommended for invalids and puerperal or menstruating women). They also differ in the use of animals (or animal parts) to treat diseases. In fact, it seems that more species of fish are recommended in periods of illness, puerperium, or menstruation than there are medicinal species of fish. These results contrast with the use of plants, where we frequently find an especially well-defined category of "medicinal plants," which are taken in the form of an infusion or syrup, for example (Begossi et al., 2002; see Chapter 11 by Hanazaki et al., this volume).

Though the first records of the consumption of fish (such as the *caraúna [G. brasiliensis]* and *amoré-guaçú [C. taiacica]* being recommended for invalids) are from Piso's expedition in the 1600s, it seems likely that the consumption of particular fish species to treat illness predates the arrival of the Portuguese in Brazil.

Finally, the importance of nonpiscivorous fish in recommendations for the ill indicates that the prey's diet might be a relevant factor in the choice of the food forbidden for invalids and menstruating or puerperal women. The diet of the prey might influence its toxicity and digestibility, and therefore its acceptability as food for humans in a weakened physical state. These findings suggest a need for additional research on the toxins in freshwater and coastal fish and on fish digestibility according to the species' position within the food chain. Further, we should examine the conditions in which humans are likely to prefer larger, meatier fish or smaller, possibly more digestible fish. These questions would increase our knowledge of human nutrition, health behavior, and environmental interaction.

REFERENCES

Araújo, A.M. (1979). *Medicina rústica*, Third edition. São Paulo: Editora Nacional.

Begossi, A. (1989). Food diversity and choice and technology in a Brazilian fishing community (Búzios Island, São Paulo State). Doctoral dissertation, University of California, Davis.

Begossi, A. (1992). Food taboos at Búzios Island (SE Brazil): Their significance and relation to folk medicine. *Journal of Ethnobiology* 12 (1): 117-139.

Begossi, A. (1998). Food taboos: A scientific reason? In Prendergast, H.D.V., N.L. Etkin, D.R. Harris, and P.J. Houghton (Eds.), *Plants for food and medicine.* Symposium, "Plants for Food and Medicine," Joint Meeting of the Society of Economic Botany and the International Society of Ethnopharmacology, July 1-6, 1996, Imperial College, London. Kew: Royal Botanic Gardens.

Begossi, A. and F.M. de S. Braga (1992). Food taboos and folk medicine among fishermen from the Tocantins River. *Amazoniana* 12 (1): 101-118.

Begossi, A. and J.L. Figueiredo (1995). Ethnoichthyology of southern coastal fishermen: Cases from Búzios Island and Sepetiba Bay (Brazil). *Bulletin of Marine Science* 56: 711-717.

Begossi, A. and J.C. Garavello (1990). Notes on the ethnoichthyology of fishermen from the Tocantins River (Brazil). *Acta Amazonica* 20: 341-351.

Begossi, A., N. Hanazaki, and N. Peroni (2000). Knowledge and use of biodiversity in Brazilian hot spots. *Environment, Development, and Sustainability* 2 (3-4): 177-193.

Begossi, A., N. Hanazaki, and R.M. Ramos (2004). Food chain and the reasons for fish food taboos among Amazonian and Atlantic Forest fishers (Brazil). *Ecological Applications* 4: 334-343.

Begossi, A., N. Hanazaki, and J. Tamashiro (2002). Medicinal plants in the Atlantic Forest (Brazil): Knowledge, use, and conservation. *Human Ecology* 30: 281-299.

Begossi, A., H.F. Leitão-Filho, and P.J. Richerson (1993). Plant uses at Búzios Island (SE Brazil). *Journal of Ethnobiology* 13 (2): 233-256.

Begossi, A., R.A.M. Silvano, B.D. Amaral, and O. Oyakawa (1999). Uses of fish and game by inhabitants of an extractive reserve (Upper Juruá, Acre, Brazil). *Environment, Development and Sustainability* 1: 1-21.

Beltrão Marques, V.R. (1999). *Natureza em Boiões. Medicinas e boticários no Brasil setecentista.* Campinas: Editora da Unicamp.

Campos, E. (1967). *Medicina popular do nordeste. Superstições, crendices e meizinhas,* Third edition. Rio de Janeiro: Edições Cruzeiro.

Costa-Neto, E. and J.G.W. Marques (2000). Faunistic resources used as medicines by artisanal fishermen from Siribinha Beach, State of Bahia, Brazil. *Journal of Ethnobiology* 20: 93-109.

Etkin, N.L. and T. Johns (1998). "Pharmafoods" and "nutraceuticals": Paradigm shifts in biotherapeutics. In Prendergast, H.D.V., N.L. Etkin, D.R. Harris, and P.J. Houghton (Eds.), *Plants for food and medicine,* pp. 3-16. Symposium, "Plants for Food and Medicine," Joint Meeting of the Society of Economic Botany and the International Society of Ethnopharmacology, July 1-6, 1996, Imperial College, London. Kew: The Royal Botanic Gardens.

Ferreira, J.G., J.A.S. Zuanon, and G.M. dos Santos (1998). *Peixes comerciais do médio Amazonas, Região de Santarém.* Brasília DF: Pará. Edições IBAMA, MMA.

Figueiredo, J.L. (1977). *Manual de peixes marinhos do sudeste do Brasil. I-Introdução. Cações, raias e quimeras.* São Paulo: Museu de Zoologia, Universidade de São Paulo.

Figueiredo, J.L. and N.A. Menezes (1980). *Manual de peixes marinhos do sudeste do Brasil.* III. Teleostei (2). São Paulo: Museu de Zoologia, Universidade de São Paulo.

Figueiredo, J.L. and N.A. Menezes (2000). *Manual de peixes marinhos do sudeste do Brasil.* III. Teleostei (5). São Paulo: Museu de Zoologia, Universidade de São Paulo.

Freire, L. (1939). *Grande e novíssimo dicionário da língua Portuguesa.* Rio de Janeiro: Editora A Noite.

Hanazaki, N. and A. Begossi (2000). Fishing and niche dimension for food consumption of Caiçaras from Ponta do Almada (Brazil). *Human Ecology Review* 7 (2): 52-62.

Hanazaki, N., J.Y. Tamashiro, H.F. Leitão-Filho, and A Begossi (2000). Diversity of plant uses in two Caiçara communities from Atlantic Forest coast, Brazil. *Biodiversity and Conservation* 9: 597-615.

Handa, S.S. (1998). The integration of food and medicine in India. In Prendergast, H.D.V., N.L. Etkin, D.R. Harris, and P.J. Houghton (Eds.), *Plants for food and medicine,* pp. 57-68. Symposium, "Plants for Food and Medicine," Joint Meeting of the Society of Economic Botany and the International Society of Ethnopharmacology, July 1-6, 1996, Imperial College, London. Kew: The Royal Botanic Gardens.

Kormondy, E.J. and D.E. Brown (1998). *Fundamentals of human ecology.* Englewood, NJ: Prentice Hall.

Marques, J.G.W. (2001). *Pescando pescadores*, Second edition. São Paulo: NUPAUB-Núcleo de Apoio a Pesquisa sobre Populações Humanas e Áreas Úmidas Brasileiras, Universidade de São Paulo.

Maués, R.H. (1990). *A Ilha encantada. Núcleo de altos estudos Amazônicos.* Belém: Universidade Federal do Pará.

Menezes, N.A and J.L. Figueiredo (1980). *Manual de peixes marinhos do sudeste do Brazil.* III. Teleostei (3). São Paulo: Museu de Zoologia, Universidade de São Paulo.

Menezes, N.A and J.L. Figueiredo (1985). *Manual de peixes marinhos do sudeste do Brazil.* III. Teleostei (4). São Paulo: Museu de Zoologia, Universidade de São Paulo.

Piso, G. (1658). *História natural e médica da India Ocidental* (1957 edition). Rio de Janeiro: Departamento de Imprensa Nacional.

Porter, R. (1997). *Medicine: A history of healing.* New York: Marlowe and Company.

Ribeiro, L. (1971). *Medicina no Brasil colonial.* Rio de Janeiro: Editorial Sul Americana.

Rossato, S., H.F. Leitão-Filho, and A. Begossi (1999). Ethnobotany of Caiçaras of the Atlantic Forest coast (Brazil). *Economic Botany* 53 (3): 377-385.

Santos, G.M., M. Jegu, and B. Merona (1984). *Catálogo de peixes comerciais do médio Tocantins.* Manaus: Centrais Elétricas do Norte (Eletronorte), Conselho Nacional de Desenvolvimento Científico e Tecnológico [CNPq], Instituto Nacional de Pesquisas da Amazônia (INPA).

Seixas, C. and A. Begossi (2001). Ethnozoology of Caiçaras from Aventureiro, Ilha Grande. *Journal of Ethnobiology* 21 (1): 107-135.

Silvano, R.A.M., N. Hanazaki, and A. Begossi (2002). Biodiversity and use of fishes at the São Paulo coast (Brazil). Paper presented at the Healthy Ecosystems Healthy People Conference, Washington DC.

Chapter 11

Edible and Healing Plants in the Ethnobotany of Native Inhabitants of the Amazon and Atlantic Forest Areas of Brazil

Natalia Hanazaki
Nivaldo Peroni
Alpina Begossi

INTRODUCTION

Ethnobotany deals with the way people incorporate plants into their cultural traditions and customary practices (Balick and Cox, 1997) or, according to Alcorn (1995), with the dynamics of the system of which plant use and plant management are a part.

An important approach of ethnobotany is to apply quantitative methods (Martin, 1995; Alexiades, 1996; Phillips, 1996). Quantification in ethnobotany is a useful tool, as long as it is used to address particular ethnobiological questions (Phillips, 1996). One of the advantages of quantitative methods is that they yield comparable data, either through systematic and replicable data collection or under an etic and an ethic research orientation (Zent, 1996). In this sense, ethnobotanical studies often deal with predefined categories of use,

We are grateful to two Brazilian agencies: FAPESP, for financial support for fieldwork and a doctoral scholarship (N. Hanazaki), and CNPq, for a research grant (A. Begossi) and a doctoral grant (N. Peroni). We thank Jorge Y. Tamashiro from Departamento de Botanica (UNICAMP), who identified the botanical material, and Silvia Rossato, who collected ethnobotanical data at Araguaia River. Last, but not least, we are very grateful to all the interviewees who kindly collaborated in this research.

in order to have comparable data from different surveys and to understand the importance of the plant resources for a given population.

Though predefined use categories have advantages, researchers using them frequently ponder how to construct categories that fully correspond to those of the informants. Classic examples of such categories are food plants and medicinal plants (Phillips, 1996). Although a real distinction exists between these categories among many native communities and for many plant species (Moerman, 1994), this division is not always crisp. Many species are undoubtedly considered as medicinal—clearly used to cure illnesses, diseases, or a given type of debilitation. However, some species straddle two or more categories at the same time. Bennett and Prance (2000) argue that the dichotomy between food and medicine can be largely absent among indigenous and rural populations. Several plants used for food are also important medicinal resources, and vice versa. In this context, the emic concepts of health, disease, and illness should vary from the etic ones (cf. Pike, 1993 and Harris, 1976). Thus, in some extreme situations, the food plants can be considered as medicinal plants, even if their unique medicinal role is to satiate hunger.

Underlying these previously constructed categories a gradient of management and domestication can be observed for each species. The terms wild, weed, cultivated, and domesticated are widely discussed in the literature and represent a continuum of the human-plant relationships (see De Wet and Harlan, 1975; Rindos, 1984; Harris, 1989; Harlan, 1992; Logan and Dixon, 1994; Clement, 1999).

In this continuum, a key group of plants lies in the wild-weed gradient. In spite of the fact that wild plants cannot invade habitats permanently disturbed by humans (De Wet and Harlan, 1975), the complex wild-weed species represent the individuals of a population that can tolerate some degree of disturbance and move back and forth on this continuum (Harlan, 1992). Another problem related to the continuous nature of human modifications of plant habitats is the difficulty of defining whether a given species is native to the area. This is especially relevant for plants from the Amazon region, because human influence in Amazonian forests is historical and intense (Balée, 1994) and includes many intermediate stages of human modification and utilization of plants in different stages of interaction. A corollary to this is that the concept of a pristine forest is not appropriate for a great part of the Amazon basin (Balée, 1994), and what is a wild plant today could once have been a weed. The questions raised when dealing with predefined and rigid categories are also the consequence of the frozen-in-time nature of the snapshot of these dynamic processes.

Ethnobotanical surveys conducted in different parts of Brazil (e.g., Amorozo and Gély, 1988; Figueiredo et al., 1993, 1997; Rossato et al., 1999; Begossi et al., 2001, 2002; Hanazaki et al., 2000; Albuquerque and Andrade, 2002) have shown that local knowledge of plant resources is important when discussing plants used for various purposes, such as medicine, food, and handicrafts. In this chapter we explore the plants useful as both food and medicine in three areas of Brazil: the Atlantic rain forest, the Araguaia River (Brazilian savanna), and the Negro River (Amazon forest).

Etkin (1994) has discussed the limitations of a perspective of plant use based mainly on the maximization of caloric sources; he stressed the need to consider other potential uses, such as the nutritional and pharmacological ones. Such a perspective, expanded by Etkin (1994), is implicit when dealing with predefined categories of "food" or "medicine," which frequently obscure less conspicuous features of plants. In this study, we analyze these overlapping features of plant species, which are reflected in overlapping categories of use.

STUDY SITE AND METHODS

Data were collected in three areas with different environmental and vegetation characteristics. During 1997 and 1998, 96 interviews were performed among riverine people from the Araguaia River, living between Aragarças and São Félix do Araguaia (11° 37'-15° 53' S and 50° 40'-52° 12' W). We covered a stretch of river approximately 900 km long, interviewing people living on both banks but excluding Indian tribes and the inhabitants of urban sites, such as cities. At each settlement we sampled 50 percent of the houses. Note that some interviews were performed in areas of cerrado vegetation (Brazilian savanna), which have been appreciably altered by cattle ranching and large soybean farms.

In the Amazon region, we conducted 73 interviews with riverine people from the Negro River, between Ponta Negra and the Unini River (01° 54'-3° 04' S and 60° 06'-61° 30' W), from 2000 to 2001. We covered approximately 300 km of the lower course of the Negro

River and part of the lower course of the Unini River, interviewing people living on the right bank, but excluding towns. In communities with more than ten houses and in communities located at the mouth of small tributaries *(igarapés)* the sample included 50 percent of the houses on the river bank. The Negro is a black-water tributary of the Amazon, flowing through an area of *igapó* (flooded forest) and *terra firme* forest (areas not periodically flooded) (Hueck, 1972).

In the Atlantic Forest region, data were collected through interviews with the local inhabitants of nine communities. Several northern communities from this part of the coast of São Paulo State (23° 15'-23° 45' S and 44° 45'-45° 00' W) were included in this study: Puruba, Picinguaba, Sertão do Puruba, Casa de Farinha, Ilha da Vitória (Rossato et al., 1999), Almada, and Camburí (Hanazaki et al., 2000). The southern communities from the coast of São Paulo State (24° 50'-24° 55' S and 47° 45'-47° 55' W) included in this study were Pedrinhas and São Paulo Bagre (Hanazaki, 2001). We interviewed 264 inhabitants between 1991 and 1999. On average, the number of families in these communities is 35; the range is from 13 (Ilha da Vitória) to 70 families (Picinguaba and Camburí). On the coast of São Paulo State the Atlantic rain forest is reasonably intact, despite recent changes due to increased tourism and urbanization.

Despite the regional differences, all interviewees shared some features regarding their main economic activities. The riverine and coastal populations we studied depended largely on fishing, either for direct subsistence or for commercial purposes. These people live in rural areas, and their degree of contact with urban centers varies with the distance from the cities and the transport facilities. The people in the Amazon region are generally called Caboclos, and those in the Atlantic Forest region are generally called Caiçaras. Both the Caboclos and the Caiçaras are people of mixed origin, descended from Europeans, Amerindians, and Africans (Willems, 1975; Wagley, 1976; Mussolini, 1980; Parker, 1985).

We accessed all the communities in the Atlantic Forest region except Ilha da Vitória by car. Most of the communities have public primary schools and public transport to the urban centers. The houses and communities along the Negro and the Araguaia were reached by boat, but some localities on the banks of Araguaia can also be reached by car. In the Araguaia and Negro River areas, especially the latter, the houses were simpler than in the Atlantic Forest area. In the

Araguaia and Negro River areas the bigger settlements have a public primary school. Transportation to the urban centers is mainly by boat. Medical assistance varies from place to place; most places are visited infrequently by the public health care service. In the Negro and Araguaia areas we observed frequent visits by government workers to control malaria.

The interviews were done individually with male and female adults, after we had asked the local inhabitants whether they were willing to participate in the research. Based on a semistructured research protocol (open-ended questionnaires), we asked them questions about their socioeconomic activities, about fishing, and about three broad, predefined categories of known and used plants: plants for medicine, plants for food, and plants for handicrafts and construction. Botanical material was collected and herborized for identification. Some common species were identified in field. The taxonomic identification was done by the late Hermógenes F. Leitão-Filho (Unicamp, Campinas), Jorge Y. Tamashiro (Unicamp, Campinas), and Olga Yano (Instituto Botânico, São Paulo). The botanical material collected was deposited at the Herbarium of the Campinas University (UEC). The field identification of some common species was checked against the literature (Lorenzi et al., 1996; De Souza et al., 1997; Lorenzi, 1998). The plant origins were based on Brücher (1989), Rehm and Espig (1991), Piperno and Pearsall (1998), and Clement (1999).

The management intensity was classified into four broad categories: plants with little or no management (Mi_0); plants facilitated by human management (Mi_1); plants infrequently cultivated (Mi_2); and plants frequently cultivated (Mi_3). Both "cultivated" and "managed" refer to human activities. Note that the term "cultivated" refers to species that are planted in prepared land or sown in prepared beds (Etkin, 1994), while "managed" refers to species that are influenced by some degree of alteration of the environment. Just as constructed categories of use do not reflect the continuum of plant uses, the categories of management intensity do not reflect the continuum of plant management; some species, therefore, straddle categories.

RESULTS AND DISCUSSION

In total there were 433 interviews. In these interviews, 85 plants mentioned were used both for food and for medicine (see Appendix). Two of the 85 species were not considered in this analysis because they are bought in markets and not produced locally (*A. sativum* and *Myristica fragrans* Houtt.).

The interviews along the Araguaia River yielded 24 plants used both for food and medicine, and the Negro River interviews yielded 19. In both cases, these figures represented 18 percent of all the total number of plants mentioned in each area. In the Atlantic Forest, approximately half (48 percent) of the species mentioned were used both for food and for medicine (see Table 11.1). The proportions of plants used only for food, only for medicine, and for both food and medicine in the three areas were statistically different ($\chi^2 = 25.57$ with 4 degrees of freedom, $p < 0.01$). A chi-square test on the proportions for the Araguaia and Negro rivers revealed that these proportions did not differ statistically ($\chi^2 = 0.27$, with 3 degrees of freedom, $p < 0.01$). However, although the proportions in the three areas were statistically different, in all three areas the average number of plants used for both food and medicine was similar (0.25 plants per interview for Araguaia, 0.26 for Negro, and 0.23 for Atlantic Forest).

In spite of the environmental and other differences between the three areas (Amazon forest, Atlantic Forest, and Brazilian savanna) seven species were used both as food and medicine in all three areas. Three of these species are introductions that are widely used in Brazil and elsewhere in the world, both as food and as medicine: mango

TABLE 11.1. Number of interviews in each area, and number of plants mentioned only as food plants, mentioned only as medicinal plants, and, post hoc, found to have been mentioned as both. Figures in parentheses indicate the average number of plants mentioned per interview in each area.

	Araguaia River	Negro River	Atlantic Forest
Number of interviews	96	73	264
Number of plants mentioned			
Food	132 (1.37)	107 (1.46)	128 (0.48)
Medicinal	133 (1.38)	98 (1.34)	221 (0.84)
Food and medicinal	24 (0.25)	19 (0.26)	62 (0.23)

(*Mangifera indica* L.), orange [*Citrus sinensis* (L.) Osbeck], and lemon (*Citrus limon* L. Burm.). These species are economically important in Brazil (Mors and Rizzini, 1966; Joly and Leitão-Filho, 1979). A further three species are native and also widely used in other parts of Brazil: jatobá (*Hymenaea courbaril* L.), guava (*Psidium guajava* L.), and cashew (*Anacardium occidentale* L.) (Mors and Rizzini, 1966). All six of these species have in common that their edible part is the fruit, whereas the medicinal part may be their bark, shoots, or leaves. The seventh species, garlic (*Allium sativum* L.), is an exception: its bulb is widely used as a condiment and as a medicine.

As well as recording whether the plants mentioned were native or introduced, we also recorded their management intensity and the environment from which they are collected. Over half (53 percent) of the 83 species mentioned that were used both for food and medicine were introduced; 47 percent were native. The similarity of these percentages indicates that the people depend on both native and introduced resources for food and medicine.

Interestingly, according to Bennett and Prance (2000), surveys of food plants tend to ignore wild species (Etkin, 1994), while surveys of medicinal plants tend to ignore introduced ones. In this context, Bennett and Prance (2000) noted that the widespread use of introduced plants is partly due to the medicinal value of plants whose primary use is for food. This is true of many edible fruit species, such as mango, papaya (*Carica papaya* L.), black mulberry (*Morus nigra* L.), avocado (*Persea americana* Mill.), and orange.

Native species used for food and medicine included fruits such as inharé [*Licania gardnerii* (Hook.) Fritsch]; pequí (*Caryocar brasiliense* Cambess.); and curriola (*Cissus spinosa* Cambess.) in the Araguaia area and açaí (*Euterpe precatoria* Mart.); beribá [*Rollinia mucosa* (Jacq.) Baill.]; murici (*Mauritia flexuosa* L.); and uichí [*Endopleura uchi* (Huber) Cuatrec.] in the Negro area. In the Atlantic Forest area, the native species included araçá (*Psidium cattleianum* Sabine); bacuparí [*Garcinia gardneriana* (Planch & Triana) Zappi]; cambucá (*Marlierea edulis* Nied); jabuticaba [*Myrciaria floribunda* (West. & Wild) Berg.]; and pitanga [*Eugenia pitanga* (O. Berg) Kiaersk.]. (See Appendix.)

Figure 11.1 schematically illustrates the different management categories. The different contexts represented in Figure 11.1 can be

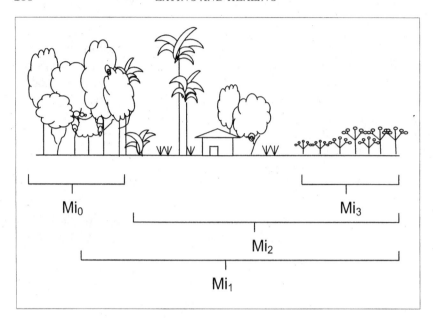

FIGURE 11.1. Schematic representation of areas where plants for food and medicine occur. Mi_0 = plants with little or no management; Mi_1 = plants facilitated by human management; Mi_2 = infrequently cultivated plants; and Mi_3 = frequently cultivated plants. See text for further details.

defined as a spatial and temporal mosaic, in which Mi_2 and Mi_3 are frequently located near the houses. However, Mi_3 can be inside Mi_2 and Mi_1. In some situations, Mi_3 can be located inside Mi_0, because many frequently cultivated plants are associated with swidden cultivation systems (Denevan and Padoch, 1987; Peroni and Hanazaki, 2002). Plants with little or no management occur in the forested areas, while plants facilitated by human management can occur in a broad range of environments, including forested areas that have undergone some manipulation (e.g., the forest-fallows). Infrequently cultivated plants generally occur near the houses, in the backyards, orchards, swidden plots, or in anthropogenic environments such as along paths, trails, and small roads.

    We will now contrast similar environments with some particular features. A swidden plot is an area of 0.5 to 1.0 ha, where some crops are frequently integrated into an agricultural system based on shifting cultivation (Conklin, 1954; Denevan and Padoch, 1987; Fox et al.,

2000; Begossi et al., 2001; Peroni and Hanazaki, 2002). The species cultivated in swidden plots are used for subsistence and sometimes are sold. In spite of this, through the plot or along its edges it is common to find some infrequently cultivated species, as well as some species facilitated by human management or by human activity.

An orchard is a smaller area, usually located in the backyards of the houses, where some species are frequently or infrequently cultivated on a smaller scale than in swidden plots, always for direct subsistence. In the backyards we often found some species facilitated by human activity or infrequently cultivated, such as fruit trees.

More than half of the species mentioned as both food and medicine are infrequently cultivated (see Figure 11.2). Eighty percent of these species are introductions. They include edible fruits (such as orange, papaya, and avocado) and other species of widespread use among many cultures throughout the world, such as sugarcane (*Saccharum officinarum* L.), onion (*Allium cepa* L.), tomato (*Lycopersicon esculentum* Mill.), rosemary (*Rosmarinus officinalis* L.), and beans (*Phaseolus vulgaris* L.).

The species facilitated by human management included some introduced ones (20 percent) with weedy habits (e.g., *Amaranthus*

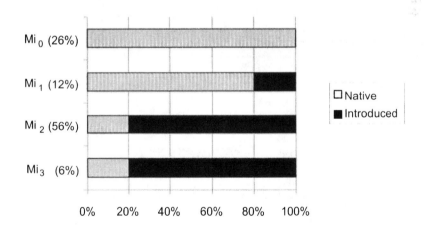

FIGURE 11.2. Management intensity of 83 plants mentioned as food and medicine in Araguaia River, Negro River, and Atlantic Forest coast, Brazil. Mi_0 = plants with little or no management; Mi_1 = plants facilitated by human management; Mi_2 = infrequently cultivated plants; and Mi_3 = frequently cultivated plants. See text for details.

viridis L.) or ubiquitous distribution (*Typha* sp.). Species with weedy habits that grow wholly or predominantly in sites disturbed by human activity (Etkin, 1994) can be an important food resource to some cultures, as exemplified by the noncultivated edible greens (Bye, 2000). We observed that in the Atlantic Forest area the use of these species as a food resource is very sporadic.

There is broad correspondence between the species with little or no management and the species occurring in forested areas (see Figure 11.3). In a general sense, a parallel correspondence occurs between the infrequently cultivated species and the species found in the backyards (Y, Figure 11.3), as well as between the frequently cultivated species and the species in the swidden plots (P, Figure 11.3). Examples of this latter group are the introduced watermelon [*Citrullus lanatus* (Thumb.) Matsum. & Nakai], squash (*Cucurbita* spp.), and beans. However, the chief species cultivated in swidden plots is cassava (*Manihot esculenta* Crantz) (Peroni and Hanazaki, 2002), which is a native of the lowlands of South America. Cassava is the main source of carbohydrates in the Negro River area, but in the Araguaia and Atlantic Forest areas it has lost its importance, having been replaced by rice.

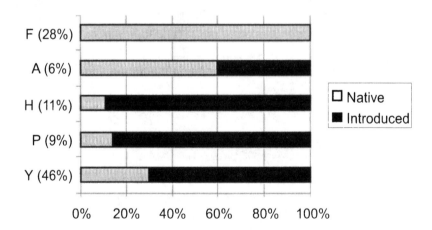

FIGURE 11.3. Environments of 83 plants mentioned as food and medicine in Araguaia River, Negro River, and Atlantic Forest coast, Brazil. F = forest; A = anthropogenic environment; H = orchard; P = plots (swiddens); Y = yards. See text for details.

Other plants used both for food and medicine are infrequently cultivated in orchards, such as leafy vegetables [e.g., *Nasturtium officinalis* R. Br., *Hipochaeris brasiliensis* (Less.) Benth., *Brassica oleracea* L.] as well as plants used as spices and condiments [e.g., onion, *A. cepa* L.; and parsley, *Petroselinum crispum* (Mill.) A.W. Hill.]. Logan and Dixon (1994) opined that with the shrinking of dietary breadth, many agricultural societies may have increasingly favored the use of spices, many of which are also used medicinally. Furthermore, the spices and condiments add palatability to the diet. According to Johns (1994), the sensory preferences in the diet can play an important role in choosing nutrient sources, pharmacological sources, and cultural markers.

It is important to stress that 80 percent of the species cultivated (which in turn represent 62 percent of the plants mentioned) have been introduced (Figure 11.2) and are present in manipulated environments (Figure 11.3). To be maintained over time, these species have required human manipulation of environments for the purpose of cultivation. We can suggest several interrelated hypotheses to explain why more introduced species are cultivated than native ones. For example, besides the strong influence of the Portuguese economy during colonial times and the strong influence of external demands regarding what is cultivated where, local inhabitants such as the Caiçaras (Atlantic Forest) and the Caboclos (Amazon) are of mixed origin and have a mixed cultural heritage. The legacy of this is visible today as cultivated plants of different origins. In Brazil, the introduction of species such as coffee, sugarcane, and orange followed an economic strategy of monocultures (Crosby, 1986). This kind of agriculture modified many native landscapes, changing large tracts of Brazilian territory. These processes have negative impacts for local people, contributing to many introduced species supplanting native ones. Associated with these factors, the high number of introduced cultivated species may be the result of the genetic erosion of local species that followed the decline of the indigenous people after 1492 (Clement, 1999). The historical loss of species and the ethnobotanical knowledge of the indigenous people could explain the current low number of native species cultivated by people of mixed origin, such as the Caiçaras and Caboclos.

Analyzed from an evolutionary perspective, the domestication process allows for a detailed examination of human-plant interactions that can be overlooked when these interactions are frozen or closed off in categories of use. The domestication processes have an evolutionary nature, showing many degrees of intermediate conditions and stages (Harlan, 1995). Along this gradient, humans alter the genetic structure of useful plant populations, modifying their distribution and abundance through management. However, modifications in distribution and abundance suggest modifications in the environments where these species occur or, in other words, not only in the management of cultivated landscapes but also in the managed landscapes where plants are collected and extraction takes place. At any given moment, the human-plant interaction is the result of a gradual process of increasing management intensity, as well as of increasing management of the environment of the species (Clement, 1999). Despite the paradigms that situate domestication as a coevolutionary process with blurred categories (Rindos, 1984) and assume the importance of caloric content in the progressive and intensifying human-plant interaction (Harris, 1989), in the discussion of domestication it is of paramount importance to include plants with pharmacological potential, in order to really understand the continuum of human-plant interactions (Etkin, 1994). Cases in which the dichotomy between what is used for food and what is used for medicine is absent should be considered carefully.

Though the Brazilian mixed-origin populations we studied make a real distinction between plants that are both edible and medicinal, we cannot ignore the richness of plants mentioned as used only for food and only for medicine, especially in Araguaia River and Negro River areas (Table 11.1). The knowledge of medicinal plants among the Caiçaras from the Atlantic Forest also shows the importance of introduced plants with a pharmacological role (Begossi et al., 2002). Among the medicinal species mentioned by at least 10 percent of 449 interviewees, Begossi and colleagues (2002) found that the species mentioned most often were used solely for medicine (e.g., *Melissa officinalis* L., *Lippia citriodora* H.B.K., *Coleus barbatus* Benth, *Chenopodium* spp., *Foeniculum vulgare* Gaertn.), while plants widely used also for food included the introduced orange and the native guava and *Eugenia uniflora* L., both with only 10 percent of mentions.

CONCLUSIONS

Our analysis of the continuous human-plant interactions revealed the paramount importance of the plants used both for food and for medicine, in spite of the fact that Caiçaras and Caboclos do distinguish many species used only as edible resources or only as medicinal resources.

Plants used for food and medicine are a relevant group of resources, and studying them can reveal important particularities of the human-plant interaction. Here, we discussed data from different environments in different parts of Brazil (Amazon forest, Brazilian savanna, and the southeastern coast of the Atlantic Forest). These resources are used by human populations sharing some similarities: their mixed origin and their main economic activities. Against this background of differences and similarities we observed a general trend when considering plants used for both food and medicine. Most of the species have edible fruits, but frequently their shoots, roots, or leaves are used as medicine. Although some plants are collected from the forest, the majority of these species depend to some degree on the anthropogenic environment (i.e., are favored by management or by cultivation). We confirm earlier predictions that some species are medicinal, but that some species straddle the categories of food and medicine.

APPENDIX

Species mentioned as food and medicine in 433 interviews in Araguaia River, Negro River, and Atlantic Forest coast, Brazil. Mi = management intensity: 0 = plants with little or no management, 1 = plants facilitated by human management, 2 = plants infrequently cultivated, 3 = plants frequently cultivated. Env = environment; F = forest; A = anthropogenic areas; Y = backyards; P = swidden plots (see text for further details); nat = native; int = introduced; na = plants bought in markets; * = identified from the literature (Lorenzi, 1998; Lorenzi et al., 1996; De Souza et al., 1997).

Botanical family	Species	Vernacular name	Status	Mi	Env
Araguaia River					
Anacardiaceae	*Anacardium occidentale* L.	Cajú	nat	2	Y
Anacardiaceae	*Mangifera indica* L.	Manga	int	2	Y

Botanical family	Species	Vernacular name	Status	Mi	Env
Apocynaceae	*Hancornia speciosa* Gomez	Mangaba	nat	0	F
Arecaceae	*Syagrus oleraceae* (Mart.) Becc.	Guariroba	nat	0	F
Caesalpiniaceae	*Hymenaea courbaril* L.	Jatobá	nat	0	F
Caesalpiniaceae	*Tamarindus indica* L.	Tamarindo	int	2	Y
Caricaceae	*Carica papaya* L.	Mamão	int	2	Y
Caryocaracee	*Caryocar brasiliense* Cambess.	Pequi	nat	0	F
Chrysobalanaceae	*Licania gardnerii* (Hook.) Fritsch	Inharé*	nat	0	F
Cucurbitaceae	*Citrullus lanatus* (Thumb.) Matsum. & Nakai	Melancia	int	3	P
Cucurbitaceae	*Cucurbita moschata* Duchesne	Abóbora	int	3	P
Liliaceae	*Allium cepa* L.	Cebola	int	2	H
Liliaceae	*Allium sativum* L.	Alho	int	na	na
Moraceae	*Morus nigra* L.	Amora	int	2	Y
Myrtaceae	*Psidium guajava* L.	Goiaba	nat	1	Y
Oxalidaceae	*Averrhoa carambola* L.	Carambola	int	2	Y
Poaceae	*Saccharum officinarum* L.	Cana	int	2	Y
Rubiaceae	*Genipa americana* L.	Jenipapo	nat	0	F
Rutaceae	*Citrus aurantifolia* Swingle	Lima	int	2	Y
Rutaceae	*Citrus limon* L. Burm.	Limão	int	2	Y
Rutaceae	*Citrus sinensis* (L.) Osbeck	Laranja	int	2	Y
Solanaceae	*Lycopersicon esculentum* Mill.	Tomate	int	2	H
Verbenaceae	*Vitex polygama* Cham.	Taromã	nat	0	F
Vitaceae	*Cissus spinosa* Cambess.	Curriola	nat	0	F

Botanical family	Species	Vernacular name	Status	Mi	Env
Negro River					
Anacardiaceae	*Anacardium occidentale* L.	Caju	nat	2	Y
Anacardiaceae	*Mangifera indica* L.	Manga	int	2	Y
Annonaceae	*Annona muricata* L.	Graviola*	nat	2	Y
Annonaceae	*Duguetia* sp.	Azeitona	nat	0	F
Annonaceae	*Rollinia mucosa* (Jacq.) Baill.	Beribá	nat	2	Y
Apocynaceae	*Couma utilis* Muell. Arg.	Sorva	nat	0	F
Arecaceae	*Euterpe precatoria* Mart.	Acaí	nat	2	Y
Arecaceae	*Geonoma* spp.	Ubim*	nat	0	F
Arecaceae	*Mauritia flexuosa* L.	Muricí*	nat	1	F
Caesalpiniaceae	*Hymenaea courbaril* L.	Jatobá	nat	0	F
Humiriaceae	*Endopleura uchi* (Huber) Cuatrec.	Uichi Liso*	nat	0	F
Lauraceae	*Persea americana* Mill.	Abacate	int	2	Y
Lecythidaceae	*Bertholletia excelsa* Humb. & Bonpl.	Castanha	nat	1	F
Liliaceae	*Allium sativum* L.	Alho	int	na	na
Myrtaceae	*Psidium guajava* L.	Goiaba	nat	1	Y
Passifloraceae	*Passiflora nitida* Humb. & Bonpl.	Maracujá	nat	2	Y
Rutaceae	*Citrus aurantifolia* Swingle	Lima	int	2	Y
Rutaceae	*Citrus limon* L. Burm.	Limao	int	2	Y
Rutaceae	*Citrus sinensis* (L.) Osbeck	Laranja	int	2	Y
Atlantic Forest Coast					
Amaranthaceae	*Amaranthus viridis* L.	Caruru	int	1	A
Anacardiaceae	*Anacardium occidentale* L.	Caju	nat	2	Y

Botanical family	Species	Vernacular name	Status	Mi	Env
Anacardiaceae	*Mangifera indica* L.	Manga	int	2	Y
Anacardiaceae	*Schinus terebinthifolius* Raddi	Aroeira	nat	1	Y
Apiaceae	*Petroselinum crispum* (Mill.) A.W. Hill.	Salsa	int	2	H
Arecaceae	*Bactris setosa* Mart.	Tucum	nat	0	F
Arecaceae	*Euterpe edulis* Mart.	Palmito	nat	0	F
Asteraceae	*Hypochaeris brasiliensis* (Less.) Benth.	Almeirão	nat	2	H
Bignoniaceae	*Tynnanthus elegans* Miers	Cipó cravo	nat	0	F
Bixaceae	*Bixa orellana* L.	Urucum	int	2	Y
Brassicaceae	*Brassica oleracea* L.	Couve	int	2	H
Brassicaceae	*Nasturtium officinale* R. Br.	Agrião	int	2	H
Caesalpiniaceae	*Hymenaea courbaril* L.	Jatobá, jataí	nat	0	F
Caricaceae	*Carica papaya* L.	Mamão	int	2	Y
Chenopodiaceae	*Beta vulgaris* L.	Beterraba	int	2	H
Clusiaceae	*Garcinia gardneriana* (Planch. & Triana) Zappi	Bacupari	nat	0	F
Commelinaceae	*Commelina* sp.	Treporava	nat	0	F
Convolvulaceae	*Ipomoea batatas* L.	Batata doce	int	3	P
Cucurbitaceae	*Cucumis sativus* L.	Pepino	int	2	Y
Cucurbitaceae	*Cucurbita pepo* L.	Abóbora	int	3	P
Cucurbitaceae	*Sechium edule* (Jacq.) Sw.	Chuchu	int	2	Y
Euphorbiaceae	*Manihot esculenta* Crantz	Mandioca	nat	3	P
Fabaceae	*Cajanus cajan* (L.) Millsp	Feijão guando	int	2	Y
Fabaceae	*Phaseolus vulgaris* L.	Feijão	int	3	P

Botanical family	Species	Vernacular name	Status	Mi	Env
Lamiaceae	*Mentha × piperita* L.	Hortelã	int	2	H
Lamiaceae	*Ocimum campechianum* Willd.	Manjericão	int	2	Y
Lamiaceae	*Ocimum gratissimum* L.	Alfavaca	int	2	Y
Lamiaceae	*Ocimum tenuiflorum* L.	Alfavaca Cravo	int	2	Y
Lamiaceae	*Rosmarinus officinalis* L.	Alecrim	int	2	Y
Lauraceae	*Persea americana* Mill.	Abacate	int	2	Y
Liliaceae	*Allium cepa* L.	Cebola	int	2	Y
Liliaceae	*Allium sativum* L.	Alho	int	na	na
Malvaceae	*Morus nigra* L.	Amora	int	2	Y
Menispermaceae	*Abuta* sp.	Buta	nat	0	F
Musaceae	*Musa acuminata* Colla	Banana	int	2	P
Myristicaceae	*Myristica fragrans* Houtt.	Nanoscada	int	na	na
Myristicaceae	*Myristica sebifera* Sw.	Bacuíba	nat	0	F
Myrtaceae	*Eugenia aquea* Burm.	Jambro	int	2	Y
Myrtaceae	*Eugenia brasiliensis* Lam.	Gumixama	nat	0	F
Myrtaceae	*Eugenia pitanga* (O. Berg) Kiaersk.	Pitanga	nat	2	Y
Myrtaceae	*Marlierea edulis* Nied.	Cambucá	nat	0	F
Myrtaceae	*Myrciaria floribunda* (West. & Wild) Berg	Jabuticaba	nat	2	Y
Myrtaceae	*Psidium cattleianum* Sabine	Araçá	nat	1	Y
Myrtaceae	*Psidium guajava* L.	Goiaba	nat	1	Y
Myrtaceae	*Syzygium cumini* (L.) Skeels	Jambolão	int	2	Y

Botanical family	Species	Vernacular name	Status	Mi	Env
Oxalidaceae	*Averrhoa carambola* L.	Carambola	int	2	Y
Passifloraceae	*Passiflora edulis* Sims.	Maracujá	nat	2	Y
Poaceae	*Cymbopogon citratus* (DC.) Stapf.	Capim cidró	int	2	Y
Poaceae	*Saccharum officinarum* L.	Cana	int	2	Y
Poaceae	*Zea mays* L.	Milho	int	2	P
Punicaceae	*Punica granatum* L.	Romã	int	2	Y
Rosaceae	*Eriobotrya japonica* Lindl.	Ameixa	int	2	Y
Rosaceae	*Pyrus communis* L.	Pêra	int	2	Y
Rosaceae	*Rubus* sp.	Morango	nat	1	A
Rubiaceae	*Borreria verticillata* G.F.W.Mey.	Bassora	nat	1	A
Rubiaceae	*Coffea arabica* L.	Café	int	2	Y
Rutaceae	*Citrus limon* (L.) Burm.	Limão	int	2	Y
Rutaceae	*Citrus sinensis* (L.) Osbeck	Laranjeira	int	2	Y
Solanaceae	*Capsicum baccatum* L.	Combarí	int	2	Y
Solanaceae	*Solanum tuberosum* L.	Batata	int	2	H
Typhaceae	*Typha* sp.	Taboa	int	1	A
Zingiberaceae	*Costus spiralis* Roscoe	Cana do brejo	nat	1	A

REFERENCES

Albuquerque, U.P.A. and L.H.C. Andrade (2002). Uso de recursos vegetais da caatinga: O caso do agreste do estado de Pernambuco (Nordeste do Brasil). *Interciencia* 27 (7): 336-346.

Alcorn, J. (1995). The scope and aims of ethnobotany in a developing world. In Schultes, R.E. and S. von Reis (Eds.), *Ethnobotany* (pp. 23-39). Portland: Dioscorides Press.

Alexiades, M.N. (1996). *Selected guidelines for ethnobotanical research: A field manual*. New York: New York Botanical Garden.

Amorozo, M.C.M. and A. Gély (1988). Uso de plantas medicinais por Caboclos do Baixo Amazonas, Barcarena, Pará. *Boletim do Museu Paraense Emilio Goeldi—Série Botânica* 4: 47-130.

Balée, W. (1994). *Footprints of the forest: Ka'apor ethnobotany—The historical ecology of plant utilization by an Amazonian people*. New York: Columbia University Press.

Balick, M.J. and P.A. Cox (1997). *Plants, people and culture*. New York: Scientific American Library.

Begossi, A., N. Hanazaki, and N. Peroni (2001). Knowledge and use of biodiversity in Brazilian hot spots. *Environment, Development and Sustainability* 2 (3-4): 177-193.

Begossi, A., N. Hanazaki, and J.Y. Tamashiro (2002). Medicinal plants and the Atlantic Forest (Brazil): Knowledge, use and conservation. *Human Ecology* 30 (3): 281-299.

Bennett, B.C. and G.T. Prance (2000). Introduced plants in the indigenous pharmacopoeia of northern South America. *Economic Botany* 54 (1): 90-102.

Brücher, H. (1989). *Useful plants of neotropical origin and their wild relatives*. Berlin: Springer-Verlag.

Bye, R.A. (2000). Quelites—Ethnoecology of edible greens—Past, present, and future. In Minnis, P.E. (Ed.), *Ethnobotany: A reader* (pp. 197-213). Norman: University of Oklahoma Press.

Clement, C. (1999). 1492 and the loss of Amazonian crop genetic resources. I. The relation between domestication and human population decline. *Economic Botany* 53 (2): 188-202.

Conklin, H.C. (1954). An ethnoecological approach to shifting agriculture. *Transactions of the New York Academy of Science* 17 (2): 133-142.

Crosby, A.W. (1986). *Ecological imperialism: The biological expansion of Europe, 900-1900*. Cambridge: Cambridge University Press.

De Souza, A.G.C., N.R. Sousa, S.E.L. da Silva, C.D.M. Nunes, A.C. Canto, and A.A. Cruz (1997). *Fruit trees of the Amazon region*. Brasília: Embrapa-Serviço de Produção de Informação.

De Wet, J.J.M. and J.R. Harlan (1975). Weeds and domesticates: Evolution in the man made habitat. *Economic Botany* 29: 99-107.

Denevan, W.M. and C. Padoch (1987). Swidden-fallow agroforestry in the Peruvian Amazon. *Advances in Economic Botany* 5: 1-107.

Etkin, N.L. (1994). *Eating on the wild side*. Tucson: University of Arizona Press.

Figueiredo, G.M., H.F. Leitão-Filho, and A. Begossi (1993). Ethnobotany of Atlantic Forest coastal communities: Diversity of plant uses in Gamboa (Itacuruçá Island, Brazil). *Human Ecology* 21 (4): 419-430.

Figueiredo, G.M., H.F. Leitão-Filho, and A. Begossi (1997). Ethnobotany of Atlantic Forest coastal communities: II. Diversity of plant uses at Sepetiba Bay (SE Brazil). *Human Ecology* 25 (2): 353-360.

Fox, J., D.M. Troung, A.T. Rambo, N.P. Tuyen, L.T. Cuc, and S. Leisz (2000). Shifting cultivation: A new old paradigm for managing tropical forests. *BioScience* 50 (6): 521-528.

Hanazaki, N. (2001). Ecologia de Caiçaras: Uso de recursos e dieta. Doctoral thesis in ecology. Campinas, Brazil: IB/UNICAMP.

Hanazaki, N., J.Y. Tamashiro, H.F. Leitão-Filho, and A. Begossi (2000). Diversity of plant uses in two Caiçara communities from Atlantic Forest Coast, Brazil. *Biodiversity and Conservation* 9: 597-615.

Harlan, J.R. (1992). *Crops and man*, Second edition. Madison: American Society of Agronomy, Crop Science Society of America.

Harlan, J.R. (1995). *The living fields: Our agricultural heritage*. Cambridge: Cambridge University Press.

Harris, D.R. (1989). An evolutionary continuum of people-plant interaction. In Harris, D.R. and G.C. Hillman (Eds.), *Foraging and farming: The evolution of plant exploitation*. London: Unwin Hyman.

Harris, M. (1976). History and significance of the emic/etic distinction. *Annual Review of Anthropology* 5: 329-350.

Hueck, K. (1972). *As florestas da América do Sul*. Brasília: UnB, Brasília.

Johns, T. (1994). Ambivalence to the palatability factors in wild food plants. In Etkin, N.L. (Ed.), *Eating on the wild side* (pp. 46-61). Tucson: University of Arizona Press.

Joly, A.B. and H.F. Leitão-Filho (1979). *Botânica econômica: As principais culturas Brasileiras*. São Paulo: Hucitec-Edusp.

Logan, M.H. and A.R. Dixon (1994). Agriculture and the acquisition of medicinal plant knowledge. In Etkin, N.L. (Ed.), *Eating on the wild side* (pp. 25-45). Tucson: University of Arizona Press.

Lorenzi, H. (1998). *Árvores Brasileiras*, Volume 2. São Paulo: Ed. Platarum.

Lorenzi, H., H.M. Souza, J.T. Medeiros-Costa, L.S.C. Cerqueira, and N. von Behr (1996). *Palmeiras do Brasil, nativas e exóticas*. São Paulo: Ed. Platarum.

Martin, G.L. (1995). *Ethnobotany: A methods manual*. London: Chapman & Hall.

Moerman, D.E. (1994). North American food and drug plants. In Etkin, N.L. (Ed.), *Eating on the wild side* (pp. 166-181). Tucson: University of Arizona Press.

Mors, W.B. and C.T. Rizzini (1966). *Useful plants of Brazil*. San Francisco: Holden-Day Inc.

Mussolini, G. (1980). *Ensaios de antropologia indígena e Caiçara*. Rio de Janeiro: Paz e Terra.

Parker, E.P. (1985). *The Amazon Caboclo: Historical and contemporary perspectives*. Studies on Third World Societies, 32. Williamsburg: College of William and Mary Department of Anthropology.

Peroni, N. and N. Hanazaki (2002). Current and lost diversity of cultivated varieties under swidden systems in Brazilian Atlantic Forest. *Agriculture, Ecosystems & Environment* 92 (2-3): 171-183.

Phillips, O.L. (1996). Some quantitative methods for analyzing ethnobotanical knowledge. In Alexiades, M.N. (Ed.), *Selected guidelines for ethnobotanical research: A field manual*. New York: The New York Botanical Garden.

Piperno, D.R. and D.M. Pearsall (1998). *The origins of agriculture in the lowland neotropics*. San Diego: Academic Press.

Rehm, S. and G. Espig (1991). *The cultivated plants of the tropics and subtropics*. Weikersheim, Germany: Verlag Josef Margraf.

Rindos, D. (1984). *The origins of agriculture: An evolutionary perspective*. Orlando: Academic Press.

Rossato, S.C., H.F. Leitão-Filho, and A. Begossi (1999). Ethnobotany of Caiçaras of the Atlantic Forest coast (Brazil). *Economic Botany* 53 (3): 377-385.

Wagley, C. (1976). *Amazon town: A study of man in the tropics*. Oxford: Oxford University Press.

Willems, E. (1975). *Latin American culture*. New York: Harper & Row.

Zent, S. (1996). Behavioral orientations toward ethnobotanical quantification. In Alexiades, M.N. (Ed.), *Selected guidelines for ethnobotanical research: A field manual* (pp. 199-239). New York: New York Botanical Garden.

Chapter 12

Food Medicines in the Bolivian Andes (Apillapampa, Cochabamba Department)

Ina Vandebroek
Sabino Sanca

INTRODUCTION

Wild and domesticated or semidomesticated plants are a versatile resource for many rural, traditional, or indigenous communities worldwide and are often used in overlapping contexts, including nutrition, health, firewood, construction material, hygiene, cosmetics, handicrafts, and as ornamentals (Etkin, 2002). A particularly interesting relationship exists between food and medicinal plants, since the borderline between food and medicine is sometimes diffuse (Bennett and Prance, 2000). Hence, food plants are often used as medicines, and vice versa. Furthermore, in many cases the food use of a plant cannot be separated from its medicinal action (Bonet and Vallès, 2002). A continuum has been described, ranging from plants that are exclusively used as food, through multipurpose food medicinals, to predominantly medicinal plants (Pieroni et al., 2002).

It seems to be difficult, however, to provide an unambiguous definition of either food or medicine. According to Moerman (1996), foods can be understood by observing the behavior "eating or drinking," whereas "medicine" refers to the intention with which the plant

The present research was funded by the Institute for the Promotion of Innovation through Science and Technology in Flanders (IWT), Belgium, by means of a postdoctoral grant to Ina Vandebroek. The authors thank the traditional healers and community members from Apillapampa and the local NGO Fepade for logistic support. The Centro de Biodiversidad y Genética from the Universidad Mayor de San Simón, Cochabamba, was the local counterpart during execution of the project.

273

is used. Hence, a person consuming a plant with the intent to relieve a stomachache is medicating, not eating. However, at the same time, the species being consumed may have a nutritional value, as is the case with passion fruit (*Passiflora* spp.): its fruits are eaten but can also be consumed to treat hepatic colic, as will be discussed.

The top five plant families in terms of medicinal species are the Asteraceae, Apiaceae, Ericaceae, Rosaceae, and Ranunculaceae (Moerman, 1996). These families contain more medicinal species than would be predicted by chance (based on their relative sizes; for instance, the Asteraceae is a very large family containing many species). The plant families with the fewest medicinal species are the Fabaceae, Cyperaceae, and Poaceae. The five most important families in terms of species people use for food are Liliaceae, Rosaceae, Ericaceae, Apiaceae, and Chenopodiaceae; the least important families are Rubiaceae, Scrophulariaceae, and Cyperaceae. Hence, the Asteraceae family has little overlap of food and medicinal species, but the overlap is large in Rosaceae and Ericaceae. The Scrophulariaceae, Rubiaceae, and Cyperaceae are underutilized for food as well as for medicines, whereas the Fabaceae and Poaceae tend to be underutilized as medicines (Moerman, 1996).

In this chapter, we report on the food aspects of medicinal plants used by Quechua healers from the Bolivian Andes. During interviews the healers were asked to report "other uses" for each medicinal plant species. They spontaneously named food applications several times. This allowed us to explore the gray area of multipurpose medicinal and food plants.

STUDY AREA

Apillapampa is situated in the Cochabamba Department, Capinota Province, at an altitude of 3,250 m, 17° 51'S (latitude) and 66° 15'E (longitude). At the nearby village of Capinota, which is at a lower altitude (2,380 m) the mean annual temperature is 18°C and the mean annual precipitation is 524 mm. In Apillapampa, the temperatures are lower and the precipitation greater, due to the higher altitude.

We collected medicinal plants at altitudes ranging from 2,800 to 3,900 m. In this range there are two ecological units: the *prepuna* (from 2,000-2,300 to 3,100-3,300 m) and the *puna* (from 3,100-3,300 to 3,900-4,000 m). The prepuna is a transitional zone, considered to be the upper part of the dry inter-Andean valleys in the broadest sense. The true valleys are below about 2,000 m (Navarro and Maldonado, 2002). For a more detailed description of the vegetation of the research area, see Vandebroek and colleagues (2004). Briefly, the vegetation has undergone significant human disturbance and is therefore mainly secondary. It is characterized by shrubs of various heights *(chaparrales* and *matorrales)* and grasses. In the prepuna part, the climax vegetation (free of anthropogenic disturbance) is *Kageneckia lanceolata* Ruiz & Pav. and *Schinus molle* L. On soils with a high degree of erosion the vegetation is *Dodonea viscose* Jacq. and *Baccharis dracunculifolia* D.C. *(matorrales* of 1 to 2 m). In the puna, the study area has a climax vegetation of *Polylepis besseri* Hieron. and *Berberis commutata* Eichler and a degraded vegetation of grassland.

ETHNOGRAPHIC DATA

Apillapampa is a community of around 2,500 Quechua-speaking inhabitants (430 families) who have been living in villagelike settlements (ex-haciendas) since the colonial period (Fepade, 1998). The population is agrarian and keeps livestock (sheep, goats, cows). Most people grow crops without irrigation and adapt their farming to the altitudinal zonation. The principal crops are wheat, potato, and maize. They are cultivated mainly for home consumption. One quarter of the produce is sold. Livestock are considered a source of savings and their dung is used as fertilizer. When harvests are poor, meat is used as source of protein (Fepade, 1998). The constraints to crop production are severe erosion (resulting in degraded soils) and a low ratio of cropland to grassland and nonarable land (Fepade, 1998). In order to improve the weak economic situation, there is constant and dynamic out-migration, essentially of men. The result is a sharp increase in the labor pressure on the women who are left behind (Fepade, 1998). Consequently, some traditional tillage practices are abandoned, which aggravates the decreases in yield. This in turn may contribute to a poor diet and hence increase susceptibility to disease.

In spite of the permanent loss of cultural values and practices worldwide (Cox, 2000) and in the present study area (Fepade, 1998), in Apillapampa there is still a tradition of collective behavior, called *ayni:* members of the community collaborate to build houses, harvest crops, and repair roads. Rituals such as *k'owa,* the worshipping of Mother Earth *(Pachamama),* are still part of daily life. Another important aspect of culture that has been maintained is traditional medicine. Traditional healers or medicine men, called *naturistas* or *curanderos* depending on their hierarchical level, are closely related to community members and are regarded as advisers. They are usually the first persons to be consulted about health, family, livestock, crops, and travel (Fepade, 1998). Eight traditional healers of Apillapampa are united in a semiformal organization, called *AMETRAC (Asociación de Médicos Traditionales),* which was founded in 1994. Health care is also provided by a primary health care service that is operated on weekdays by a bilingual (Spanish, Quechua) nurse and a medical doctor from outside the community.

METHODOLOGY

Agreements and Permits

Before the start of research, meetings were held with members of AMETRAC, during which the project was presented and the objectives discussed. AMETRAC's approval was formalized in a written agreement. Thereafter, a permit for fieldwork was obtained from the Bolivian Ministry of Sustainable Development and Planning in La Paz (General Directory of Biodiversity).

Fieldwork

Medicinal plant species were collected during field trips with traditional healers in the dry (July to October 2000) and rainy (January to April 2001) seasons. Four to five voucher specimens of each species were collected for botanical identification. Subsequently, GPS (Garmin 12XL) coordinates and altitude (Thomming) measurements were taken. Plant characteristics were photographed (Minolta 600si Classic with 28-80 mm zoom lens) and noted, together with the ecological conditions of the collection site. Voucher specimens were pressed, dried, and identified at a later stage according to standard herbarium procedures in the *Herbario Nacional Forestal Martin Cárdenas* in Cochabamba, in which they have been deposited, and the *Herbario Nacional de Bolivia* in La Paz. Upon return from the plant collection trips, semistructured interviewing was conducted in the primary health care service of the community with each of eight traditional healers (the healers' background is described in Vandebroek et al., 2004). During the interviews, the drying plant specimens were shown to each interviewee to stimulate answers. The healers were asked about local plant names, the precise use of the species as a remedy to treat named illness(es), the plant parts used, the mode of application, the dosage and treatment regime, the restrictions on use (for pregnant women and children), other uses (all categories, including food, forage, firewood, construction material and working tools, ornamental, ritual, coloring agent), the plant habitat, the perceived abundance, and plant ecology.

RESULTS AND DISCUSSION

In total, 180 medicinal plants were collected during the research. About a quarter (23 percent) of these species are also used as food, to supplement the regular diet. Table 12.1 shows the species with food applications and also the uses other than for medicine or consumption.

Fifteen percent of all species collected have no other use besides their medicinal application. Among the other uses frequently mentioned for medicinal plants are firewood and forage. The minor uses reported are coloring agent, raw material for tools, construction material, ornamental, handicrafts, and use in rituals.

Table 12.2 shows the proportion of species per plant family that are used both as food and as medicine, in relation to the total number of medicinal species collected from that family. Only data on the most abundant families in the sample are shown (Asteraceae, Fabaceae, Solanaceae, and Lamiaceae). The table shows a substantial overlap of medicinal and food plants in the Lamiaceae and Fabaceae species. Five of the nine Lamiaceae species collected have overlapping uses, in comparison with 29 percent of the Fabaceae, 17 percent of the Asteraceae, and 8 percent of the Solanaceae. As has been pointed out in the literature, the Fabaceae contains a fair number of food species and the Lamiaceae produces a wide range of aromatic volatile oils, including menthol and thymol, which are appreciated by local peo-

TABLE 12.1. Food uses and other applications of medicinal plant species collected in Apillapampa, Cochabamba Department (*N* = 43 species).

Voucher number	Local name	Plant family	Scientific name	Nonmedicinal uses	Plant part used for medicinal purposes
IV89	Khuchi kuruta	Alstroemeriaceae	*Alstroemeria pygmaea* Herb.	Food (tubers eaten), forage	—
IV46	Yuyu/jatago (w)	Amaranthaceae	*Amaranthus hybridus* L.	Food (leaves eaten as spinach), forage	Leaves, seeds
IV35	Molle	Anacardiaceae	*Schinus molle* L.	Food (refreshing beverage, alcoholic beverage from fruits), firewood, construction wood	Branches, leaves
JBC49	Jamaskia	Asteraceae	*Baccharis torricoi* spec. ined.	Food (lejia), forage, coloring agent	Aerial parts
ET11	Kuti, chiñi michi michi	Asteraceae	*Chuquiraga parviflora* (Griseb.) Hieron.	Food (coffee), firewood, forage	Branches, flowers, leaves
JBC53	Chiñi t'ola, k'itachiñi t'ola	Asteraceae	*Helogyne straminea* (D.C.) B.L. ROB	Food (lejia), firewood, forage	Branches
IV66	Leche leche (w)	Asteraceae	*Sonchus asper* (L.) Hill	Food (leaves eaten in salads)	Whole plant, exudate, leaves, roots
IV5	Leche leche (w)	Asteraceae	*Sonchus oleraceus* L.	Food (leaves eaten in salads), forage	Whole plant, exudate, leaves
IV147	Kuru suyko (w)	Asteraceae	*Tagetes minuta* L.	Food (condiment), forage	Flowers, leaves
IV7	Suyko (w)	Asteraceae	*Tagetes multiflora* Kunth	Food (condiment)	Whole plant, branches, roots

Code	Local name	Family	Scientific name	Use	Parts used
IV138	Anis anis, k'ita anis (w)	Asteraceae	*Tagetes pusilla* H.B. & K.	Food (alcoholic beverage, condiment, flavored tea), forage	Whole plant, aerial parts, flowers, leaves
IV106	Graniso t'ika	Begoniaceae	*Begonia baumannii* Lemoine	Food (tubers used for preparation of cheese), forage, ritual (brings rain)	Whole plant, roots
IV79	Nina nina	Berberidaceae	*Berberis boliviana* Lechler	Food (sweet fruits eaten), forage	Branches
JBC17	Churisik'e	Berberidaceae	*Berberis commutata* Eichler	Food (fruits eaten), coloring agent, firewood	Branches, flowers, leaves, spines
IV6	Mostaza (w)	Brassicaceae	*Brassica rapa* L.	Food (roots eaten), forage	Flowers, leaves, roots
IV128	Isikira, tisikira, sitikira	Cactaceae	*Cleistocactus buchtienii* Backeb.	Food (fruits eaten, lejia), forage	Spines; juice from stem
IV88	Waraqo	Cactaceae	*Echinopsis obrepanda* (Salm-Dyck) K. Schum. Var. calorubra	Food (fruits eaten), forage	Juice from stem, roots
JBC33	Tuna (c)	Cactaceae	*Opuntia ficus-indica* (L.) Mill.	Food (fruits eaten, alcoholic beverage, jam), fodder	Stem (pads)
IV129	Ulala	Cactaceae	*Trichocereus tunariensis* Cárdenis	Food (fruits eaten), forage (spines removed)	Spines; juice from stem
IV24	Sano sano	Ephedraceae	*Ephedra americana* Humb. & Bonpl. ex Willd.	Food (coffee), forage, firewood	Whole plant, branches, flowers, leaves, roots, seeds

TABLE 12.1. *(continued)*

Voucher number	Local name	Plant family	Scientific name	Nonmedicinal uses	Plant part used for medicinal purposes
JBC18	Tarwi (c)	Fabaceae	*Lupinus mutabilis* L.	Food (fruits eaten cooked and rinsed), forage	Whole plant, flowers, leaves, fruits
IV61	Alfa, alfa alfa (c)	Fabaceae	*Medicago sativa* L.	Food (sauce, leaves eaten in salads), fodder	Branches, flowers, leaves, shoots
IV15	K'ita alfa, trebol amarillo (w)	Fabaceae	*Melilotus indicus* (L.) All.	Food (leaves eaten in salads), forage	Whole plant, branches, flowers, leaves
IV13	Thaqo	Fabaceae	*Prosopis laevigata* (Humb. & Bonpl. ex Willd.) M.C. Johnst.	Food (fruits eaten, refreshing beverage), firewood, forage	Whole plant, leaves, stems, fruits, seeds
IV48	Janukara/aujilla (w)	Geraniaceae	*Erodium cicutarium* (L.) L'Her. Ex Aiton	Food (leaves eaten in salads), forage	Whole plant, roots, leaves
IV90	Chiñi oregano, pampa oregano	Lamiaceae	*Hedeoma* cf. *mandoniana* Wedd.	Food (condiment), forage	Whole plant
JBC39	Aya muña	Lamiaceae	*Minthostachys andina* (Britton ex Rusby) Epling	Food (flavored tea, refreshing beverage, condiment), forage	Whole plant, branches, flowers, leaves
JBC60	Chumu chumu	Lamiaceae	*Salvia haenkei* Benth.	Food (tea from sweet flowers), firewood, forage	Whole plant, branches, flowers, leaves
IV135	Chumu chumu rosado	Lamiaceae	*Salvia orbignaei* Benth.	Food (tea from sweet flowers), forage, firewood	Branches, flowers, leaves
IV31	Chiñi muña	Lamiaceae	*Satureja boliviana* (Benth.) Briq.	Food (condiment)	Whole plant, branches, flowers, leaves

Code	Local name	Family	Scientific name	Use	Parts used
JBC6	Chiñi jamillo	Loranthaceae	*Ligaria cuneifolia* (Ruiz & Pav.)	Food (lejia)	Flowers, leaves
ET8	Llave	Loranthaceae	*Tripodanthus acutifolius* (Ruiz & Pav.) Tiegh	Food (flavored tea, alcoholic beverage), firewood, forage, ornamental	Branches, flowers, leaves
IV91	Awayunku	Oxalidaceae	*Oxalis eriolepis* Wedd.	Food (sweet tubers eaten)	–
IV98	Awayunku	Oxalidaceae	*Oxalis pinguiculacea* R. Knuth	Food (stems used to make cheese, sweet tubers eaten)	–
ET39	Tumbo (c)	Passifloraceae	*Passiflora mollissima* (Kunth) Bailey	Food (fruits eaten, alcoholic beverage from fruits), forage	Fruits, flowers
JBC38	Locoste (c)	Passifloraceae	*Passiflora umbilicata* (Griseb.) Harms	Food (fruits eaten)	Leaves
JBC23	Durasno (c)	Rosaceae	*Prunus persica* (L.) Batsch	Food (fruits eaten), firewood, construction wood	Buds with leaves, flowers
JBC32	Roda (c)	Rutaceae	*Ruta graveolens* L.	Food (condiment)	Whole plant, aerial parts, branches, flowers, leaves, roots
JBC46	Chiri molle	Rutaceae	*Zanthoxylum coco* Gillies ex Hook. F. & Arn.	Food (coffee), firewood, forage	Branches, flowers, leaves, fruits
IV154	Pampa chumu chumu	Scrophulariaceae	*Castilleja pumila* (Benth.) Wedd.	Food (sweet flowers sucked), forage	Whole plant

281

TABLE 12.1. (continued)

Voucher number	Local name	Plant family	Scientific name	Nonmedicinal uses	Plant part used for medicinal purposes
IV93	Okururo	Scrophulariaceae	Mimulus glabratus H.B.K.	Food (leaves eaten in salads), forage	Whole plant, leaves
IV73	Chuli chuli	Solanaceae	Salpichroa tristis Miers var. tristis	Food (sour fruits eaten), forage, firewood	Fruits
IV133	K'ita uva (w)	Verbenaceae	Lantana fiebrigii Hayek	Food (sweet fruits eaten), firewood	Branches
IV59	Verbena (w)	Verbenaceae	Verbena hispida Ruiz & Pav.	Food (refreshing beverage from flowers), forage	Whole plant, flowers

Note: (w) indicates weed species growing in agricultural fields; (c) indicates cultivated species.

TABLE 12.2. Percentage of species collected per family that are used both as a medicine and as a food.

Family	Total number of species collected	Number of species used as both medicine and food
Lamiaceae	9	5 (56%)
Fabaceae	14	4 (29%)
Asteraceae	42	7 (17%)
Solanaceae	12	1 (8%)

Note: Only the four most abundant families are shown in relation to the family size (total number of species collected).

ples for their therapeutic value as well as for their culinary use as condiments and aromatic teas. The Asteraceae, however, is a very large family in which food plants are underrepresented by comparison with medicinal plants. Finally, the Solanaceae contain a variety of quite toxic species, which might restrict their use as foods (Moerman, 1996).

Medicinal Foods: Food Plants with Medicinal Value

Several species collected during the study are cultivated food plants. Most of these are cultivated for their fruits, such as *Opuntia ficus-indica* (L.) Mill., *Prunus persica* (L.) Batsch, *Passiflora umbilicata* (Griseb.) Harms, and *Passiflora mollissima* (Kunth) Bailey. *Lupinus mutabilis* L. is a native crop of the Central Andes, cultivated as a pulse. It was an important crop in pre-Columbian times that lost its importance after the arrival of the Spanish. Its seeds contain a toxic alkaloid, so special treatment is needed to extract this chemical before the seeds are safe to eat. The treatment entails boiling the seeds and then washing them for several days in running water.

Ruta graveolens L. is also cultivated. Its leaves are used as a condiment in meals, although several informants stated that the species has a bad odor. Therefore, we suspect that it is primarily cultivated for its use as a medicine, as is the case in Catalonia (Agelet et al., 2000). Several species collected during our research are used to feed livestock: *Medicago sativa* L. is cultivated as fodder, and after their spines have been removed the cultivated *Opuntia ficus-indica* and wild Cactaceae (*Cleistocactus buchtienii* Backeb., *Trichocereus tunariensis* Cárdenas) are also fed to animals.

Food Medicines: Medicinal Species with Food Applications

Weeds Used As Medicines and Foods

Several weed species that grow in agricultural fields are eaten. Many are introduced species, such as *Sonchus asper* (L.) Hill, *Sonchus oleraceus* L., *Melilotus indicus* (L.) All., *Erodium cicutarium* (L.) L'her. ex Aiton, and *Brassica rapa* L. The leaves of these species are eaten raw in salads. According to our informants, the root of *Brassica rapa* contains vitamin C and is considered a famine food "when there are no vegetables on the land." In Patagonia, it is the leaves, not the root, of *Brassica rapa* that are eaten raw in salads or cooked (Ladio, 2001), while in Italy and Mexico its leaves, the young stems, and flowering tops are boiled and fried (Pieroni et al., 2002; Vieyra-Odilon and Vibrans, 2001). The literature confirms consumption of the cooked leaves of *Erodium cicutarium* (Patagonia), and of the raw or cooked leaves of *Sonchus asper* and *S. oleraceus* (Italy, Mexico) (Casas et al., 2001; Ladio, 2001; Pieroni, 2000; Pieroni et al., 2002). *Sonchus oleraceus* and *S. asper* leaves have a high concentration of nutrients, which accounts for their value as food (Guil-Guerrero et al., 1998).

Some weedy native species are also eaten, such as *Amaranthus hybridus* L., whose leaves are cooked and eaten as spinach is. According to our informants, the leaves must be cooked before the plant is flowering and are considered a source of vitamin C. They declared that this species does not grow in poor soils. *Amaranthus hybridus* is better known as a vegetable than as a medicinal plant in Peru, where it is a wild species that is sometimes cultivated for its leaves (Roersch, 1994). It is also used as a food and medicine in Mexico (Casas et al., 2001; Vieyra-Odilon and Vibrans, 2001). Other native species that are found in agricultural fields are *Tagetes pusilla* H.B. & K. and *T. multiflora* Kunth. At higher altitudes *Tagetes minuta* L. can be found. The leaves of these three species are used as a condiment in soups and main dishes. *T. minuta* is sometimes cultivated in Peru for its use as a condiment (Roersch, 1994) and in Catalonian home gardens for its medicinal use as a digestive (Agelet et al., 2000). One informant stated that flowers from the weed *Verbena hispida* Ruiz & Pav. are used to prepare a refreshing drink, but this use was not confirmed by other informants.

Modes of Consumption

Some species are consumed directly after the edible part has been cleaned, while others undergo further preparation. Direct consumption includes eating the leaves in salads, consuming the fresh fruits or raw roots or tubers, sucking the flowers because of their sweet taste, or using the plant part as a condiment in soups or main dishes. Alternatively, plant parts may be processed before consumption: boiled or braised (in the case of leafy vegetables); infused (for refreshing beverages, flavored teas, alcoholic beverages, or coffee substitutes); made into jam; used in cheese making; and burnt to make *lejía* (plant ash, which is chewed together with coca leaves).

Leaves Are Eaten Raw in Salads or Used in a Sauce

Weedy vegetables, as well as the marsh species *Mimulus glabratus* H.B.K and the cultivated *Medicago sativa,* are eaten raw in salads that are often dressed with oil. The leaves of *Mimulus glabratus* (see Figure 12.1) are also eaten raw in salads in another high-altitude area in Bolivia (Pestalozzi, 1998), in Patagonia (Ladio, 2001), and in Peru. In the latter country, the species is described as a "health-promoting food eaten in salads" (Roersch, 1994). Not only the leaves but also the shoots of *Medicago sativa* are eaten. The species is considered a source of vitamins by informants and also in the literature (Roersch, 1994). Its leaves, as well as the leaves of *Mimulus glabratus,* are also processed separately in a sauce that is useful to clean the abdomen. Consumption of the leaves of *Medicago sativa* is a remedy to treat gastritis. The weedy species *Melilotus indicus* and *Erodium cicutarium* are eaten to alleviate kidney problems.

Condiment in Soups, Salads, or Bread

The plant species used as a condiment have aromatic properties. Those on our list belong to the mint family (Lamiaceae) or sunflower family (Asteraceae); *Ruta graveolens* from the Rutaceae is also used

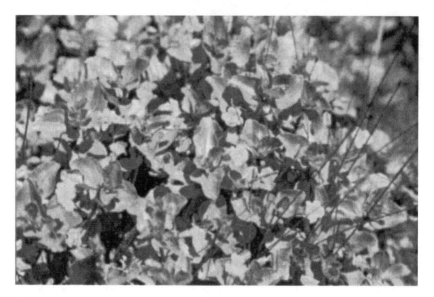

FIGURE 12.1. *Mimulus glabratus* H.B.K. (Scrophulariaceae), a marsh plant that is eaten raw in salads.

as a flavoring agent in soups or main dishes. The three plants collected from the mint family belong to three different genera: *Satureja boliviana* (Benth.) Briq., *Minthostachys andina* (Britton ex Rusby) Epling, and *Hedeoma* cf. *mandoniana* Wedd. (see Figure 12.2). Nevertheless, they all have the same local generic name *muña*, which probably reflects their similarity in taste and smell. Three members from the sunflower family that are also used as a condiment, *Tagetes minuta, T. pusilla,* and *T. multiflora,* share the same scientific genus name. However, one of them, *T. pusilla,* bears the local name *k'ita anis,* while the others are named *suyko.* Here again, the determining characteristic is the smell. *K'ita anis* has a smell that is similar to anise but different from the two other *Tagetes* species, which is why it was given a different local name. The term *k'ita* reflects its wild status. It is not cultivated.

Edible Fruits and Roots, Sweet Treats, and Jam

The plants providing edible fruits are often cultivated and have already been mentioned. However, the fruits of wild species are also

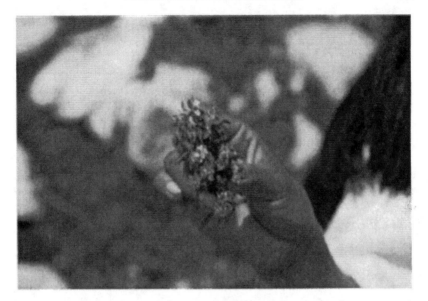

FIGURE 12.2. *Hedeoma* cf. *mandoniana* Wedd. (Lamiaceae), an aromatic species that is used as a condiment in main dishes.

consumed. Among these are Cactaceae fruits [*Echinopsis obrepanda* (Salm-Dyck) K. Schum. Var. calorubra, *Cleistocactus buchtienii* Backeb., *Trichocereus tunariensis* Cárdenas], fruits of Berberidaceae *(Berberis commutata* Eichler, *Berberis boliviana),* the sour fruits of *Salpichroa tristis* (Miers) A.T. Hunziker (Solanaceae), the dark purple fruits of *Lantana fiebrigii* Hayek (Verbenaceae), and the pods from the small Andean tree *Prosopis laevigata* (Humb. & Bonpl. ex Willd.) M.C. Johnst. (Fabaceae). Informants indicated that it is usually children who eat the fruits from wild plant species. In Patagonia, the fruits from *Berberis heterophylla* Juss. are eaten raw or processed (Ladio, 2001). In the Bolivian highlands, the mature sweet and sour fruit of *Salpichroa glandulosa* (Hook.) Miers, which has a taste comparable to that of grapes, is peeled and eaten raw (Pestalozzi, 1998). In Peru, too, the fruits of different species of the genus *Salpichroa* are eaten (Roersch, 1994). Finally, *Prosopis laevigata* is used both as an edible and as a medicinal species in Mexico (Casas et al., 2001).

The tubers of *Oxalis eriolepis* Wedd., *Oxalis pinguiculacea* R. Knuth (Oxalidaceae) and *Alstroemeria pygmaea* Herb. (Alstroemeriaceae) are sweet and are eaten raw. According to informants, the tubers of *Oxalis* spp. are sweeter than those of *Alstroemeria pygmaea*. In Mexico, *Oxalis* spp. are considered edible, although it was not stated whether the tuber is used (Casas et al., 2001). Although according to our informants *Oxalis eriolepis* has no medicinal use, its leaves are chewed in Peru to treat flu and gingivitis, while a tea made from the whole plant is drunk to relieve stomachache (Roersch, 1994). In Patagonia, the rhizome of *Alstroemeria patagonica* Phillipi is eaten raw or cooked (Ladio, 2001).

Nectar from the flower tube of *Castilleja pumila* (Benth.) Wedd. (Scrophulariaceae) is sucked by children as a sweet treat. This use has been confirmed in another Andean community in Bolivia (Pestalozzi, 1998). Jam is made from one species only: the fruits of *Opuntia ficus-indica*.

Refreshing Beverages, Flavored Teas, Substitutes for Coffee, and Alcoholic Beverages

Castilleja pumila (Scrophulariaceae) has a sweet taste and is locally named *pampa chumu chumu*. Two other species (*Salvia haenkei* Benth. and *Salvia orbignaei* Benth.) have the local generic name *chumu chumu*, although they belong to the Lamiaceae instead of the Scrophulariaceae (see Figure 12.3). The flowers of these latter species are also appreciated for their sweet taste and are used to prepare a tea that is drunk during meals. The similarity in taste may be the basis for their shared local name. A tea can also be prepared from an aromatic species such as *Tripodanthus acutifolius* (Ruiz & Pav.) Tiegh (Loranthaceae). This species has a rich flavor according to informants and hence is drunk in tea or in an alcoholic beverage made from its leaves. Alcoholic beverages are also prepared from fruits of *Passiflora mollissima*, *Opuntia ficus-indica*, and *Schinus molle* L. (Anacardiaceae). *Schinus molle* is a typical resinous tree from the Andes. Its fruits are sweet and are mixed with water to prepare a refreshing drink. An alcoholic beverage prepared from the fruits is called *chicha de molle*. In ancient Peru, *Schinus molle* was cultivated for its fruits to prepare *chicha*. However, when consumed in excessive quantities the fruits are toxic (Roersch, 1994). In Mexico, *Schinus molle* is used as an edible as well as a medicinal species (Casas et al., 2001). Finally, three species from different families collected in Apillapampa are "drunk as coffee," according to informants. These

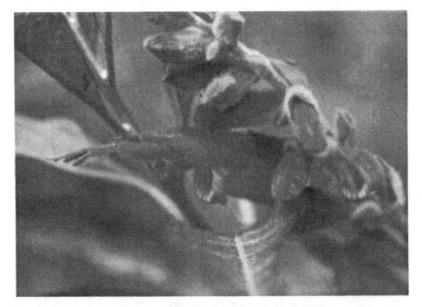

FIGURE 12.3. *Salvia haenkei* Benth. (Lamiaceae). The sweet flowers of this species are used to prepare a warm beverage.

are *Ephedra americana* Humb. and Bonpl. ex Willd (Ephedraceae), *Zanthoxylum coco* Gillies ex Hook. f. & Arn. (Rutaceae), and *Chuquiraga parviflora* (Griseb.) Hieron. (Asteraceae). In another high-altitude community in Bolivia, *Ephedra* cf. *rupestris* Benth. is boiled in water to make a pleasant-tasting red drink (Pestalozzi, 1998).

Ingredients to Make Cheese

One popular use mentioned by all informants is the use of the tubers of *Begonia baumannii* Lemoine (Begoniaceae) for the preparation of cheese. For this, the tubers are washed, chopped, and then put in the milk to make it curdle. Subsequently, the tubers are removed and the milk is further processed into cheese. According to informants, it is the juice from the tubers that is important in this preparation because it has a sour taste like lemon. Another species used to curdle milk, though less often than *Begonia baumannii* (see Figure 12.4), is *Oxalis pinguiculacea*. Again, the juice of its stems has a sour taste and is used to prepare cheese. In Patagonia, the leaves of

Oxalis adenophylla Gill. ex Hook & Arn. are used as lemon substitutes to make juices (Ladio, 2001). In Peru, the local name for *Oxalis* spp. is *chupo,* which probably derives from *chupar* and indicates the use of the plant, since children like to suck its stems (Roersch, 1994).

Plant Ash Chewed Together with Coca (Erythroxylum coca) *Leaves*

Coca insalivation is still widely practiced in contemporary Bolivia as a means to maintain a high working pace without getting tired or to make long journeys on foot without becoming hungry or thirsty. Often, coca leaves are chewed together with plant ash, or *lejía,* or in more urban settings with sodium bicarbonate ($NaHCO_3$) of commercial origin. Plant ash consists of alkaline substances. When chewed together with coca leaf, these substances are primarily responsible for the transformation of alkaloids to free bases, which allows a better extraction of these plant alkaloids and hence enhances the physiolog-

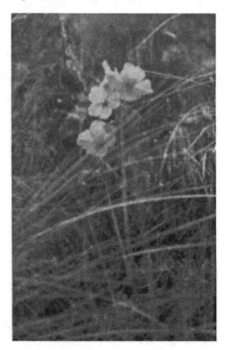

FIGURE 12.4. *Begonia baumannii* Lemoine (Begoniaceae). The tuber of this species contains a sour juice that serves to curdle milk.

ical effect of *Erythroxylum coca* (Hilgert et al., 2001). In Apilla-pampa, *lejía* is prepared from three species, *Cleistocactus buchtienii* Backeb. (Cactaceae), *Ligaria cuneifolia* Ruiz & Pav. (Loranthaceae), and *Baccharis torricoi* spec. ined. (Asteraceae). The stem (trunk) of *Cleistocactus buchtienii* Backeb. is first dried and then converted into ash. In Argentina, the species used to provide ash for coca insali-vation are different. They belong to the Asteraceae (two species), Amaranthaceae (two species), and Poaceae (one species) (Hilgert et al., 2001).

Correspondence Between Plant Parts Used for Medicine and Food

Table 12.1 shows which plant parts from each species are used for medicinal and food purposes. They have been grouped into the fol-lowing categories to allow a better comparison between food and me-dicinal uses: (1) whole plant, (2) aerial part, (3) fruit, (4) root, and (5) unknown. The aerial part includes the bark, branches, leaves, flowers, or spines, and excludes any part of the fruit. For the majority (69 per-cent) of the species in Table 12.1, the same plant part is used for both food and medicinal applications. Table 12.3 shows the proportion of plant parts used within the categories of medicine or food. In nearly all (90 percent) of the 40 species considered in this table, the aerial part is used for medicinal applications; the next most important cate-gory is the whole plant (45 percent of species). For food applications, the aerial part is also predominantly used (53 percent of species), fol-lowed by fruits (35 percent of species). Data from native North Americans show that medicinal uses are associated with aerial parts; and, to a lesser extent, with roots and the whole plant, while fruits (and to a lesser extent aerial parts) are primarily used for food applications (Moerman, 1996).

Along the Food-Medicine Continuum

At the far left of the food-medicine continuum are plant species primarily used as foods in Apillapampa, with no reported medicinal applications. These are *Alstroemeria pygmaea, Oxalis pinguicula-cea,* and *Oxalis eriolepis.* The roots of these plants are eaten raw. The latter two species were collected during field trips with healers to

TABLE 12.3. Proportion of plant parts of the 40 species used for food and/or medicine, expressed as percentages.

Plant part	% used for food	% used for medicine
Whole plant	3	45
Aerial part[a]	53	90
Fruit	35	18
Root	5	20
Unknown	10	0
Total[b]	106	173

[a]Aerial part includes bark, branches, leaves, flowers or spines, but excludes any part of the fruit

[b]The totals exceed 100 percent because often different parts of the same species are used (total number of species on which the calculation is based is 40).

inventorize the medicinal plants from Apillapampa, but during subsequent interview sessions in the village the healers stated unanimously that these species were only eaten for their sweet tubers. The far right of the continuum is made up of "pure" medicinal plants with no reported food applications in Apillapampa. These constitute 77 percent of all medicinal species collected in the present study. In-between is a gray area of medicinal foods and food medicines.

Passiflora mollissima provides a good example of a medicinal food, since its fruits are eaten and drunk in juices or processed in an alcoholic beverage, while its juice is also used to treat hepatic colic and to alleviate the effects of a hangover. Examples of food medicines are *Melilotus indicus* and *Erodium cicutarium:* their leaves are eaten raw as a salad, with the addition of oil, to treat kidney problems. The leaves of *Medicago sativa* are also eaten in a salad to treat gastritis. In these cases, the food use of a plant cannot be separated from its medicinal action. Actually, it is the *mode* of usage that can blur the borders between a food and a medicinal plant, since plants that are eaten directly or drunk as a juice may be considered a food or a food-medicine. Aromatic plants used as a condiment in dishes represent another interesting group. Although they may not be deliberately used for their medicinal value, their presence in the often-heavy meals may be more than just culinary, since they also increase the digestibility of these meals. Furthermore, their positive effect on the digestive system is confirmed by their explicit medicinal use as a carminative to relieve pain and swelling of the abdomen, liver problems, vomiting, and hepatic colic (our findings and Roersch, 1994).

Medicinal Plant Uses As Food Reported in the Literature

When reviewing the literature, not only were we able to confirm the majority of our own results on food applications of medicinal plants, but we also came across food uses of medicinal plants from our inventory that were not reported in Apillapampa. For example, the small tubers of *Solanum acaule* Bitter are eaten in Peru (Roersch, 1994). In Mexico, *Anoda cristata* (L.) Schltdl is eaten (Rendón et al., 2001), while *Malva parviflora* L. and *Polygonum aviculare* L. are ingredients for a green chili sauce and *Chenopodium ambrosioides* L. is used as a condiment (Vieyra-Odilon and Vibrans, 2001). The nectar of the flowers of *Mutisia orbignyana* Wedd. is sucked by children in Bolivia (Pestalozzi, 1998). *Dianthus caryophyllus* L., *Chenopodium ambrosioides,* and *Plantago lanceolata* L. are used to prepare homemade liquors in Catalonia (Bonet and Vallès, 2002). In Patagonia and Italy, the leaves and aerial parts of *Stellaria media* (L.) Vill. are eaten raw in salads or cooked in soups (Ladio, 2001). Also in Italy, the young whorls of *Capsella bursa-pastoris* (L.) Medik. are boiled and fried, while the leaves of *Plantago lanceolata* are boiled and mixed with other greens in soups (Pieroni, 2000; Pieroni et al., 2002). It is interesting that all these species, except *Mutisia orbignyana,* are weeds on agricultural fields and that most have been introduced into Bolivia. These additional food applications increase the food potential of our medicinal inventory from 23 to 28 percent. Although we do not claim that our medicinal inventory is complete, this percentage is similar to others reported in the literature. In the culturally important plant flora of Native North America, for example, 29 percent of the utilized species are used as both foods and drugs (Moerman, 1996). In rural Hausaland in Nigeria, 26 percent of local semiwild plant species in the pharmacopoeia also serve dietary needs (Etkin, 2002).

CONCLUSION

Four main findings came from our research. First, the food uses of medicinal plants reported in Apillapampa agree with literature data from Bolivia, Peru, Patagonia, Mexico, Catalonia, and Italy. Second, as eleven of 43 species with overlapping food and medicinal uses are weeds on agricultural fields and seven species are cultivated, the wild food/medicinal species account for 58 percent. Third, the ranking of families according to the proportion of overlapping medicinal and food applications (in relation to the total number of collected medicinal plants) is Lamiaceae > Fabaceae > Asteraceae > Solanaceae. Finally, the aerial plant parts (bark, branches, leaves, flowers, or spines) are used most frequently for food applications, as well as for medicinal uses. However, use of fruits ranks second for food purposes, while use of the whole plant ranks second for medicinal applications.

REFERENCES

Agelet, A., M.A. Bonet, and J. Vallès (2000). Homegardens and their role as a main source of medicinal plants in mountain regions of Catalonia (Iberian Peninsula). *Economic Botany* 54 (3): 295-309.

Bennett, B.C. and G.T. Prance (2000). Introduced plants in the indigenous pharmacopoeia of northern South America. *Economic Botany* 54 (1): 90-102.

Bonet, M.A. and J. Vallès (2002). Use of non-crop food vascular plants in Montseny biosphere reserve (Catalonia, Iberian Peninsula). *International Journal of Food Sciences and Nutrition* 53: 225-248.

Casas, A., A. Valiente-Banuet, J.L. Viveros, J. Caballero, L. Cortés, P. Dávila, R. Lira, and I. Rodríguez (2001). Plant resources of the Tehuacán-Cuicatlán Valley, Mexico. *Economic Botany* 55 (1): 129-166.

Cox, P.A. (2000). Will tribal knowledge survive the millennium? *Science* 287: 44-45.

Etkin, N.L. (2002). Local knowledge of biotic diversity and its conservation in rural Hausaland, Northern Nigeria. *Economic Botany* 56 (1): 73-88.

Fepade (Fundación Ecuménica Para el Desarrollo) (1998). *Diagnostico del distrito Apillapampa.* Cochabamba, Bolivia: Fepade.

Guil-Guerrero, J.L., A. Giménez-Giménez, I. Rodríguez-García, and M.E. Torija-Isasa (1998). Nutritional composition of Sonchus species (*S. asper* L., *S. oleraceus* L. and *S. tenerrimus* L.). *Journal of the Science of Food and Agriculture* 76: 628-632.

Hilgert, N., S. Reyes, and G. Schmeda-Hirschmann (2001). Alkaline substances used with coca (*Erythroxylum coca,* Erythroxylaceae) leaf insalivation in northwestern Argentina. *Economic Botany* 55 (2): 325-329.

Ladio, A.H. (2001). The maintenance of wild edible plant gathering in a Mapuche community of Patagonia. *Economic Botany* 55 (2): 243-254.

Moerman, D.E. (1996). An analysis of the food plants and drug plants of native North America. *Journal of Ethnopharmacology* 52: 1-22.

Navarro, G. and M. Maldonado (Eds.) (2002). *Geografía ecológica de Bolivia. Vegetación y ambientes acuáticos.* Cochabamba, Bolivia: Centro de Ecología Simón I. Patiño-Departamento de Difusión.

Pestalozzi, H.U. (Ed.) (1998). *Flora ilustrada altoandina. La relación entre hombre, planta y medio ambiente en el Ayllu Majasaya Mujlli (Prov. Tapacarí, Departamento. Cochabamba, Bolivia).* La Paz, Bolivia: Herbario Nacional de Bolivia.

Pieroni, A. (2000). Medicinal plants and food medicines in the folk traditions of the upper Lucca Province, Italy. *Journal of Ethnopharmacology* 70: 235-273.

Pieroni, A., S. Nebel, C. Quave, H. Münz, and M. Heinrich (2002). Ethnopharmacology of *liakra:* Traditional weedy vegetables of the Arbëreshë of the Vulture area in southern Italy. *Journal of Ethnopharmacology* 81: 165-185.

Rendón, B., R. Bye, and J. Núñez-Farfán (2001). Ethnobotany of *Anoda cristata* (L.) Schl. (Malvaceae) in central Mexico: Uses, management and population differentiation in the community of Santiago Mamalhuazuca, Ozumba, State of Mexico. *Economic Botany* 55 (4): 545-554.

Roersch, C. (Ed.) (1994). *Plantas medicinales en el sur Andino del Perú.* Koenigstein: Koeltz Scientific Books.

Vandebroek, I., P. Van Damme, L. Van Puyvelde, S. Arrazola, and N. De Kimpe (2004). A comparison of traditional healers' medicinal plant knowledge in the Bolivian Andes and Amazon. *Social Science & Medicine* 59: 837-849.

Vieyra-Odilon, L. and H. Vibrans (2001). Weeds as crops: The value of maize field weeds in the valley of Toluca, Mexico. *Economic Botany* 55 (3): 426-443.

Chapter 13

Gathering of Wild Plant Foods with Medicinal Use in a Mapuche Community of Northwest Patagonia

Ana H. Ladio

INTRODUCTION

In aboriginal populations, wild plant use constitutes a distinctive manifestation of cultural identity that reflects the characteristics of local environment, the history, and the belief system of the people (Wetterstrom, 1978; Thornton, 1999; Ladio and Lozada, 2003a). In this context, the inclusion of wild plant foods in people's diets is deeply linked not only to their nutritional needs but also to the mitigation of their health problems; these needs are integrated and they cannot be easily separated, as is currently done in occidental society. It was Schultes and von Reis (1995) who suggested this aspect, indicating that in native classifications, the distinction between edible or medicinal plants is very infrequent. The study I describe here was done in a Mapuche community of Argentina. I will evaluate similarities and differences between edible and medicinal wild plant use, using distinct levels of analysis such as botanical, ecological, and socio-cultural.

In ethnobotanical studies, the most investigated level of analysis has been the species; when explaining patterns in wild plant use, little attention has been paid to botanical families and their evolutionary

This research was supported by the Consejo Nacional de Investigaciones Científicas y Técnicas (CONICET), the Universidad Nacional del Comahue of Argentina (grant 082), and the FONCYT (grant PICT 01-06429). I also wish to thank Laura Acevedo and the Hueché Foundation for their invaluable field assistance. Special gratitude is expressed to the families from Cayulef for their kind hospitality.

relationships (Gottlieb and Borin, 2002). It has been proposed that the selection of plants for food or medicine by humans has a strong chemical-taxonomical base (Gottlieb, 1982; Gottleib and Stefanello, 1991; Gottlieb et al., 1996; Gottlieb and Borin, 2002). The plant families used for food purposes are predominantly primitive in evolutionary terms, whereas the medicinal plants are from advanced families. The diversity of phytochemical compounds increases gradually with evolution (Gottlieb and Borin, 2002), and because of this, families of medicinal plants possess a more developed biosynthesising mechanism than families of food plants and, in consequence, contain a complex of toxic compounds. Hence, human recognition of the presence of these compounds should be crucial in the anthropogenically influenced evolution of plants brought about by different patterns of plant utilization.

From an ecological point of view, many studies have shown that, guided by complex processes, humans weigh the nutritional benefit (in terms of energy content) of food resources against the cost of searching, handling, and traveling to the gathering site (Gragson, 1993; Ladio and Lozada, 2000, 2001). Classically, it is hypothesized that foragers seek to maximize the net rate of energy capture while foraging (Smith, 1983). In addition, some edible plants with medicinal use contain antinutritional substances such as tannins, alkaloids, or glucosides that make them unpalatable or indigestible in large quantities (Hoffmann et al., 1992; Prendergast et al., 1998). The chemical defenses that plants use to protect themselves from herbivory provide medicinal applications for human populations (Howe and Westley, 1988; Moerman, 1996). Therefore, the selection by humans of wild plants with different uses (food, medicine, or both) could be related to maximizing energy and minimizing antinutritional sustances and could lead to differential patterns of gathering.

Finally, in terms of a sociocultural level of analysis, the use of edible and medicinal plants is principally passed on from individual to individual by social transmission (Alcorn, 1995; Gispert and Gómez Campos, 1986). People learn by doing as well as by observing others, although they also learn from personal experience and motivations such as illness situations or food shortages. In this context, since time immemorial humans have acquired their plant knowledge via experimentation, and this wisdom has been transferred to their descendants and disseminated to and among other individuals.

Nevertheless, knowledge of plants and their use variants are not equally likely to be acquired by human groups (Boesch and Tomasello, 1998). It is generally thought that the different opportunities to learn about edible and medicinal plants are closely related to age and sex roles, because the division of labor between men and women generates a physical separation of the natural world they interact in (Boster, 1985; Garro, 1986; Zent and López-Zent, 2003; Begossi et al., 2002). In this context, gender differentiation within an aboriginal population could be proposed, given that women are generally more involved in the health care of the family than are men. In contrast, knowledge of food plants seems to be equally distributed between the sexes (Ladio and Lozada, 2003b).

Many studies on aboriginal communities have shown that knowledge of wild plants increases with age (Caniago and Siebert, 1998; Benz et al., 1994, 2000; Ladio and Lozada, 2001). This relationship has been largely used to describe the processes of erosion of traditional knowledge and to find possible causes. Nevertheless, this traditional knowledge is not lost in the same way; some plant information is lost more easily, depending principally on its generality and adaptability to new situations (Brodt, 2001). For example, younger generations tend to abandon ancestral practices and refocus their interest on manufactured products. However, in poor communities, not all the wild resources are equally replaceable, especially if industrial drugs are less easily obtainable than manufactured foods. Moreover, the use of medicinal plants is associated with perceptions of the different diseases and their distinct causes (natural or supernatural) and with a perception that these ailments can be suppressed only by these traditional species and not by substitutes.

The aim of the study described here was to quantitatively compare the pattern of using wild plants with edible and medicinal properties in a rural Mapuche community by using different approaches. Five hypotheses were formulated:

1. In addition to the plants used solely as remedies, many of the wild edible plants people know and use in their diets also have medicinal uses.
2. These wild edible plants with medicinal uses belong to different botanical families than the plants that are used solely for food.

3. The plant-gathering patterns for plants that have both food and medicinal uses will differ from the patterns used to gather edible plants only.
4. The knowledge of wild food and medicinal plants varies with gender; women know more about food and nonfood plants with medicinal application than men do.
5. Though personal knowledge of wild edible plants is decreasing in the younger generation, this is not true of personal knowledge of medicinal plants.

The Mapuche People

At present, the Mapuche people are the most important aboriginal group inhabiting the Andean and extra-Andean Patagonia of Argentina and Chile (Donoso and Lara, 1996). The Mapuche communities living in the province of Neuquén (northwest Patagonia, Argentina) have been characterized as descendants of primary gatherers of the temperate *Araucaria araucana* (Mol.) C. Koch forests (*pehuén* forests) (Mösbach, 1992; Ladio, 2002). These ancient dwellers used to base their subsistence on the *pehuén* seeds as a staple food and on the hunting of the *guanaco (Lama guanicoe)* and *rhea (Pterocnemia pennata)* (Aagesen, 1998). As the *guanaco* and *rhea* have become scarce, the transhumance circuits to obtain *pehuén* seeds and other wild plants have prevailed in the Mapuche families who have settled in rural areas in and around the *Araucaria araucana* forest (Ladio, 2001). In these poor and isolated communities wild plants are utilized regularly, since their high nutritional and vitamin content and their medicinal properties make them particularly important for the subsistence of the Mapuche, constituting an essential component of their material and spiritual life system (Ladio, 2002).

In spite of the profound social and economic changes the Mapuche have undergone, the plant-gathering tradition persists in their communities (Ladio, 2001). Horses, sheep, and cattle were brought to the area by Spanish settlers, and as early as the seventeenth century the Mapuches had incorporated them into their economy. The Mapuche subsequently became cattle farmers. Hence, they adapted their transhumance circuits to the *pehuén* forests, also moving their livestock for grazing. Since the late nineteenth century, the majority of Mapuche communities have been forced to live in reservations on land ceded by the government, principally in the semiarid Patagonian steppe (extra-Andean Patagonia), far away from the *pehuén* forest or with difficult access to this traditional environment (Ladio, 2002).

Case Study: The Cayulef Community

This aboriginal community is composed of 40 families in two locations: La Costa (near the Catan-lil river) and El Salitral (30 km away). All these families live in very poor socioeconomic conditions, lacking electricity, telephone, running water, and a sewage system. They inhabit precarious single-room houses with almost no furniture and earth floors. The primary energy source for cooking and heating is fuel wood, which is mainly collected from the surroundings. Access to both areas is difficult because the few existing dirt roads are impassable for most of the year and there is no regular transport service. Cayulef's nearest urban populations are Las Coloradas and Junín de los Andes, located more than 100 km away. Most of the adults are illiterate or semiliterate, and the children attend two nearby rural schools where they receive the state-endorsed education in Spanish. At the time of the study, 68 percent of the Cayulef people spoke the Mapuche language (Ladio and Lozada, 2003b). Livestock raising (sheep, goats, and horses) is the primary source of their income. The exogenous products most widely used in their diets are potatoes, onions, *yerba maté* (an herb tea from northeastern Argentina), sugar, flour, and lard. No professional health care is available in the community and the nearest public hospitals are located in Las Coloradas and Junín de los Andes. The majority of the community carry out their own medical practices in their domestic ambit, but sometimes they consult the *machi* or *yerbatera* (always a woman). These are the most highly regarded "medical practitioners," especially when the health problems are related to soul illness or supernatural factors.

STUDY AREA

The Cayulef community is located in northwestern Patagonia, in the Argentine province of Neuquén (39° 70' S and 70° 60' W). Phytogeographically, the region belongs to the Patagonian steppe. The study area receives strong westerly winds and has a mean annual temperature of 8°C, a mean maximum temperature of 14.1°C, and a mean minimum temperature of 2.4°C. The mean annual precipitation of 300 mm is concentrated in autumn and winter (Barros et al., 1983).

The vegetation cover, which is herbaceous and bushy, is mostly composed of *Stipa speciosa* Trin. et Ruprecht, *Festuca pallescens*

(St. Yves) Parodi, *Mulinum spinosum* (Cav.) Pers., *Haplopappus pectinatus* Phil., *Senecio filaginoides* D.C., and *Nassauvia glomerulosa* (Lag.) Don (Cabrera, 1976; Cabrera and Willink, 1980). These species are never taller than 2 m. There are also isolated specimens of *Schinus o'donelli* Barkley, the largest plant in the area, and *Berberis heterophylla* Juss. The only trees are *Salix fragilis* L., planted near houses to serve as windbreaks. In the vicinity of the houses, corrals, and roads grow many exotic weeds, such as *Erodium cicutarium* (L.) L'Hérit., *Bromus tectorum* L., *Hordeum murinum* L., *Capsella bursa-pastoris* (L.) Med., *Brassica rapa* L., *Diplotaxis tenuifolia* (L.) D.C., *Plantago lanceolata* L., *Chenopodium album* L., *Rumex acetosella* L., *Lactuca serriola* L., and *Taraxacum officinale* Weber. In addition, outside the settlements, in hills and mountains, thorny cushion-shaped or crust plant forms withstand the low temperatures and the strong winds of the area, including *Azorrella monanthos* Clos in Gay, *Adesmia corymbosa* Clos, *Tetraglochin alatum* var. patagonicum (Gill. ex Hook), *Nardophyllum obtusifolium* Hooker et Arnott, *Junellia* spp., *Ephedra ochreata* Miers., *Chuquiraga straminea* Sanwith, and *Anarthrophyllum rigidum* (Gill.) Benth. In rocky soil the species commonly found are *Diposis patagonica* Skottsberg, *Oxalis adenophylla* Gill. ex Hook & Am., *Sisyrinchium arenarium* Poepp., and so on. Near the Catan-lil River, the most common plants are hydrofilous: *Juncus* spp., *Carex* spp., *Phragmites australis* (Cav.) Trin. Ex Steud., *Mimulus glabratus* H.B.K., and exotic species such as *Medicago lupulina* L., *Trifolium repens* L., *Taraxacum officinale* Weber, *Nasturtium officinale* R. Brown, and *Stellaria media* (L.) Villars. At present, the total area is grazed intensively by both caprine and ovine livestock (Ladio, 2002).

METHODS

During the summer of 1999, one person from each Cayulef family (32 in total) was interviewed using a semistructured questionnaire. At each location the people were randomly selected: 15 (47 percent) people from La Costa and 17 (53 percent) from El Salitral. The Cayulef people also participated in the collection of plants for the specimen vouchers and in the assignation of their local names. To check the botanical affiliations, in the interviews I used the species occurring principally near the community (within 2 km walking distance), in addition to plant photographs and other herbarium specimens from the different gathering sites utilized by these people. The following information was recorded (some was categorized: see Table 13.1): exclusively edible plants, edible plants with medicinal use, and exclusively medicinal plants (all these as known and used nowadays, per person, and in total for the community); gathering sites; time taken to travel to the collecting site; amount gathered; and method of preparation (handling time). This last variable was obtained by totaling the time spent searching, gathering, cleaning, peeling, and cooking edible resources. A nutritional plant classification was included by considering the energy content of the plants, as was done in Ladio and Lozada (2000). In addition, the plants were classified into native and exotic categories. The age and sex of the people interviewed were also recorded. Eighteen women and 14 men participated. Only one of the women was a plant specialist, considered to be a *machi* by the population.

Plants were pressed and dried at the Ecotono Laboratory at the Universidad Nacional del Comahue. Botanical nomenclature follows Correa (1969-1999) and Marticorena and Quezada (1985).

The importance of the species mentioned was estimated from the number of people who mentioned each plant and the use percentage per species. This last index (one of the most commonly used in ethnobotanical literature) considers the proportion of plants mentioned by their local names (using the scientific name in the analysis) with respect to the total number of interviewees. Note that all the species mentioned by people in the free listing were always corroborated by means of the reported gathering behavior.

Statistical Analysis

The knowledge and use of edible and medicinal plants were analyzed through parametric tests and, when the data were not normally distributed, by nonparametric tests. The Fisher Exact Test was performed to ascertain if the richness of wild edible plants used nowadays depends on their medicinal utilization (Agresti, 1996). This test was also applied to elucidate differences in the botanical families of plants with or without medicinal use. The number of edible plants (medicinal and nonmedicinal) and the exclusively medicinal plants mentioned per person was compared by using the Kruskal-Wallis test

TABLE 13.1. Ecological variables applied to the analysis of the use of wild edible plants by the community of Cayulef.

Ecological variable	Category	Description
Energy content	1	Leaves and shoots (5.8 g carbohydrates and 2.8 g protein / 100 g)
	2	Roots (11.4 g carbohydrates and 3.18 g protein / 100 g)
	3	Fruits and legumes (30.7 g carbohydrates and 2.3 g protein / 100 g)
	4	Seeds (38 g carbohydrates and 4.5 g protein / 100 g)
Handling time	1	Leaves and raw fruit (< ½ h / 100 g)
	2	Leaves and cooked fruit (> ½ h < 1 h / 100 g)
	3	Roots and small raw fruit (>1 h < 1 ½ h / 100 g)
	4	Roots and small cooked fruit (>1 ½ h < 2 h / 100 g)
	5	Raw or cooked seeds (> 2 h / 100 g)
Distance to gathering site	1	Less than 100 m
	2	Between 100 m and 5 km
	3	More than 5 km
Quantity collected per trip	1	Nothing
	2	Less than 5 kg
	3	Between 5 and 50 kg
	4	More than 50 kg
Traveling time to the gathering site	1	Less than 1h
	2	Between 1 and 2 h
	3	Between 2 h and 1 day
	4	More than 1 day

Note: All categories of variables were obtained from interviewees. Energy content was estimated by averaging the known values of carbohydrates and proteins of several plant species from: Duke (2001), Sundriyal and Sundriyal (2001), Schmeda-Hirschmann, Razmilic, Gutierrez, et al. (1999), Schmeda-Hirschmann, Razmilic, Reyes, et al. (1999). Elias and Dykeman (1990), and Schmidt-Hebbel and Pennacchiotti Monti (1985). Distances and travel time to the gathering site were obtained from interviews and refer solely to the outward journey.

with a significance level of 0.05 (Agresti, 1996). The relationship between age and the number of plants mentioned per person was investigated by using simple linear regression analysis. Moreover, given the categories of data (see Table 13.1), I used the Mann Whitney test for the comparison of: people's age, gender, distance to gathering site, traveling time, quantity of plants collected, and nutritional content, in relation to the medicinal value of plants.

RESULTS

Use of Edible Plants with Additional Medicinal Applications

The Cayulef interviewees mentioned a total of 36 wild edible resources, comprising 33 edible wild plants, three types of edible fungi, and two plants that I was unable to taxonomically identify. Twenty-five of these plants are still consumed today (see Table 13.2). Many of the edible plants were mentioned only once by a person; of these, 13 species are known, but are not consumed nowadays. Of the total of 38 plants mentioned, 24 (63 percent) are also used as medicine by the population. They include both native and exotic resources (the latter principally of European origin): see Table 13.2. Nevertheless, the proportion of edible plants with medicinal use that people know (24 species) and consume (17 species) is not significantly different from the edible plants without medicinal properties known (12 species) and utilized (8 species) (Fisher Test, $p > 0.05$).

The exotic herb *menta (Mentha piperita)* and the native fruit plant *michay (Berberis heterophylla)* were the plants used most frequently in the local diets: 75 percent of the interviewees used them. The remaining most frequently used wild products are leafy plants. They include the native *culle colorado (Oxalis adenophylla)* (44 percent), and also the exotic watercress locally known as *berro (Nasturtium officinale)*, the exotic *achicoria (Taraxacum officinale)*, and the native *nalca (Gunnera tinctoria)* (Table 13.2). Most of these species are eaten raw in salads or boiled in water with other vegetables.

A great number of these edible plants are used for illness associated with fever and pains; gastrointestinal problems (diarrhea, stomachache, and hepatic disorders); respiratory diseases (colds, lung pains); and urinary diseases (kidney pains) (Table 13.2). Hot infu-

TABLE 13.2. Edible and medicinal plants mentioned by families from the Mapuche community of Cayulef (*N* = 32 interviewees).

Species	Local name (* in Mapudungum)	O	Number informants	Percent -age	Food use	Part used	Medicinal use	Part used
Berberis heterophylla Juss.	Michai*	N	24	75	Snack, jam, juice	F	—	—
Mentha piperita L.	Menta, hierba buena	E	24	75	Seasoning in *maté*, a herb infusion from northeastern Argentina	L	Stomachache, fever, nausea, digestive	L
Oxalis adenophylla Gill. Ex Hook Am.	Culle* colorado	N	14	44	Snack, juice as lemon substitute	L, R	Fever, colds	L, R
Nasturtium officinale R. Brown	Huentrai,* berro	E	13	41	Salads	L	Hepatic troubles	L
Taraxacum officinale Weber	Huentrai,* Achicoria	E	12	37.5	Salads	L	Hepatic troubles, depurative	L
Gunnera tinctoria (Mol.) Mirbel	Pangue,* nalca*	N	8	25	Salads, jam	L	Lung problems, bone problems	R
Ephedra ochreata Miers.	Cuparra,* sulupe rojo, caman*	N	7	22	Snack	F	Sweaty feet	L
Apium australe Thouars	Nolquín,* apio silvestre	N	6	19	Seasoning in *puchero*, a native dish with other vegetables and meat	L	Cough, fever, kidney pain	L, R
Diposis patagonica Skottsberg	Yocón-llocúm*	N	6	19	Roasted on hot rocks, boiled or mashed as a potato substitute	R	Fever	R

Species	Common name	Status	No.	%	Use	Part	Medicinal use	L/R
Schinus o'donelli Barkey	Molle, michi*	N	6	19	Snack, beverages	F	Toothaches	L
Muehlenbeckia hastulata (Sm.) Johnst.	Quilo,* quineo,* zarparrilla	N	4	12.5	Snack	F	Rheuma	L
Oxalis valdiviensis Bernéoud in Gay	Culle* amarillo	N	4	12.5	Snack, juices as lemon substitute	L	Fever	L
Araucaria araucana (Mol.) C. Koch	Pehuén,* araucaria	N	3	9	Cooked, toasted, boiled, or roasted on hot rocks to make cakes, soups, or *empanadas*, traditional pastries	S	—	—
Eryngium paniculatum Cavanilles et Dom.	Chupalla*	N	3	9	Snack	R	Hepatic and renal problems	R
Rumex acetosella L.	Cascacheu,* alcacheu,* romaza	E	3	9	Snack, salads	L	Wounds, vulnerary	L
Arjona tuberosa Cavanilles	Papita de los arenales, macachin	N	2	6	Snack, boiled or mashed as potato substitute	R	—	—
Chenopodium album L.	Trel-trum,* quinhuilla	E	2	6	Cooked in *pucheros*	L	—	—
Tristagma patagonicum (Bak.) Traub.	Chaleo*	N	2	6	Cooked in *puchero* as onions	R	Childbirth	R
?	Chaquira	?	1	3	Snack	R	—	—

307

TABLE 13.2. *(continued)*

Species	Local name (* in Mapudungum)	O	Number informants	Percent -age	Food use	Part used	Medicinal use	Part used
Erodium cicutarium (L.) L'Hérit.	Cachú loica,* loica-cachu,* alfilerillo	E	1	3	Snack, cooked in *pucheros*	L	Hepatic and kidney disorders	L
Austrocactus patagonicus (Web.) Backeberg	Chupasangre, fruto de la barda	N	1	3	Snack	L	—	—
Malus sylvestris Mill.	Manzana silvestre	E	1	3	Jam, cakes, juices, raw as fruit	F	—	—
Matricaria matricarioides (Less.) Porter	Manzanilla	E	1	3	Seasoning in cakes or in *maté*	L	Stomachache	L
Sanicula graveolens Poepp. ex D.C.	Cilantro silvestre	N	1	3	Seasoning in soups, salads, or *puchero*	L	—	—
Stellaria media (L.) Villars.	Quiroi, quilloi*	E	1	3	Salads	L	Fever	L
Aristotelia chilensis (Mol.) Stuntz	Maqui,* clon*	N	1	0	Snack, jam, not used nowadays	F	Diarrhea	L
Azorella monanthos Clos in Gay	Leña de piedra	N	1	0	Cooked on hot rocks like potato, not used nowadays	R	Lung problems, pulmonia	L, R
Caiophora patagonica (Speg.) Urban et Gilg.	Ortiga blanca	N	1	0	Boiled as potato, not used nowadays	R	Kidney problems, infections, hepatitis	R

Species	Common name	Origin	No.	Food use	Part	Medicinal use	Part
?	Cochilo	?	0	Snack, not used nowadays	R	—	—
Cyttaria hookeri Berk.#	Fruto del ñire*	N	1	Snack, cooked in puchero	F	—	—
Cyttaria hariotti Lisch.#	Llao-llao*	N	1	Snack, salads with sliced apples, not used nowadays	F	—	—
Brassica rapa L.	Napor,* repollo del campo	E	1	Salads, cooked in pucheros or fritters, not used nowadays	L	—	—
Phragmites australis (Cav.) Trin. Ex Steud.	Carrizo	E	1	Boiled or roasted as potato, not used nowadays	R	Childbirth	R
Maihueniopsis darwinii var. hickenii (Brit.) Kiesling	Chupasangre	N	1	Snack, not used nowadays	R	Bone problems	F
Maytenus boaria Mol.	Maitén*	N	1	Salads, not used nowadays	L	Internal pain	L
Mimulus glabratus H.B.K.	Placa*	N	1	Salads, not used nowadays	L	—	—
Lycoperdon spp.*	Polvera	N	1	Cooked in pucheros, not used nowadays	F	—	—
Ribes cucullatum Hook. et Arn.	Parrillita	N	1	Snack, jelly, not used nowadays	F	Liver, blood disorders	L

Note: 0: plant origin (N: native, E: exotic). Number of informants who mentioned the species as useful. Percentage (number of mentions of each species/total number of interviewees). Part used, F: fruit or fruit bodies of fungus; L: leaves, flowers, or stems; R: roots, rhizomes, or bulbs; S: seeds. ? = plant taxonomically unidentified; # = fungi species.

sions are the preferred method of administering these medicines. All these plants have only familiar use: people of the community do not sell wild plants.

The Cayulef people collect these wild plants in three distinctive gathering sites or ecological environments:

1. *Andean forest:* This highland corresponds to the Andean valleys, which include small forests of *Araucaria araucana (pehuén)* located in ranches (of non-Mapuche property) more than 50 km away from their dwellings.
2. *Steppe:* These lands constitute their present territory, where the Cayulef community has settled.
3. *Around dwellings:* These anthropogenic environments include trails, roads, and corrals, where exotic weeds are very common. More details about these gathering sites are in Ladio (2001, 2002).

Botanical Families of Edible Medicinal and Nonmedicinal Wild Plants

The edible wild species mentioned by the Cayulef people belong to 26 different plant families: 12 are edible species without medicinal use and 18 correspond to food plants with medicinal applications (Figure 13.1, a and b). A significant difference (Fisher Test, $p > 0.05$, Figure 13.1, a and b) exists between the botanical families in the proportions of edible medicinal and nonmedicinal species. The most important families of edible medicinal plants are Umbelliferae (with four species), Compositae (with two species), and Oxalidaceae (also with two species). In contrast, the most important families of edible nonmedicinal plants are Cyttariaceae (fungi, with two species) and other representative families such as Araucariaceae, Berberidaceae, and Rosaceae. The majority of families include only one medicinal or nonmedicinal species.

Use of Exclusively Medicinal Plants

The Cayulef people use a relatively large variety of medicinal plants, comprising 77 wild species. The ten most mentioned plants are *carqueja* [*Baccharis linearis* (R. et Pav.) Pers.], mentioned by 8 percent of the interviewees; *cachanlahue* [*Centaurium cachanlahuen*

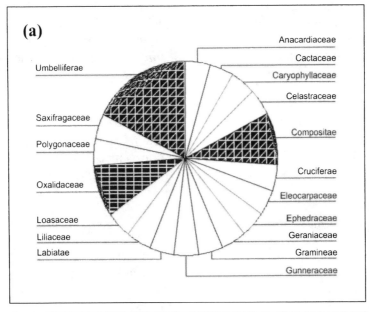

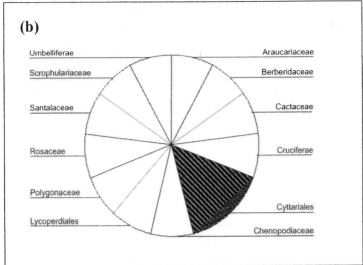

FIGURE 13.1. Botanical families of wild food plants and fungus mentioned by Cayulef people, (a) with medicinal use and (b) without medicinal use. Shaded segments indicate the most important families (with more than one species for these uses).

(Mol.) Rob.], mentioned by 5 percent; *pañil* (*Buddleja globosa* Hope) and *paico* (*Chenopodium ambrosioides* L.), both mentioned by 3 percent; *ñanculahuen* (*Valeriana carnosa* Sm.), *limpia plata* (*Equisetum bogotense* H.B.K.), and *cola da caballo* (*Equisetum giganteum* L.), all mentioned by 2 percent; and *siete venas* (*Plantago lanceolata* L.), *Quinchamalium chilense* Brong., and *malvarrubia* (*Marrubium vulgare* L.), all mentioned by 1 percent. As was found for wild edible plants, these resources included both native and exotic species. These results will not be described in detail here, because the main focus of this chapter is the dichotomy between the use of wild food plants and those with additional medicinal applications.

Comparison of Patterns of Gathering Medicinal and Nonmedicinal Plants

No significant difference was found between distance and travel time spent gathering wild edible plants with medicinal use and nonmedicinal plants (Mann Whitney test, $p > 0.05$, Figure 13.2, a and b). Therefore, the collection of plant foods with or without medicinal use shares the same gathering sites. However, edible wild plants with medicinal use are collected in smaller quantities than plants without additional medicinal use (Mann Whitney test, $p < 0.05$, Figure 13.2 c). Moreover, the handling time spent by the Cayulef people in searching and processing wild plants with medicinal use was significantly less than the time spent in searching and processing exclusively food plants (Mann Whitney test, $p < 0.05$, Figure 13.2 d). Compared with nonmedicinal plants, the plants with medicinal use have a significantly lower nutritional value in terms of energy content (Mann Whitney test, $p < 0.05$, Figure 13.2 e). No significant differences were found between the mean age of the Cayulef people who knew the additional medicinal use of wild plants and those who did not (Mann Whitney test, $p > 0.005$, Fig. 13.2 f).

Gender and the Use of Wild Plants

In general, the people of Cayulef mentioned a similar richness of total edible and medicinal species per person, demonstrating a wide knowledge of plant properties (Mann Whitney Test, $p = 0.76$, Figure 13.3). However, knowledge of medicinal plants varied more per person than knowledge of edible plants (women 13 ± 10 and men 12 ± 9,

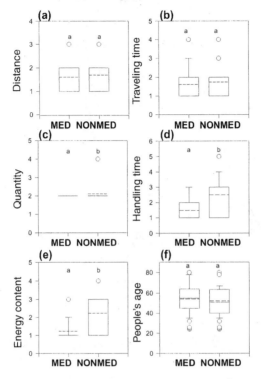

FIGURE 13.2. Comparison between edible medicinal (MED) plant and edible nonmedicinal (NONMED) plant use in the Cayulef community in relation to (a) distance to gathering site; (b) traveling time; (c) quantity collected; (d) handling time; (e) energy content; and (f) people's age. Median and mean ± SE values are depicted. When a line is depicted in the graph, this means that only one category of the variable was mentioned. Categories and descriptions of ecological variables are shown in Table 13.1. Different letters correspond to significant differences ($p < 0.005$).

see Figure 13.3). It is important to note that edible plants, whether medicinal or not, were mentioned in a similar proportion by both sexes (Figure 13.3). No significant differences were found between sexes in the total number (i.e., medicinal plus nonmedicinal) of wild edible plants known per person (Kruskal-Wallis test, $p = 0.492$), the edible nonmedicinal plants (Kruskal-Wallis test, $p = 0.139$), or the edible plants with medicinal use (Kruskal-Wallis test, $p = 0.716$, Figure 13.3). In addition, no significant difference was found between

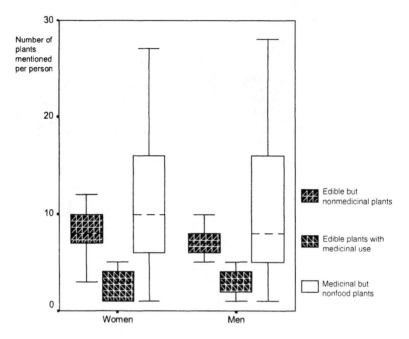

FIGURE 13.3. Wild plant knowledge per person between sexes in Cayulef community (N = 32 interviewees). Mean ± SE values are depicted.

sexes in the number of medicinal plants (i.e., nonfood) known per person (Kruskal-Wallis test, $p = 0.261$, Figure 13.3).

Age and the Use of Wild Plants

The mean age of the interviewees was 50 years (range 24 to 80 years). The total number of wild edible plants known increased significantly with the age of the interviewee (simple linear regression, F = 15.4, $p < 0.05$, see Figure 13.4). Moreover, age was found to be significantly related both to the number of exclusively food plants mentioned (simple linear regression, F = 10.3, $p < 0.05$, Figure 13.4) and to the plants mentioned that are both edible and medicinal (simple linear regression, F = 6.5, $p < 0.05$, Figure 13.4). No significant relationship was found between the total number of nonedible medicinal plants known per person and interviewee's age (simple linear regression, F = 2.8, $p = 0.107$).

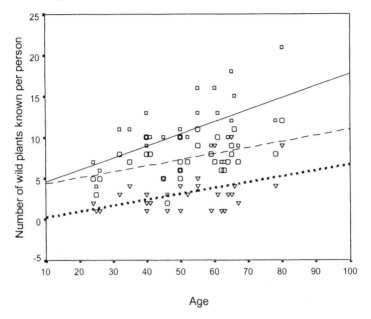

FIGURE 13.4. Regression between age and the number of wild edible plants known by the Cayulef people ($N = 32$), distinguished into (---) number of edible but nonmedicinal plants mentioned per person ($R^2 = 0.23$); (•••)number of edible plants with medicinal use mentioned per person ($R^2 = 0.19$); and (—) the total sum of edible medicinal and nonmedicinal plants mentioned per person ($R^2 = 0.30$).

DISCUSSION

The present study on wild plant use shows that in the Cayulef community the selection of edible and medicinal plants is influenced by botanical, ecological, and sociocultural aspects that lead to distinct patterns of species use and to a different risk of losing knowledge in future generations.

The first hypothesis was confirmed; Cayulef people know and use a variety of wild edible plants, some of which are also utilized as medicine. This indicates a substantial overlap of edible and medicinal species (63 percent). Moerman (1998) also found this pattern for food and medicinal plants used by natives of North America, though there the overlap was only 30 percent. These medicinal foods amplify the opportunities to cure illness and improve the well-being of families at the same time. This fact indicates that there is an ample exploitation of wild resources that does not result in people generating unconnected categories of uses; on the contrary, it results in an advantageous amalgamation of knowledge.

The second hypothesis was also upheld. The wild food species with medicinal and nonmedicinal utilization belong to diverse botanical families that are distinct from the botanical families of the exclusively edible species. In light of the results obtained by Gottlieb et al. (2002), chemiotaxonomical differences can be proposed: the plants utilized as food by the Cayulef people belong to primitive families of angiosperms such as Rosaceae, Celastraceae, Myrtaceae, and Saxifragaceae, or to less-advanced families of nonangiosperms (Araucariaceae and Ephedraceae). In contrast, the families of edible plants utilized as medicine (both native and exotic species) correspond principally to Compositae, Labiatae, Caryophyllaceae, and so on, which are more advanced in evolutionary terms. These findings suggest the existence of a systematic and evolutionary pattern in wild plant use, but more investigations might be conducted in the future in order to further explore this.

As was found in other studies (Prance and Plana, 1998; Moerman, 1996), a great proportion of the wild edible plants collected by the Cayulef people are exotic greens that also have medicinal properties. This might be related to the fact that the acquired knowledge of native plants has blended with knowledge from Spanish colonists (Citarella, 1995). This has led to exotic plants being included in the Mapuche diet as well as in their medicines. For example, the frequently used exotic leafy plants such as mint *(M. piperita)*, watercress *(Nasturtium officinale)*, and dandelion *(Taraxacum officinale)* are an important source of vitamins and minerals as well as essential remedies for digestive problems.

The results also confirm the third hypothesis, which was that plants that are both edible and medicinal have different gathering patterns. The gathering of these plants with medicinal usage is associated with shorter distances travelled and a shorter handling time. Moreover, shrubs and herbs with both usages have a low nutritional content in terms of energy and are gathered in small quantities. This pattern of use seems to be related to minimizing time and energy and to reducing the intake of large quantities of the antinutritional substances present in many medicinal plants.

Notwithstanding, the energy cost-benefit consideration should be treated with care, given that factors other than protein and calories have significant importance in human diets, as indicated previously. The need to incorporate vitamins and minerals is also essential, and these are usually provided by edible greens (Laferriere, 1995; Nordeide et al., 1996). In this chapter, the nonenergy nutritional contribution has been ignored. Future research would be needed to analyze this aspect of the use of edible resources.

The analysis done from an ecological point of view provides another perspective that confirms that the use of wild edible plants by the Cayulef people is declining. Most at risk is the gathering of edible forest plants with low nutritional content in terms of energy and without medicinal use. In their current environment, denied access to traditional gathering sites, the people might forget some plants, resulting in an unrecoverable loss of plant lore.

The fourth hypothesis was rejected: no differences were found between the sexes in knowledge of edible and medicinal plants. The explanation could be that both men and women share the same activity and they go to the same gathering environments. Both sexes know a similar number of wild plants. As was found by Begossi and colleagues (2002), the use of medicinal wild plants does not seem to be concentrated among women, though some women have a very wide knowledge of medicinal plants and are key elements in retaining this wisdom in the community.

In the past, whole families travelled to the Andean forests to move their livestock and gather wild plants (Ladio, 2002). Nowadays they stay near their dwellings and the steppe year-round. The Cayulef people said they did so as a consequence of territorial conflicts with adjoining non-Mapuche property owners who impede them from trespassing and gaining access to the *Araucaria araucana* forests. It seems likely that this reduces the opportunities both sexes have to learn about wild edible plants, because without these transhumance circuits (far from any urbanization) families are in less contact with their traditional environments (Ladio and Lozada, 2003b).

In addition, as found in other studies (Caniago and Siebert, 1998; Benz et al., 2000), knowledge of edible plants (medicinal and non-medicinal use) increased with age in the Cayulef community, but the number of medicinal plants per person did not vary with age. This confirms the fifth hypothesis. Manufactured products may be largely replacing traditional wild food, but the indigenous health system is less at risk. The community is located in an isolated region where the difficult communication with urban and medicinal centers might favor the persistence of indigenous medicines. Most indigenous populations of the region have *machis* (female shamans) who are at the top of their hierarchy in the whole community (San Martín, 1983; Houghton and Manby, 1985; Citarella, 1995). Hence, alterations in the small-scale dynamics of the population, such as the death of these knowledgeable people, might cause changes or losses in the use of medicinal wild plants.

The results of this study have implications for the conservation of Mapuche plant lore. Edible and medicinal plants have distinct attributes in terms of taxonomic affiliations, which lead to a distinct pattern of use. These attributes are specific and strongly depend on the conservation of the plant diversity in the area, especially in the protection of shared gathering sites, where both edible and medicinal plants are collected. In addition, it is urgent that free access to these sites should also be provided by the government. Finally, elders and knowledgeable women should be considered and included in local projects of cultural revival, because they serve as an important vehicle for the transmission and maintenance of these valuable resources for younger generations.

REFERENCES

Aagesen, D.L. (1998). Indigenous resource rights and conservation of the monkey-puzzle tree (*Araucaria araucana*, Araucariaceae): A case study from southern Chile. *Economic Botany* 52 (2): 146-160.

Agresti, A. (1996). *An introduction to categorical data analysis.* New York: John Wiley and Sons, Inc.

Alcorn, J.B. (1995). The scope and aims of ethnobotany in a developing world. In R.E. Shultes and S. von Reis (Eds.), *Ethnobotany: Evolution of a discipline.* Portland: Dioscorides Press.

Barros, V., V. Cordon, C. Moyano, R. Mendez, J. Forguera, and O. Pizzio (1983). *Cartas de precipitación de la zona oeste de las provincias de Río Negro y Neuquén. Primera contribución.* Cinco Saltos, Argentina: Universidad Nacional del Comahue. Fac. de Ciencias Agrarias.

Begossi, A., N. Hanazaki, and J. Tamashiro (2002). Medicinal plants in the Atlantic Forest (Brazil): Knowledge, use, and conservation. *Human Ecology* 30 (3): 281-299.

Benz, B.F., E.J. Cevallos, M.F. Santana, A.J. Rosales, and M.S. Graf (2000). Losing knowledge about plant use in the Sierra de Manantlan Biosphere Reserve, Mexico. *Economic Botany* 54 (2): 183-191.

Benz, B.F., M.F. Santana, R. Pineda, E.J. Cevallos, L. Robles, and D. de Niz (1994). Characterization of meztizo plant use in the Sierra de Manantlan, Jalisco-Colima, México. *Journal of Ethnobiology* 14 (1): 23-41.

Boesch, C. and M. Tomasello (1998). Chimpanzee and human cultures. *Current Anthropology* 39 (5): 591-614.

Boster, J.S. (1985). "Requiem for the omniscient informant": There is life in the old girl yet. In Dougherty, J.W.D. (Ed.), *Directions in cognitive anthropology*. Urbana and Chicago: University of Illinois Press.

Brodt, S. (2001). A systems perspective on the conservation and erosion of indigenous agricultural knowledge in Central India. *Human Ecology* 29 (1): 99-120.

Cabrera, A.L. (1976). *Regiones fitogeográficas Argentinas*. Fac. 1. Enciclopedia Arg. de la Agricultura y Jardinería. Tomo II. Buenos Aires: Editorial Acme S.A.C.I.

Cabrera, A.L. and A. Willink (1980). *Biogeografía de América Latina*. Monografía no. 13. Washington, DC: Secretaría General de la Organización de los Estados Americanos.

Caniago, I. and S.F. Siebert (1998). Medicinal plant ecology, knowledge, and conservation in Kalimantan, Indonesia. *Economic Botany* 52 (3): 229-250.

Citarella, L. (1995). *Medicinas y Culturas en la Araucanía*. Trafkin. Programa de atención primaria en salud. Cooperación Italiana. Chile: Ed. Sudamericana.

Correa, M.N. (1969, 1971, 1978, 1984, 1988, 1998, 1999). *Flora Patagónica*. Partes 1, 2, 3, 4, 5, 7, and 8. Bs. As. Argentina. Colección Científica del Instituto Nacional de Tecnología Agropecuaria.

Donoso, C. and A. Lara (1996). Utilización de los bosques nativos en Chile: Pasado, presente y futuro. In Armesto, J., C. Villagrán, and M.K. Arroyo (Eds.), *Ecología de los bosques nativos de Chile*. Santiago, Chile: Editorial Universitaria.

Duke, J.A. (2001). *Handbook of phytochemical constituents of GRAS herbs and other economic plants*. Boca Ratón, FL: CRC Press, Inc.

Elias, T.S. and P.A. Dykeman (1990). *Edible wild plants: A North American field guide*. New York: Sterling Publishing Co.

Garro, L.C. (1986). Intracultural variation in folk medical knowledge: A comparison between curers and noncurers. *American Anthropologist* 88: 351-370.

Gispert, M. and A. Gómez Campos (1986). Plantas medicinales silvestres: El proceso de adquisición, transmisión y colectivización del conocimiento vegetal. *Biótica* 11 (2): 113-125.

Gottlieb, O. (1982). Ethnopharmacology versus chemosystematics in the search for biologically active principles in plants. *Journal of Ethnopharmacology* 6: 227-238.

Gottlieb, O. and M.R. Borin (2002). Shamanism or science? *Anais da Academia Brasileira da Ciencias* 74 (1): 135-144.

Gottlieb, O., M.R. Borin, and B.M. Bosisio (1996). Trends of plant use by humans and nonhuman primates in Amazonia. *American Journal of Primatology* 40: 189-195.

Gottlieb, O., R.M. Boris, and N.N. de Brito (2002). Integration of ethnobotany and phytochemistry: Dream or reality? *Phytochemistry* 60: 145-152.

Gottlieb, O. and M.E. Stefanello (1991). Comparative ethnopharmacology: A rational method for the search of bioactive compounds in plants. *Anales de la Academia Brasilera de Ciencias* 63 (1): 23-31.

Gragson, T.L. (1993). Human foraging in lowland South America: Patterns and process of resource procurement. *Research in Economic Anthropology* 14: 107-138.

Hoffmann, A., C. Farga, J. Lastra, and E. Veghazi (1992). *Plantas Medicinales de Uso Común en Chile*. Santiago, Chile: Fundación Claudio Gay.

Houghton, P.J. and J. Manby (1985). Medicinal plants of the Mapuche. *Journal of Ethnopharmacology* 13: 89-103.

Howe, H.F. and L.C. Westley (1988). *Ecological relationships of plants and animals*. New York: Oxford University Press.

Ladio, A.H. (2001). The maintenance of wild edible plants gathering in a Mapuche community of Patagonia. *Economic Botany* 55 (2): 243-254.

Ladio, A.H. (2002). Las plantas comestibles en el noroeste Patagónico y su utilización por las poblaciones humanas: Una aproximación cuantitativa. Doctoral thesis. Universidad Nacional del Comahue.

Ladio, A.H. and M. Lozada (2000). Edible wild plant use in a Mapuche community of northwestern Patagonia. *Human Ecology* 28 (1): 53-71.

Ladio, A.H. and M. Lozada (2001). Non-timber forest product use in two human populations from NW Patagonia: A quantitative approach. *Human Ecology* 29 (4): 367-380.

Ladio, A.H. and M. Lozada (2003a). Comparison of edible wild plant diversity used and foraging strategies in two aboriginal communities of NW Patagonia. *Biodiversity and Conservation* 12 (5): 937-951.

Ladio, A.H. and M. Lozada (2003b). Recolección de productos no maderables del bosque Andino Patagónico y su relación con la práctica de la trashumancia en una comunidad Mapuche del NO de la Patagonia. Quito, Ecuador: *Ponencias del Congreso Iberoamericano de Desarrollo y Medio Ambiente*.

Laferrière, J.E. (1995). A dynamic nonlinear optimization study of mountain Pima subsistence technology. *Human Ecology* 23 (1): 1-27.

Marticorena, C. and M. Quezada (1985). Flora vascular de Chile. *Gayana Botanica* 42 (1-2): 1-157.

Moerman, D.E. (1996). An analysis of the food plants and drug plants of native North America. *Journal of Ethnopharmacology* 52: 1-22.

Moerman, D.E. (1998). Native North American food and medicinal plants: Epistemological considerations. In Prendergast, H.D.V., N.L. Etkin, D.R. Harris, and P.J. Houghton (Eds.), *Plants for food and medicine*. Kew: Royal Botanic Gardens.

Mösbach, E.W. (1992). *Botánica indígena de Chile*. Museo Chileno de Arte Precolombino. Santiago: Editorial Andrés Bello.

Nordeide, M.B., A. Hatløy, M. Følling, E. Lied, and A. Oshaug (1996). Nutrient composition and nutritional importance of green leaves and wild food resources in an agricultural district, Koutiala, in Southern Mali. *International Journal of Food Sciences and Nutrition* 47: 455-468.

Prance, G.T. and V. Plana (1998). The use of alien plants in tropical South American folk medicines. In Prendergast, H.D.V., N.L. Etkin, D.R. Harris, and P.J. Houghton (Eds.), *Plants for food and medicine*. Kew: Royal Botanic Gardens.

Prendergast, H.D.V., N.L. Etkin, D.R. Harris, and P.J. Houghton (Eds.) (1998). *Plants for food and medicine*. Kew: Royal Botanic Gardens.

San Martín, J.A. (1983). Medicinal plants in central Chile. *Economic Botany* 37 (2): 216-227.

Schmeda-Hirschmann, G., I. Razmilic, M.I. Gutierrez, and J.I. Loyola (1999). Proximate composition and biological activity of food plants gathered by Chilean Amerindians. *Economic Botany* 53 (2): 177-187.

Schmeda-Hirschmann, G., I. Razmilic, S. Reyes, M.I. Gutierrez, and J.I. Loyola (1999). Biological activity and food analysis of *Cyttaria* spp. (Discomyetes). *Economic Botany* 53 (1): 30-40.

Schmidt-Hebbel, H. and I. Pennachiotti Monti (1985). *Tabla de composición química de alimentos Chilenos*. Fac. Ccias. Químicas y Farmacéuticas. Santiago, Chile: Universidad de Chile Editorial Universitaria.

Schultes, R.E. and S. von Reis (Eds.) (1995). *Ethnobotany: Evolution of a discipline*. Portland, OR: Dioscorides Press.

Smith, E.A. (1983). Anthropological applications of optimal foraging theory: A critical review. *Current Anthropology* 24 (5): 625-651.

Sundriyal, M. and R.C. Sundriyal (2001). Wild edible plants of the Sikkim Himalaya: Nutritive values of selected species. *Economic Botany* 55 (3): 377-390.

Thornton, T.F. (1999). Tleikw Aaní, the "berried" landscape: The structure of Tlingit edible fruit resources at Glacier Bay, Alaska. *Journal of Ethnobiology* 19 (1): 27-48.

Watterstrom, W. (1978). Cognitive system, food patterns, and paleoethnobotany. In Ford, R.I. (Ed.), *The nature status of ethnobotany*. Anthropological Papers Nro. 67. Ann Arbor, MI: University of Michigan.

Zent, S. and E. López-Zent (2003). Ethnobotanical convergence, divergence, and change among the Hotï of the Venezuelan Guayana. In Maffi, L. and T. Carlson (Eds.), *Ethnobotany and conservation of biocultural diversity. Advances in economic botany series*. Bronx, NY: New York Botanical Garden Press.

Chapter 14

Dietary and Medicinal Use of Traditional Herbs Among the Luo of Western Kenya

Charles Ogoye-Ndegwa
Jens Aagaard-Hansen

INTRODUCTION

The use of herbs both as food and medicine is widespread among African communities. Long ago, Price (1939) emphasized the significance of traditional food items in the context of changing conceptions of food and food habits and underscored the fact that the changing of food habits is accompanied by new infections and deficiencies. Etkin and Ross made similar observations about a West African community. They write:

> The Hausa of Africa eat many kinds of leafy vegetables at the end of the rainy season, the time of greatest risk of malaria infection. These are food plants, but they also may treat malaria, for laboratory investigation shows that they increase red blood cell oxidation. (Etkin and Ross, 1983, p. 188)

As well as being used as food, most traditional vegetables may have medicinal potential. Plants and plant material gathered from the

This study was conducted within the framework of the Nyang'oma Research Training Site (NRTS) with funding from the Danish Bilharziasis Laboratory (DBL). We acknowledge the support from Mbeka Primary School, particularly Mr. Donnic Abudho and the 1998-2001 grade six pupils; the local community; the area educational authorities; the National Museum of Kenya; and the local nongovernmental organization "Care for the Earth" for their support of this study.

wild (including weeds) have received little attention in terms of their potential value as high-nutrient foods in rural communities. To achieve enhanced food and nutrition security, especially among vulnerable, rural communities, emphasis has been placed on the establishment of kitchen gardens and campaigns to promote the consumption of traditional food items (Ogoye-Ndegwa et al., 2002). In rural settings, traditional vegetables often double as food and medicine, but the dual functions have received little attention.

It has been observed that the application of a food-based–systems approach is useful as a measure to help increase the number of foods rich in micronutrients. This approach involves "the development of a community garden and small household plots, containing many indigenous plant species, as a practical and a sustainable solution" (Leemon and Samman, 1998, p. 24). Ferguson and colleagues (1993) employed a food-based systems approach in Ghana and Malawi in an intervention program aimed at increased zinc bioavailability. The strategy involved encouraging more consumption of locally available indigenous foods and changing the local food-processing techniques by introducing fermentation. Similar studies, for example, in rural Bangladesh (Bloem et al., 1996), have shown that an increase in the volume of fruits and vegetables grown in home gardens led to an increased intake of vitamin A among women. Solon and colleagues (1979) state that there is a correlation between home gardens and increased vitamin A intake and weight for height among malnourished Philippine children. Kumar (1978) reported a positive relationship between a garden project in southern India and the nutritional status of children of weaning age.

The decline in the consumption of traditional vegetables in rural areas has negative implications for the food and nutrition security of the populace. Some of the traditional vegetables from rural settings find a market in towns, where they are sold rather expensively in big hotels and restaurants. The decline in their consumption in the rural areas is not just a matter of accessibility and affordability, but also reflects their familiarity and the related perception that they are not palatably enticing (Ogoye-Ndegwa and Aagaard-Hansen, 2003). Familiarity does not imply abundance over long periods, but rather having been in the people's diet for a long time, and hence lacking appeal to curious consumers with changing food habits.

Decline in the use of traditional plant foods is attributed to changing food preferences, agricultural development, and increasing population pressure on land, which are inevitably leading to the decreased diversity and abundance of wild vegetables and other foodstuffs (Lepofsky et al., 1985). As some families consume the traditional vegetables because they have no alternative due to their extremely low purchasing power, the vegetables are consumed in large volumes, when in season (Ogoye-Ndegwa and Aagaard-Hansen, 2003).

Food and culture are interwoven. In almost all societies, changing food habits has had a close relationship with changes in cultural practices. Thus, among the Luo, the consumption of traditional food items is declining with the introduction of new food items. This has nutritional implications, especially if the traditional food items could be major sources of micronutrients to most families. Traditional food items have been reported to have a high nutrient content (Behar, 1976; FAO, 1968) and, therefore, encouraging them in the people's diet would be a good measure to achieve food and nutrition security.

Food has been studied from a biocultural perspective that combines both nutritional and anthropological approaches in the understanding of food use and consumption. From a nutritional point of view, this perspective relates people's food preferences and habits to the functioning of the physical body. Eating practices are viewed in terms of how good or bad they are for the development of the human body. Beneficial practices are to be encouraged, while the adverse ones are to be discouraged. The approach views food as "emerging from a natural basis for the human diet which is guided by both genetic predispositions and culturally structured preferences" (Lupton, 1996). Fieldhouse (1998, p. 19) goes beyond the scope of nutritional anthropology, and maintains that a comprehensive food-habit research "invites the curious eyes of historians, geographers, sociologists and folklorists among others." A comprehensive study of nutrition, therefore, calls for cross-disciplinary cooperation, focusing not only on the health aspects of food but also paying equal attention to the cultural elements regarding food (Cattle, 1977; Fieldhouse, 1998; Freedman, 1977; Krondl and Boxen, 1975).

Culture comprises value systems (or sets of value systems), and the dominant values will influence how particular foods and feeding habits are viewed. This creates a common and shared understanding of preferences; for example, by classifying food as good or bad. Food depicts status and is a marker of social difference. Usually, the type of food eaten or the way it is prepared indicates the social status. New food items have often been associated with affluence and prestige (Barthes, 1997). The way food is distributed and shared is guided by customs and rules that underlie social values and structure (Meigs, 1997) as well as power differentials (Sen, 1992). However, in addition to these structural factors, personal variations may be found based on different individual positions.

In pluralistic African medical systems, herbs play a major role in treating illnesses. Geissler and colleagues have made extensive studies on this subject among the Luo, and they conclude that "it is astonishing how well the healers' and the mothers' plant knowledge is in agreement with each other" (2002, p. 47). By this statement they refer to the different categories of herb users: the "professional" healers and the mothers who mainly treat members of their own family. Interestingly, it seems that Luo children themselves have significant knowledge of medicinal plants (Prince et al., 2001) and that they frequently treat themselves for various ailments without consulting adults (Geissler et al., 2000). Their knowledge about medicinal plants was often acquired in informal and experiential ways (Prince et al., 2001; Prince and Geissler, 2001). Hedberg and Staugård (1989) have studied similar pharmacopoeia of medicinal herbs in Botswana.

The present chapter aims at describing how plants are and have been used for dietary as well as for medicinal purposes among the Luo in western Kenya.

MATERIALS AND METHODS

Study Area

The study was conducted among the Luo in Bondo District, Nyanza Province, in western Kenya in a community along the shores of Lake Victoria. The main rainy season is between January and May when the land is cultivated; usually, a shorter period of rain occurs in October and November. The Lake Victoria basin receives an average annual rainfall of 750 to 1,000 mm. The area varies in altitude from 1,140 to 1,300 m and experiences temperatures varying between a minimum of 14 and 16°C and a maximum of 26 to 30°C (Survey of Kenya cited in Geissler, 1998, pp. 27-28). The landscape is characterized by homesteads dispersed through the bush. The soil is mostly black cotton soil with rock outcrops.

Study Population

The Luo—estimated to number about 3 million—are one of the largest ethnic groups in Kenya. Their main occupation is subsistence farming, with maize, sorghum, millet, and cassava the main staple food crops. The Luo, who were originally predominantly pastoralists, still keep a substantial number of goats, cows, and poultry. Sheep and donkeys are also quite common. In addition, petty trade, fishing, and migratory work supplement the household economy. All in all, the population is impoverished and consequently vulnerable to drought periods and a decline in agricultural produce and cash income. The majority of the population is affiliated with the Anglican Church of Kenya, the Roman Catholic Church, or the Seventh-Day Adventists, though there are several smaller syncretic sects as well.

The study population comprised about 3,000 people, from whom key informants were purposively sampled. The key informants chosen were elderly males and females that were knowledgeable about traditional modes of subsistence. The main local primary school of the area, with about 500 pupils, formed a central element of the study. A teacher from the school joined the team as coresearcher and other collaborators were selected from the pupils in grade six, based on their outspokenness, inquisitiveness, willingness to participate, and ability to neatly record research data.

Study Design and Data-Collection Methods

The study was conceptualized as action research, in which the researchers, the teacher, and grade six pupils in a local primary school simultaneously engaged in different horticultural and research activities. By action research, we mean an endeavor that uses research as a tool to improve the living conditions of a given population in a concrete way, with their active involvement in at least some stages of the process. Grade six was selected as the "research class," as this group would already have been taught most of the relevant material on horticulture according to the Kenyan national curriculum.

The first phase, the findings of which are presented here, was comprised of three different activities. The main part was a cross-sectional survey done by the researchers as well as the pupils. It was an exploration of traditional food items (in particular, vegetables) in order to make a complete inventory for the community. Second, field walks were conducted with key informants, in order to sample plants. Third, the botanical names of 29 of the plants were identified. Many of the data on dietary use have previously been reported (Ogoye-Ndegwa and Aagaard-Hansen, 2003). A botanical study is presently exploring the botanical taxonomy, toxicology, and micronutrient content of the vegetables (Orech, personal communication).

Phase two of the project, which is ongoing, focuses on the integration of selected traditional vegetables in the agricultural teaching and school gardening of a local primary school and the dissemination of the study findings to relevant groups in the surrounding community (Ogoye-Ndegwa et al., 2002). However, this falls outside the scope of the present chapter.

The first section of the study described here was carried out with 27 key informants, who were elderly people knowledgeable of traditional modes of subsistence, particularly regarding traditional vegetables. Using semistructured interviews, data were collected on the physical characteristics of the herbs, their ecological distribution, procurement, preparation or cooking, seasonality, medicinal uses, and underlying perceptions and practices. As a supplement, the research pupils wrote down all the names of traditional vegetables they knew in their area and compared the information with that of the key informants. Follow-up verification was then done among some key informants by means of visits to the relevant habitats, collecting samples of traditional vegetables, and cross-checking for identical plants with different names. Subsequently, a final list was made. The exact botanical nomenclature of 29 of the 72 plants was then ascertained.

RESULTS

Ethnic Taxonomy, Distribution, and Procurement

Although most of the plants were identified by common Luo names, some terms are specific to the region or even to a household. Some of the plants have two or three names, and usually the informants were not aware that others use different terms for the same species.[1]

The most complex answers were responses to the question, "What does it look like?" A description of the physical appearance of a plant entails a comparison with another plant. Typical is a comparison of three very similar vegetables: "*kabich samba* resembles *kandhira,* but has smaller leaves than sukuma wiki."[2] Thus, reliable identification had to be based on samples of the various plants (Ogoye-Ndegwa and Aagaard-Hansen, 2003).

Initial interviews with the 27 key informants produced 112 names of traditional vegetables. On cross-checking, it appeared that there were several cases of duplication (i.e., different names for the same plant). For example, *amondi (Talinum portulacifolium)* had also been mentioned as *alonde.* A collection of samples revealed that the two are actually the same, except that the two names are area-specific: *alonde* being the name in a neighboring division and *amondi* the name in the study area. The informant was a woman from the neighboring area who married in the study area. After complete cross-checking by collecting samples, the list comprised 72 traditional vegetables (annuals, biennials, and perennials); subsequently, 29 of these were taxonomically identified.

The plants studied thrive in four distinct habitats: in kitchen gardens, in the bush, along the lakeshores or riverbanks, and on fallow farmlands. The bulk of the traditional vegetables, about 58, are believed to be undomesticable and thrive in the wild. Fifteen of the plants on the list have been domesticated and are cultivated in kitchen gardens. These are vegetables such as *akeyo (Gynandropsis gynandra), osuga (Solanum nigrum), mito madongo (Crotalaria brevidens),* and *boo (Vigna unguiculata,* cowpea). The rest, although domesticated, are rarely consumed as vegetables but are cultivated for their seeds, fruits, or roots rather than for the leaves. They include *it pilu* pilu (leaves of the chile plant), *it nyanya* (tomato leaves), *it rabuon* (potato leaves), *it omuogo* (cassava leaves), *susa* (pumpkin leaves), *it kipoyo* (papaya leaves), *it nyim* (simsim leaves), and *it nduma* (arrowroot leaves). Three of the vegetables can be cultivated or are collected from the wild: *apoth (Corchorus trilocularis), osuga (Solanum nigrum),* and *onyulo (Sesamum angustifolium)* (Ogoye-Ndegwa and Aagaard-Hansen, 2003).

Sixteen of the vegetables on the list thrive in the bush; most are climbers or creepers. They include *nyamit kuru (Coccinia adoensis), oriadho (Erythrococca bongensis), bwombwe matindo (Cyphostemma orondo), bwombwe madongo (Cyphosyemma nierense),* and *ndemra (Basella alba).* Plants that thrive along the shores of the lake or riverbanks number eleven, and include *it nduma* (arrowroot leaves), *atek min angasa (Dyschoriste radicans), dindi (Acalphya volkensii), nyasgumba (Ludwigia stoloniferia), oyombe (Ottelia ulvifolia), ndemra (Basella alba), nyaketh mwanda, owich, obera, aurao,* and *obwanda (Portulaca quadrifida).* Most of the plants grow on fallow farmlands and include *atipa (Asystasia mysorensis), nyatonglo (Physalis angulata), achak (Sonchus schweinfurthii),* and *nyayado (Senna occidentalis)* (Ogoye-Ndegwa and Aagaard-Hansen, 2003).

Furthermore, there are two species of edible mushrooms: *obuolo madongo* (literally, "large mushrooms") and *obuolo matindo* (literally, "small mushrooms"). *Obuolo madongo (Termitomyces schimperi* [Agaricaceae]) (Kokwaro and Johns, 1998) is the most dominant one in the study area, growing wild on old termite mounds.[3] According to some of the key informants, many of the traditional vegetables are much less common nowadays. Previously, they could easily be obtained, whereas they now have to be looked for in places far away that have not yet been cleared for human settlement or cultivation. The high population pressure on farmland means that fewer stretches of land are left uncultivated. During the rainy season, plants that grow along with cultivated crops (e.g., maize, tomatoes, or sorghum) are considered to be weeds and so are uprooted. They are usually thrown away instead of being eaten or sold, partly due to limited knowledge about traditional vegetables (Kokwaro and Johns, 1998).

Seasonality strongly determines the availability of traditional vegetables. All 72 vegetables are available during the wet season, whereas only 38 are available during the dry season. The wet season gives a wide range of choices, though only about 34 traditional vegetables are actually consumed, with the dominant ones being apoth *(Corchorus trilocularis),* boo *(Vigna unguiculata),* atips *(Asystasia mysorensis),* akeyo *(Gynandropsis gynandra),* and osuga *(Solanium nigrum).* During the wet season there are many traditional vegetables to choose from, which means that the less-preferred ones are not consumed, even though they may be abundant (Kokwaro and Johns, 1998).

The plants grow in different ecological zones, and their existence is strongly influenced by the long and short rains from February to May and October to December, respectively. Their availability is therefore limited by seasonality (Ogoye-Ndegwa and Aagaard-Hansen, 2003). All the 38 available traditional vegetables that are consumed during the lean days of the dry season may be useful for most poor, rural families. They even include some vegetables that are not regarded as "genuine" foodstuffs. Examples include *nyayado (Senna occidentalis), it nduma* (pumpkin leaves), and *it kipoyo* (papaya leaves). The few vegetables available during the dry season are consumed indiscriminately and usually in mixtures. During the dry season, women procure vegetables along the lakeshores and in the bush, where it is relatively green. However, during the wet season, many varieties of traditional vegetables are available to choose from, and they can also be procured from the kitchen gardens and the fallow farmlands next to the homes (Ogoye-Ndegwa and Aagaard-Hansen, 2003).

Culturally, it is frowned upon for a man to pick vegetables, and therefore procurement is predominantly the domain of women and girls. The availability of certain vegetables in specific procurement sites is a secret treasured by the women. In most cases, procurement takes into consideration what is enough for a meal, except for the vegetables that are cooked *aboka* (see p. 332). Except for the kitchen-garden vegetables, those that thrive in other sites can be gathered by everyone, and do not belong to any particular individual. Vegetables that grow in kitchen gardens are grown from seeds that are purposely sown there (e.g., *boo*) or from the seeds that were shed during the previous season (e.g., *akeyo*). Kitchen-garden vegetables have avoidance regulations attached to them. For example, it is believed that menstruating women, culturally considered unclean, should not enter the kitchen garden to procure them, lest the vegetables wither. At these times a woman will therefore stand at the gate, pointing out to a younger girl which vegetables to pick (Ogoye-Ndegwa and Aagaard-Hansen, 2003).

Traditionally, it was prohibited to feed on what one used as medicine, although this restriction is not strictly observed nowadays. However, the same plants are dealt with in completely different ways, depending on their intended use. Collecting them for use as vegetables can be done publicly, by groups of girls or women. Collecting them for medicinal use is an event whereby one or two leaves are picked, often in secrecy. Preparation is very different as well. Hence, women prepare the food, and the medicine must be prepared by the herbalist himself or herself, or an apprentice under his or her instructions. Medicinal plants are usually collected in very small quantities. In contrast to vegetables for food, both men and women (herbalists) can collect medicinal plants (Ogoye-Ndegwa and Aagaard-Hansen, 2003).

Dietary Use

As with procurement, it is culturally unacceptable for a man to cook. Men who cook are often referred to as "women." After the vegetables have been sorted for cooking, it is believed that they should be torn by hand, as cutting with a knife "makes them bitter." Two main methods of cooking are used: *aruda* (literally, "stirred") and *aboka* (literally, "fermented"). Vegetables that are cooked *aruda* have salt and soda (sodium carbonate) added to them and are in most cases intended for immediate consumption. Soda ash is bought from the shop or is prepared from wood ash taken from the fireplace. Water is mixed with the ash and left to settle for some time until a suspension is formed and the water "tastes like soda." This water is then used to cook the vegetable. Soda ash is meant to soften and detoxify the vegetables. However, it should be added in minimal amounts, as otherwise the dish is unpalatable. Milk may be added as well, in order to initiate fermentation. Examples of vegetables cooked this way include apoth *(Corchorus trilocularis), boo (Vigna unguiculata), atipa (Asystasia mysorensis), mito madongo (Crotalaria brevidens),* and *onyulo (Sesamum angustifolium)* (Ogoye-Ndegwa and Aagaard-Hansen, 2003).

Vegetables that are cooked *aboka* have no salt added. Instead, during an average of two days, milk is added and they are put on the fire and cooked several times. It usually takes some days before they become soft and the bitter taste disappears and they are ready for consumption. About 28 traditional vegetables are cooked *aboka.* Examples include akeyo *(Gynandropsis gynandra), osuga (Solanum nigrum),* and *alika (Amaranthus* spp.) (Ogoye-Ndegwa and Aagaard-Hansen, 2003).

However, some traditional vegetables may be cooked either *aruda* or *aboka,* and they are often cooked in mixtures. There are about eleven such vegetables, including *nyayado (Senna occidentalis), it rabuon* (potato leaves), *okuuro,* and *dindi (Acalypha volkensii).* A vegetable that is cooked *aboka* may be mixed with the ones cooked *aruda,* and if an *aruda* vegetable is the predominant one, the dish is stirred and becomes *aruda* and vice versa. For example, *it achak,* which is *aruda* when mixed with *akeyo,* may be cooked *aboka,* and when mixed with *apoth* it may be cooked *aruda* (Ogoye-Ndegwa and Aagaard-Hansen, 2003).

Whether vegetables are mixed during cooking depends on their abundance and taste. During periods of drought, traditional vegetables are usually cooked in mixtures, since they are very scarce. Some vegetables are so bitter that they have to be cooked together with others in order to reduce the bitterness and make them more palatable. Examples include *nyamand dhiang', achak (Sonchus schweinfurthii), mito madongo (Crotalaria brevidens),* and *atek min angasa (Dyschoriste radicans)* (Ogoye-Ndegwa and Aagaard-Hansen, 2003).

However, other than taste and abundance, some vegetables such as *it kipoyo* (papaya leaves) and *bwombwe matindo (Cyphostemma orondo)* are feared to be "poisonous" and should be very minimal in the mixture. For example, goats die soon after eating large quantities of *it omuogo* (cassava leaves), and it is believed that the leaves are equally dangerous for human beings, if not taken minimally. Other species of *omuogo*[4] are known to be so poisonous that those who have eaten them, usually during famine, have been reported to have died from poisoning. Some traditional vegetables, for example *nyasgumba (Ludwigia stoloniferia),* have to be boiled, followed by more than two rinses with water, with a final amount of water being added for cooking (Ogoye-Ndegwa and Aagaard-Hansen, 2003).

According to the local perceptions, vegetables compare very unfavorably with other food items such as meat or fish. Among the Luo, it is usually considered undignified to serve vegetables to a visitor. Vegetables are referred to as "the caterpillars' bed,"[5] and it is said that "the hyena cries and still leaves it untouched,"[6] (i.e., the hyena, the animal the Luo perceive as the greediest, doesn't feed on vegetables!). Though most people do not like the rather bitter taste of some traditional vegetables such as *osuga (Solanum nigrum), akeyo (Gynandropsis gynandra),* and *mito madongo (Crotalaria brevidens),* some people relish their mild bitterness (Ogoye-Ndegwa and Aagaard-Hansen, 2003).

Medicinal Use

Besides being used as food, most of the many traditional vegetables among the Luo of western Kenya are considered to be of medicinal value. Most plants are used to treat different kinds of ailments, ranging from simple wounds affecting various parts of the body to treating the more complex ailments such as *chira,* spirit possession, and the evil eye. They can also be used for love potions and protective charms.

According to the typology of Foster (1976), some are used to deal with "naturalistic" physical ailments or alleviate bodily pain such as stomachache and labor pain (see Table 14.1). Others are seen to protect against "personalistic" conditions in which harm is inflicted by others using witchcraft (see Table 14.2). Foster (1976) states that "A naturalistic system explains illness in impersonal, systemic terms . . . from such natural forces or conditions," whereas "A personalistic medical system is one in which disease is explained as due to the *active, purposeful intervention* of an *agent,* who may be human, . . . nonhuman, . . . or supernatural" (p. 775). Though simplistic, this typology will be used in this chapter to categorize the illnesses for which herbal treatment is used.

The "naturalistic" illnesses are many and varied. *Okulbat* is an illness of infants, characterized by acute swellings of the armpits and accompanied by fever. The disease is not easily diagnosed by the younger mothers during its initial stages, and the diagnostic experience of the elderly mothers is often sought. *Mbaha* is a skin condition, often accompanied by fever in infants. The condition can be spread throughout the whole body, making the infant restless and in severe pain.

"Milk teeth" is a condition suspected to be caused by human or supernatural intervention, especially in cases of numerous growths. The infant does not feed well, neither does it suckle, and it is believed that traditional treatment is the only option. The fact that an infant develops "teeth" is seen as highly abnormal, explicable only in terms of the supernatural.

Possession by spirits is accompanied by abnormal behavior; some patients even talk in tongues. Spirits can be good or bad. The good spirits are nurtured and "developed," since they eventually help in healing the possessed person. The bad spirits, however, bring suffer-

TABLE 14.1. "Naturalistic" uses of medicinal plants according to the terminology of Foster (1976). The table gives an overview of the herbs used for various disorders and in some cases mentions other herbs and substances with which they are mixed.

Herb	Disorder	Mixture
Achak	Stomachache Ang'iew	Nyaydo
Adongo nyar yuora	Abscess/boils without an "eye"	–
Akeyo	Mgongo in babies	–
Anyim	Mbaha	–
Anyulo	Constipation/cracking anus Cough	–
Apoth	Measles	Other herbs
Atek min angasa	Bunda (edema) in pregnancy	–
Atipa	Reduces labor pain	Ombok alika
Aurao	Tapeworms Akuodi (kwashiorkor) Mbaha	–
Awayo matindo	To ripen boils	Awayo madongo
Ayucha	Mbaha	Other herbs
Boo	Mbuda (edema) Stomach fullness in pregnancy	Kikuyu grass
Dindi	Mbaha Eases labor pain	–
It nduma	Boils, other airborne diseases	–
Ndemra	Mbaha Removal of placenta Measles	Water
Nyadeg dani	Leprosy Baby rashes	Oil
Nyaketh mwanda	Mbaha	–
Nyalak dede	Stomachache Worms Removal of placenta Mbaha	–
Nyamit kuru	Okulbat (swollen lymph nodes of the armpit)	Oil
Nyarag achogo	Stomachache Edema in pregnancy Difficulty in breathing	Yago leaves Cow's fat Oil, other herbs

TABLE 14.1. *(continued)*

Herb	Disorder	Mixture
Nyatigatiga	Orienyancha in infants Clean an infant's tongue for better suckling	–
Nyayado	Stomachache Worms	–
Obudo	Stomachache	–
Obuolo madongo	Worms	–
Ododo	Hima or Orip	Ombok alika, oil
Okuro	Orienyancha in infants; Delayed delivery with persistent labor pain	–
Oriadho	Stomachache Boils	–
Owich	Pulls thorns from body Cough	Kat sero (kind of salt)
Radier remo	Worms Leprosy	Oriadho, Osuga Minya, pork fat
Tungu	Removal of placenta	–

ing and diseases such as madness, *ang'iew* in children, and epilepsy. *Chira* is a state of weakness, slow wastage of the body, and maybe eventual death. It is often associated with transgression of taboos in relation to cultivation, marriage and sexuality, or disrespect for the "living dead," including disrespect for seniority. A man's disrespect for the taboos may result in *chira* affecting him, his wife, and children thereafter. Nowadays the manifestations of HIV/AIDS are often equated with *chira*.

About 65 out of the 72 plants identified in the study are used for medicinal purposes. The medicinal herbs used by the Luo are collected in various ways. Some medicinal plants are openly and widely used by ordinary people and some are secretively used and the preserve of the professional healers.

The medicinal plants are not only eaten but also quite often used to prepare solutions for bathing and massaging. The preparation of medicines is illness-specific. Some medicines are diluted to drink, some are applied on the body, and some are hidden in folds of cloth,

TABLE 14.2. "Personalistic" uses of medicinal herbs according to the terminology of Foster (1976). The table gives an overview of the herbs used for various disorders and in some cases mentions other herbs and substances with which they are mixed.

Herb	Illness	Mixture
Atek min angasa	Spirits	Ndemra leaves
Angayo	Spirits (from the lake)	–
Atipa	Spirits (sepe)	–
Buombwe matindo	Spirits	–
Dindi	Spirits	–
It onyiego	Evil eye (an infant)	–
Nyamand dhiang'	Spirits	Other herbs
Nyarag achogo	Chira	–
Nyatigatiga	Chira	–
Nyasgumba	Spirits (from the lake)	–
Nyawend agwata	Sunken, "breathing" head	–
Ododo	Chira	Ombok alika, oil
Oyombe	Spirits	–
Radier remo	Chira	Other herbs

as protective charms. The preparation of certain medicines remains a treasured secret, and only a few ingredients may be revealed by the healer. Sometimes the procedure is complex and may involve slaughtering an animal (usually a lamb), whose blood forms an important ingredient. The harvesting and preparation of the medicines is often done by an apprentice under the instructions of the healer, but this is practiced under privatized and publicized professional treatment. In certain cases, the medicines are given to the sick with instructions on how to prepare and use them (dosage). Even so, in most cases the medicines are given to the sick when mashed. This is a safeguard to ensure that it is impossible to identify an ingredient. Even so, the ability to identify medicinal ingredients does not qualify a person to use them in treatment. This explains why even the apprentices cannot treat until they receive the blessings of the healer. Some medicines are considered "useless" unless and until blessed by the "owner." Blessing entails acknowledging the source of knowledge ownership and paying for that service.

Often, the patient pays a fee, which depends on the severity and seriousness of the disease. Often a fee is charged to initiate the treatment process before the medicine is dispensed. This is called *gir bungu*, literally, "the property of the forest." Other payments follow later, depending on the improvement of the sick person.

DISCUSSION

The Luo of western Kenya live in a transitional period in which food preference undermines food and nutrition security. Presently, food consumption practices are rapidly changing, and many traditional Luo food items are considered to have low status.[7] Recently introduced vegetables such as *sukuma wiki* have assumed a superior status and are more popular and abundantly consumed by most people. Paradoxically, some Luo traditional vegetables such as *osuga (Solanum nigrum), akeyo (Gynandropsis gynandra), mito madongo (Crotalaria brevidens),* and *ododo (Amaranthus hybridus)* can be found in big hotels in urban areas.

Most of the traditional vegetables exist as weeds of agriculture and are procured from the bushland and previously cultivated farmlands, where they are gathered communally. A few grow in kitchen gardens and along the lakeshores. The fact that most of these traditional vegetables are not cultivated increases their scarcity, as many of the natural habitats are vanishing. Far fewer traditional vegetables are reported to be abundant, compared to a decade ago. Furthermore, as this knowledge is rarely passed on to the younger generation, there is a risk that it will eventually be lost.

Previous studies have shown that some of these traditional vegetables are highly nutritious (FAO, 1968). An analysis comparing some of the traditional vegetables with the recently introduced and preferred "cabbages" (which semantically includes *sukuma wiki*) shows, for example, that *ododo (Amaranthus hybridus)* is almost twice as high in calories and eight times as high in iron content. *Akeyo (Gynandropsis gynandra)* is three times as high in protein and six times as high in iron content. In addition, the comparisons of beta-carotene reveal that the traditional herbs have a clear advantage (FAO, 1968). The present study has not analyzed the vegetables' content of micronutrients or toxins in the raw form. Neither has it looked into the modifications of content that are likely to take place during the various traditional processes of preparation. However, these research questions are now being addressed (Orech, personal communication). One critical area of consideration is the determination of the toxicity as well as the nutritional content of specific plants. Although it is contended that some of these plants are highly nutritious (FAO, 1968), some of them are potentially highly toxic. This last point suggests that some of the traditional vegetables are considered poisonous if not "properly cooked" (Ogoye-Ndegwa and Aagaard-Hansen, 2003).

In sub-Saharan Africa, the bioavailability of dietary iron has been considered the most important determinant of anemia in every age group except pregnant women (Sub-Committee on Nutrition, 1997, p. 35). Horticultural approaches are increasingly recognized for their effectiveness and potential sustainability in improving not only vitamin A but also general micronutrient status (p. 33).[8] Home gardening, however, has the added advantage of contributing to women's income (p. 31). Wild plants and other wild food sources are widespread in most human societies. However, the extent to which such plants and other wild food items are consumed has not been systematically documented; neither has their nutritional significance been fully ascertained (Fleuret, 1979; Nordeide et al., 1996).

Our study has shown that a substantial number of traditional herbs (65 of the 72 on our list) are used as medicine as well as vegetables. The plants are used for a great variety of illnesses which, according to the typology of Foster (1976), fall both into the "naturalistic" and "personalistic" categories. The widespread use of medicinal herbs is in accordance with the findings of other scholars who have studied Luo medicine (Prince et al., 2001; Geissler et al., 2002). Though widely used for medicinal purposes, their chemical content and clinical effects have only been sparsely examined. Furthermore, some of the plants may have toxic effects, which should be looked into before recommendations can be made. The use of herbal medicine in Kenya is gaining wider application (for example, people are increasingly resorting to Chinese herbal treatment). A debate is currently taking place in Kenya about whether herbal medicine should be included in the mainstream national health program.

CONCLUSION

We have described how plants that mostly grow wild are used by the Luo of western Kenya partly as food items (vegetables) and partly for medicinal purposes. Most of the plants in the study are used for both dietary and medicinal purposes. Indications are strong that many of the wild herbs used as vegetables have high contents of important micronutrients such as iron and vitamin A. However, uncritical advocacy of traditional vegetables as a means of counteracting food insecurity should be cautioned, as many of them are toxic.

Many of the herbs are also used for medicinal purposes. The significance of modern medicine notwithstanding, the potential use of medicinal herbs could be further explored and those that prove to be effective could be exploited.

NOTES

1. For example, most of the pupils had named boo (*Vigna unguiculata*), *hamba, ajur,* and *manyonyo* as four separate vegetables. On validation, it was discovered that the four names refer to the growth and storage stages of a single vegetable species, *boo. Hamba* are the hard, old leaves of *boo,* whereas *ajur* refers to *boo* that has sprouted from a stump after rain has ended a dry spell. *Manyonyo* is the *boo* dried and preserved for later use. Key informants later confirmed that the four names refer to one and the same species (Ogoye-Ndegwa and Aagaard-Hansen, 2003).

2. *Dholuo* terms (the local language) are indicated in italics. However, some of the terms are borrowed from other languages, e.g., *sukuma wiki* comes from Kiswahili.

3. Mushrooms are clearly not vegetables in the strict, botanical sense.

4. *Omuogo* can generally be divided into the edible *marieba (Manihot esculenta),* which is a shrub, and the generally inedible *omuok nawi,* which grows to the size of a tree (Capen, 1998). However, during periods of food scarcity, some people harvest the tubers of *omuok nawi,* which need to be processed carefully in order to detoxify them before eating. We noted several reports of cases where people had died because of inappropriate detoxification (Ogoye-Ndegwa and Aagaard-Hansen, 2003).

5. *Otanda oyuo.*

6. *Ondiek ywak to pod weye aweya oko.*

7. It is beyond the scope of the present chapter to analyze the dynamics of the changes in the Luo culture in general and those regarding food practices in particular. See, however, Cohen and Odhiambo (1989, pp. 64-65) on the shift from millet and sorghum to white maize.

8. Though vegetables supply the nonhemoglobin type of iron, it is still the most important source of dietary iron, especially in developing countries (Sub-Committee on Nutrition, 1997, p. 39).

REFERENCES

Barthes, R. (1997). Towards a psychology of contemporary food consumption. In C. Counihan and P. van Esterik (Eds.), *Food and culture* (pp. 20-27). New York: Routledge.

Behar, M. (1976). European diets vs. traditional foods. *Food Policy* 1: 432-435.

Bloem, M.W., N. Huq, J. Gorsten, S. Burger, T. Kahn, N. Islam, S. Baker, and F. Davidson (1996). Production of fruits and vegetables at the homestead is an important source of vitamin A among women in rural Bangladesh. *European Journal of Clinical Nutrition* 50, supplement 3: S62-S67.

Capen, C.A. (1998). *Bilingual Dholuo-English dictionary.* Tucson, AZ: Carole A. Capen.

Cattle, D.J. (1977). An alternative to nutritional particularism. In T.K. Fitzgerald (Ed.), *Nutrition and anthropology in action* (pp. 35-45). Amsterdam: Van Gorcum.

Cohen, D.W. and E.S.A. Odhiambo (1989). *Siaya: The historical anthropology of an African landscape.* Nairobi: Heinemann Kenya.

Etkin, N.L. and P.J. Ross (1983). Malaria, medicine and meals: Plant use and its impact on disease. In L. Romanucci-Ross, D.E. Moerman, and L.R. Tancredi (Eds.), *The anthropology of medicine* (pp. 231-259). New York: Praeger Publishers.

Ferguson, E.L., R.S. Gibson, C. Opare-Obisau, F. Osei-Opare, C. Lamba, and S. Ounpuu (1993). Seasonal food consumption patterns and dietary diversity of rural preschool Ghanian and Malawian children. *Ecology of Food and Nutrition* 29: 219-234.

Fieldhouse, P. (1998). *Food and nutrition.* Cheltenham: Stanley Thornes Ltd.

Fleuret, A. (1979). The role of wild foliage plants in the diet. A case study from Lushoto, Tanzania. *Ecology of Food and Nutrition* 8: 87-93.

Food and Agriculture Organization (FAO) (1968). *Food consumption table for use in Africa.* Geneva: Division of Nutrition, Food and Agriculture Organization.

Foster, G.M. (1976). Disease etiologies in non-Western medical systems. *American Anthropologist* 78: 773-782.

Freedman, R.L. (1977). Nutritional anthropology: An overview. In T.K. Fitzgerald (Ed.), *Nutrition and anthropology in action* (pp. 1-23). Amsterdam: Van Gorcum.

Geissler, P.W. (1998). Geophagy among primary schoolchildren in Western Kenya. PhD thesis. University of Copenhagen.

Geissler, P.W., S.A. Harris, R.J. Prince, A. Olsen, R.A. Odhiambo, H. Oketch-Rabah, P.A. Madiega, A. Andersen, and P. Mølgaard (2002). Medicinal plants used by Luo mothers and children in Bondo District, Kenya. *Journal of Ethnopharmacology* 83: 39-54.

Geissler, P.W., K. Nokes, R.J. Prince, R.A. Odhiambo, J. Aagaard-Hansen, and J.H. Ouma (2000). Children and medicines: Self-treatment of common illnesses among Luo primary school children in western Kenya. *Social Science and Medicine* 50 (18): 1771-1783.

Hedberg. I. and F. Staugård (1989). *Traditional medicinal plants*. Gaborone, Botswana: Ipeleng Publishers.

Kokwaro, J.O. and T. Johns (1998). *Luo biological dictionary*. Nairobi: East African Educational Publishers.

Krondl. M.M. and G.G. Boxen (1975). Nutrition behaviour, food resources and energy. In M. Arnott (Ed.), *Gastronomy: The anthropology of food and food habits* (pp. 113-120). The Hague: Mouton Publishing.

Kumar, S.K. (1978). Role of the household economy in child nutrition at low incomes: A case study in Kerala. Occasional paper No. 95. Department of Agricultural Economics, Cornell University, Ithaca, NY.

Leemon, M. and S. Samman (1998). A food-based systems approach to improve the nutritional status of Australian Aborigines: A focus on zinc. *Ecology of Food and Nutrition* 10: 1-33.

Lepofsky, D., N.J. Turner, and H.V. Kuhnlein (1985). Determining the availability of traditional wild plant foods: An example of Nuxalk foods, Bella Coola, British Columbia. *Ecology of Food and Nutrition* 16: 223-241.

Lupton, D. (1996). *Food, the body and the self*. London: Sage.

Meigs, A. (1997). Food as a cultural construction. In C. Counihan and P. van Esterik (Eds.), *Food and culture* (pp. 95-106). New York: Routledge.

Nordeide, M.B., A. Hatloy, M. Folling, E. Lied, and A. Oshaug (1996). Nutrient composition and nutritional importance of green leaves and wild food resources in an agricultural district. Koutiala, in southern Mali. *International Journal of Food Sciences and Nutrition* 47: 455-468.

Ogoye-Ndegwa, C. and J. Aagaard-Hansen (2003). Traditional gathering of wild vegetables among the Luo of Western Kenya—A nutritional anthropology project. *Ecology of Food and Nutrition* 42 (1): 69-89.

Ogoye-Ndegwa, C., D. Abudho, and J. Aagaard-Hansen (2002). New learning in old organisations: Children's participation in a school-based nutrition project in western Kenya. *Development in Practice* 12 (3 and 4): 449-460.

Price, W.A. (1939). *Nutrition and physical degradation: A comparison of primitive and modern diets and their effects*. New York: Paul B. Hoeber.

Prince, R. and P.W. Geissler (2001). Becoming "one who treats": A case study of a Luo healer and her grandson in western Kenya. *Anthropology & Education Quarterly* 32 (4): 447-471.

Prince, R.J., P.W. Geissler, K. Nokes, J.O. Maende. F. Okatcha. E. Gringorenko, and R. Sternberg (2001). Knowledge of herbal and pharmaceutical medicines among Luo children in western Kenya. *Anthropology & Medicine* 8 (2/3): 211-235.

Sen, A. (1992). *Inequality re-examined*. Cambridge. MA: Harvard University Press.

Solon, F., T.L. Fernandez, M.C. Latham, and B.M. Popkin (1979). An evaluation of strategies to control vitamin A deficiency in the Philippines. *American Journal of Clinical Nutrition* 32: 1445-1453.

Sub-Committee on Nutrition (ACC/SCN) (1997). *Third report on the world nutrition situation*. Geneva: WHO.

Chapter 15

Ethnomycology in Africa, with Particular Reference to the Rain Forest Zone of South Cameroon

Thomas W. Kuyper

INTRODUCTION

Several years ago, the Africa Museum in Berg en Dal (the Netherlands) organized a special exhibition, "Herbs, Health, Healers" (De Smet, 1999), which was devoted to ethnopharmacology—the production and use of substances with medicinal properties that are derived from local flora and fauna—in Africa. In the catalog that accompanied the exhibition only incidental mention of mushrooms was made. Only one species was dealt with in detail: *Coprinus africanus*. The vernacular name of that species among the Yoruba in Nigeria is *ajeimutin,* which translates as "eat, without drinking alcohol." The same fungal species also occurs in the Central African Republic, and the Lissongo (a group of Pygmies) call this mushroom *itongomokolo:* "the mushroom that spins your head and heart when simultaneously drinking palm wine" (Heim, 1963). From both vernacular names it is clear that several African cultures know that consuming this mushroom in combination with alcohol can result in very disagreeable physical symptoms. In the northern hemisphere, it is medically known that consuming the related mushroom species *Coprinus atramentarius* in combination with alcohol gives rise to similar disagreeable symptoms. It has been suggested that the substances re-

The fieldwork in Cameroon was done jointly with Han van Dijk and Neree Awana Onguene. Their help is greatly appreciated. I also thank the Bantu and Bagyeli informants for their willingness to share information.

sponsible for this physical reaction could be used to treat alcoholism, but the fact that regular consumption of this species was found to decrease the fertility of male rats prevented its subsequent clinical trials and commercial use.

The scant attention paid to mushrooms in the Africa Museum exhibition is at first sight somewhat curious and therefore in need of an explanation. Could it be that indigenous knowledge about medicinal and other mushrooms is grossly underdeveloped compared to knowledge about plants? The African continent is in fact very rich in plant species that have been used in traditional medicine, and several of these (such as *Prunus africana*, which is used for healing prostate cancer) are already regularly used in modern medicine or appear to have great promise (such as *Ancistrocladus korupensis*, a potential drug against human immunodeficiency virus and malaria). Or, could it be that despite ample knowledge of indigenous mushrooms, their use is still restricted because mushrooms decay rapidly and cannot easily be dried and preserved in a humid climate? Or, is there extensive knowledge and use, but much of this utilization takes place in ritual and secret sessions that are not accessible to Western scientists? On a very different level, could it be possible that mushroom knowledge and utilization is extensive, but that European (and eurocentric) anthropologists have a blind spot for it?

MYCOPHILIA VERSUS MYCOPHOBIA

The possibility of research bias deserves attention. Since the work of the Wasson couple (he of American, she of Russian provenance) it has been customary and fashionable to classify cultures as *mycophobic* (mushroom avoiding) and *mycophilic* (mushroom loving). An anecdote suggests that mycophobia exists among anthropologists. During a dinner at an anthropology conference, the French anthropologist Lévi-Strauss, who had been impressed by the work of Wasson (1968), had an animated discussion with a British colleague about the issue of mycophobia and mycophilia. The British anthropologist showed his usual skepticism, being unconvinced that this classification reflects a fundamental distinction and claiming that if the British do indeed show little interest in mushrooms, it is for no other reason than that there are hardly any mushrooms in Great Britain (Lévi-Strauss, 1970).

According to Wasson (1968), mycophobia is widespread among the Anglo-Saxon linguistic group. As many nineteenth and early twentieth century anthropologists were of English or German provenance it is not surprising that these scientists had a blind spot for mushrooms. Mycophilic cultures are found among the Slavonic linguistic group, and furthermore among the Sami (Laps) and the Indians in northwestern North America and in Mexico. It is not clear whether this distinction between mycophobic and mycophilic cultures also applies to Africa. To my knowledge, the issue has never been systematically studied on that continent. However, a curious pattern has been noted among the population of African descent on the Caribbean island of Hispaniola. In francophone Haiti the Afro population is predominantly mycophilic, while in the neighboring hispanophone Dominican Republic it is predominantly mycophobic (Nieves-Rivera, 2001). This distinction may be a consequence of the different attitudes of the French and Spanish colonists and, in particular, the possible mycophobic attitude of the Roman Catholic Church.

Mycophilic cultures possess an extensive folk taxonomic knowledge in which many different mushrooms are recognized and named. They also have a wide variety of mushroom uses, including dietary, culinary, medicinal, and ritual and religious.

OVERVIEW OF MUSHROOM USE IN AFRICA

It has been proposed that the oldest traces of mushroom use in Africa date back about 9,000 to 7,000 years BP (Samorini, 1992). Rock paintings in Tassili (Algeria), and also to a lesser extent in Lybia, Egypt, and Chad, have been interpreted as showing anthropomorphic beings or masked dancing figures holding mushrooms in their right hands. Emanating from the mushroom object are two parallel lines that reach the central part of the dancer's head. These lines have been interpreted as a representation of the effect that psychotropic mushrooms have on the human mind. However, alternative interpretations of the mushroomlike symbol have also been proposed, such as an arrowhead, oar, plant, or flower. Sometimes the symbol has been undefined. In this regard it is curious that there are very few reports on the use of hallucinogenic mushrooms in Africa, even though the hallucinogenic species *Panaeolus cyanescens* and several *Psilocybe* species are not uncommon on dung in eastern and southern Africa.

The first report on hallucinogenic mushrooms in Africa is rather suspect. The famous explorer Livingstone mentioned mushrooms being used in a local meal; after eating the meal he experienced intense dreams of roast beef (Piearce, 1985). To date, the identity of the mushroom has remained speculative, and the possibility that hallucinogenic plants had been added to the meal cannot be excluded. It is also conceivable that Livingstone's dreams were induced by homesickness.

The report by Soubrillard (cited in Samorini, 1995) is questionable. Soubrillard maintains that somewhere on the Ivory Coast two mushroom species with psychotropic properties are used. One of these, *tamu*, the mushroom of knowledge, is apparently a recent discovery by the local population, while the other species, called the mushroom of action, has been known for a substantial period, even though the fungus does not have a vernacular name. Soubrillard's account of his encounter with the local healer also seems to be too unusual to believe this report at face value.

Finally there is Terence McKenna's (1992) "stoned ape" theory of human evolution, which claims that during the evolution that led to the species *Homo sapiens*, the ancestral species shifted its habitat to savanna as a consequence of climatic change; this resulted in a dietary shift. The new diet included psilocybin-containing mushrooms growing on the dung of herbivores that roamed the savanna. Consuming these fungi jumbled the experiences from the various senses and, according to McKenna, led to language. The empirical basis for this theory is extremely weak, and McKenna's theory has been dismissed by evolutionary biologists.

The almost complete absence of reports on hallucinogenic mushroom use in Africa does not indicate that Africans are not interested in natural products with psychotropic activities. Africa is well endowed with hallucinogenic plants, such as *Catha edulis* (the source of qat), *Areca catechu* (betel nut), and *Tabernanthe iboga* (De Smet, 1999). Neither should we fall into the error of assuming that a simple relation exists between mycophilic cultures and the use of hallucinogenic mushrooms.

In recent decades, interest in ethnomycology (the study of the indigenous knowledge and use of mushrooms) in Africa has increased substantially. Research, driven by curiosity, has been based on the assumption that such knowledge could contribute to food security and to better protection of Africa's wildlife resources. Mushrooms are an important source of protein; in some African cultures they are known as the meat of the poor. The nitrogen content of mushrooms usually varies from 1 to 2 percent in wood-decomposing fungi to 4 to 5 percent in ectomycorrhizal fungi. Values are even higher in species of *Termitomyces*. Not all the nitrogen is in the protein, but because the fungal cell walls contain the nitrogenous polymer chitin, the protein content can reach values of up to 20 percent of dry weight in ectomycorrhizal mushrooms and more than 30 percent in *Termitomyces microcarpus* (Parent and Thoen, 1977; Degreef et al., 1997). Often, mushrooms are considered to be a substitute for animal protein. However, mushroom proteins are somewhat more difficult to digest than animal protein, making mushrooms only a partial substitute for meat. Nevertheless, a shift toward a diet in which mushrooms play a large role could simultaneously protect wild animals that are now illegally hunted and trapped to provide bush meat for local residents and urban populations.

In eastern Africa, mushroom consumption is common and widespread (Buyck, 1994; Malaisse, 1997). It is especially important in the *miombo,* a savanna or open woodland vegetation dominated by trees of the Caesalpiniaceae that form ectomycorrhizas: mutually beneficial associations between tree roots and certain mushrooms. In this landscape, termitaria (termite mounds) are also prominent features, and mushrooms of the genus *Termitomyces,* which are cultivated by certain termites, are also a very important food. The largest representative of that genus, *T. titanicus,* has caps with a diameter of up to 100 cm. Annual mushroom consumption in these areas can vary between 15 and 30 kg fresh weight per capita. Given the strong seasonality of mushrooms, this is a very substantial amount.

MUSHROOM KNOWLEDGE AND UTILIZATION BY BANTU AND BAGYELI IN SOUTH CAMEROON

The relatively good information on mushroom knowledge and utilization in central and eastern Africa contrasts sharply with our limited knowledge about western Africa. Very little work has been done on the knowledge and utilization of mushrooms in the rain forests of this area (Heim, 1963; Oso, 1975, 1977). As part of the Tropenbos Cameroon Program, which was aimed at the protection and sustainable management of Cameroon's rain forests, studies were conducted on nontimber forest products (Van Dijk, 1999) and on the role of mycorrhizal associations for forest management (Onguene, 2000). Both studies focused on mushrooms growing in pristine and disturbed rain forests. The results of these combined studies that included questionnaires on mycological knowledge, a socioeconomic household survey, and an extensive mushroom collection and preservation effort have recently been published (Van Dijk, Onguene, and Kuyper, 2003). They are summarized following.

The fieldwork area was in southwest Cameroon, in the Congo-Guinea forest refuge, about 80 km east of the coastal town of Kribi. The area is sparsely populated (less than ten inhabitants per square kilometer), implying that as yet very little human pressure has been put on the land. No strong signs of declining soil fertility due to agricultural intensification were noted. Most of the area is covered by forest, which has been and still is being logged by domestic and foreign companies. A large part of the forest is therefore degraded. Two major groups of people co-occur in the area. The large majority (around 90 percent) of the population consists of Bantu farmers (mainly Bulu, but also Fang, Bassa, and Ngumba) who practice shifting cultivation; cocoa cash-cropping; and hunting, fishing, and gathering. Around 10 percent of the population are Bagyeli (Pygmy) hunter-gatherers, who mainly live in small settlements in the forest, although some of them have recently adopted shifting cultivation and, to a lesser extent, cocoa farming. The Bagyeli spend almost all of their lives in the forest, and mushroom collection can easily be combined with their other hunting and gathering activities. The Bantu visit the rain forest much less frequently, so are more likely to be less time efficient at searching for mushrooms in the forest. However, mushroom collection in the immediate vicinity of their agricultural plots can easily be combined with other agricultural activities. Property rights also have an impact on collecting sites. Bantus usually have property rights over the mushrooms in the immediate vicinity of their fields and plantations. The property rights on secondary forests and old fallows are more variable and depend on how far back the collective memory about land ownership extends. Mushroom collection in the pristine rain forest is essentially free (Van den Berg and Biesbrouck, 2000). The different lifestyles of the Bantu and Bagyeli result in differences in habitats in which mushrooms are collected (see Table 15.1).

Consequently, both tribes have a different mushroom diet, as different mushroom species grow in the different habitats. The Bantu diet consists mainly of saprotrophic (litter- and wood-decomposing) mushrooms, the most important being *Volvariella volvacea* and *Lentinus squarrosulus*. The Bagyeli collect mainly in undisturbed rain forest where patches dominated by ectomycorrhizal Caesalpiniaceae occur. Their diet contains a large amount of ectomycorrhiza-forming mushrooms such as *Cantharellus rufopunctatus* and several other *Cantharellus* species and *Lactarius gymnocarpus*. Species of the genus *Termitomyces* also form a major part of their mushroom diet. Table 15.2 gives an overview of the habitats of the six mushroom species that are consumed in the largest quantities.

Despite the differences in mushroom diets, mushroom consumption is very comparable: on average 1.4 kg fresh weight per person per year for Bantu, and 1.1 kg for Bagyeli. The ethnomycological survey showed extensive knowledge of mushrooms that were eaten, used for medicinal purposes, or both. During the interviews, more than 50 vernacular names for mushrooms were mentioned. To date, some 35 species have been identified (for the complete list, see Van Dijk et al., 2003), a level of mushroom knowledge comparable to that in eastern Africa, where the number of mushrooms with vernacular names usually ranges between 20 and 60. In south Cameroon, women have a much more extensive mushroom knowledge than men, at least among Bantu, although Bantu men regularly engaged in hunting also

TABLE 15.1. Habitats in the Congo-Guinea Forest Refuge where mushrooms are collected (in percent of total mushroom harvest).

Vegetation type	Bagyeli	Bantu
Primary forest	21	54
Secondary forest	32	17
Cocoa plantations	6	6
Home gardens	10	3
Young fallow, agricultural plots	31	20

Source: Data from Van Dijk et al., 2003.

TABLE 15.2. Habitats of the six most important edible mushrooms harvested in south Cameroon.

Scientific name	Amount harvested (kg)	PF	SF	CP (%)	HG	FA
Volvariella volvacea	69	6	21	16	23	34
Termitomyces sp. 1	36	81	19	–	–	–
Lentinus squarrosulus	34	15	39	2	–	44
Marasmius katangensis	15	33	67	–	–	–
Cantharellus rufopunctatus	10	87	13	–	–	–
Termitomyces sp. 2	6	79	13	–	8	–

Source: Data from Van Dijk et al., 2003.

Note: Amount of mushrooms harvested includes harvests by both Bantu and Bagyeli.

PF = primary forest; SF = secondary forest; CP = cocoa plantations; HG = home gardens; FA = young fallow and agricultural plots.

have good knowledge of mushrooms. Among the Bagyeli, men and women contribute equally to mushroom collection. Mushroom knowledge is transmitted orally from mother to child. Edible mushrooms are considered an alternative for and supplement to animal protein. Mushrooms are often added to soups of peanut *(Arachis hypogaea)*, bush mango almonds *(Irvingia gabonensis)*, and oil palm fruits *(Elaeis guineensis)*. Most mushrooms are cooked fresh; they are rarely preserved (sun-drying, smoke-drying, or salting).

Although toxic mushrooms such as *Amanita bingensis* do occasionally occur in the forest (Heim, 1940), they were not mentioned during the interviews. The local people do, however, use various criteria to judge whether mushrooms are edible or not. Mushrooms that show signs of having been eaten by rodents or snails are considered edible, whereas mushrooms with a bitter or sharp taste and mushrooms that when rubbed on the breast nipple or elbow generate irritation or itching are considered poisonous. In other parts of Africa, mushrooms are fed to chickens to assess their toxicity, and mushrooms observed to have been eaten by apes and monkeys are also considered edible. Both the Bantu and the Bagyeli consider boletes whose flesh turns blue on exposure to air as poisonous—a criterion often also encountered in popular European beliefs on mushroom toxicity. However, other boletes are also rarely eaten by the indigenous populations, but figure more prominently in the diet of mycophilous Europeans living in Africa. The apparent lack of knowledge about poisonous mushrooms not only reflects the rarity of these species, but may also be related to people's extensive knowledge of plant species containing rapidly working toxins. In Africa more than 250 plant species with very rapidly acting toxins are used on arrowheads (De Smet, 1999).

Various mushrooms in south Cameroon are used not only as food but also for medicinal purposes—but only by the Bantu farmers. *Lentinus squarrosulus* may help to heal a newborn baby's navel. *Pleurotus tuber-regium* may improve the lactation of breast-feeding women, and its sclerotium may heal heart palpitations. The cup fungi *Cookeina sulcipes* and *C. tricholoma* are used against ear inflammation, and a species of *Termitomyces* is reported to be used for the same purposes. The medicinal and ritual use of mushrooms among the Yoruba in Nigeria has been described by Oso (1975, 1977). It has been reported that species of *Termitomyces* increase sexual activity in those who take it. Consumption of *Termitomyces microcarpus*, a small white mushroom that can occur in large numbers on termitaria, is reported to bring good luck to parents wanting many children, while merchants eat it to attract more customers to their shops. Finally, in combination with several herbs, the species is used to treat gonorrhea. A much larger species of the same genus, *Termitomyces robustus*, is also reputed to increase parents' fecundity and merchants' clientele. The local population believes that in combination with alcohol and certain herbs it is used to treat *maagun*, a disease that women unknowingly attract. As a consequence of the disease, any man with whom the woman commits adultery will die.

MUSHROOMS: MEAT OF THE POOR

The Tropenbos research in south Cameroon has shown an extensive knowledge of mushrooms (over 50 species are used for food and medicine) among the local people, though the annual per capita consumption of mushrooms was quite low: 1.1 kg fresh weight for the Bagyeli and 1.4 kg for the Bantu. In contrast, in eastern Africa mushroom consumption is over ten times higher (15 to 30 kg), though mushroom knowledge is at a comparable level. How can this difference be explained? At least three factors play a role:

- In the tropical rain forest the mushrooms are often small, thin-fleshed, and prone to rapid decay. In contrast, in the miombo big, fleshy mushrooms of the genera *Amanita, Cantharellus,* and *Termitomyces* occur.
- In the rain forest, mushrooms are far less seasonal than in the miombo, where mushrooms appear in huge quantities at the onset of the rainy season. This phenological pattern affects not only when mushrooms appear but also food availability in general. In the rain forest, alternative food sources are always available to a large extent, while in the miombo, mushrooms peak at the time when other food sources such as cereals and legumes are very scarce or absent.
- In the rain forest, wildlife is still an abundant source of protein. Though the Bagyeli and Bantu consume less than 1.5 kg mushrooms per capita annually, their annual per capita consumption of meat and fish can easily amount to 100 kg. These amounts include skin, hair, bone, and other parts that we consider inedible, but it is nonetheless clear that mushroom diets can be understood only in the context of the diversity of other sources of protein and the societal value attached to these sources.

In south Cameroon, mushrooms are literally the meat of the poor. This has two implications: the first is that extensive mushroom consumption is viewed negatively, as evidence of poverty; the second is that alternative protein sources cannot be procured. One example illustrates this situation forcefully. In one of the fieldwork villages a woman living alone with her daughter, without any males, could not go hunting. What meat she and her daughter consumed consisted of rats caught around the house, meat bought or received as a gift, and mushrooms. Consequently, they ate large amounts of mushrooms (almost 20 kg per person).

This type of social prejudice against mushrooms could hamper attempts to promote the cultivation of edible mushrooms being supported by governments, foreign aid agencies, and nongovernmental organizations in various parts of Africa to make women more financially independent and empower female farmers. The data from south Cameroon suggest that such a strategy may not be successful everywhere. When mushrooms are considered to be the meat of the poor, a social stigma may be attached to their consumption, and consequently mushroom consumption will not become important as long as sufficient supply of bush meat and fish is available. This situation might not apply around the major towns of south Cameroon (Douala, Yaoundé, Limbe). Here, the price of bush meat is rising as supply begins to lag behind the demand from the ever-growing population. This creates a market niche for mushrooms. Some mushrooms are already being sold in markets, and in Limbe a small mushroom farm cultivating nonindigenous mushrooms has been set up.

Although this general conclusion on the value society attaches to mushrooms is based on only one case study and must therefore be considered as provisional, it is clear that subsequent ethnomycological studies will gain from closer integration of the natural and social sciences.

REFERENCES

Buyck, B. (1994). *Ubwoba: Les champignons comestibles de l'ouest du Burundi.* Brussels: AGCD.

De Smet, P.A.G.M. (1999). *Herbs, health and healer—Africa as ethnopharmacological treasury.* Berg en Dal: Afrika Museum.

Degreef, J., F. Malaisse, J. Rammeloo, and E. Baudart (1997). Edible mushrooms of the Zambezian woodland area; a nutritional and ecological approach. *Biotechnology, Agronomy, Society and Environment* 1: 221-231.

Heim, R. (1940). Une amanite mortelle de l'Afrique centrale. *Revue de Mycologie* 5: 22-28.

Heim, R. (1963). La nomenclature mycologique des Lissongos. *Cahiers de Maboké* 1: 77-85.

Lévi-Strauss, C. (1970). Les champignons dans la culture—A propos d'un livre de M. R.-G. Wasson, L'Homme. *Revue Française de l'Anthropologie* 10: 5-16

Malaisse, F. (1997). *Se nourrir en Forêt Claire Africaine. Approche écologique et nutritionelle.* Gembloux, Belgium: Les presses agronomiques de Gembloux.

McKenna, T. (1992). *Food of the gods—The search for the original tree of knowledge.* New York: Bantam New Age Books.

Nieves-Rivera, A.M. (2001). Origin of mycophagy in the West Indies. *Inoculum* 52 (2): 1-3.

Onguene, N.A. (2000). Diversity and dynamics of mycorrhizal associations in tropical rain forests with different disturbance regimes in South Cameroon. *Tropenbos Cameroon Series* 3: 1-167.

Oso, B.A. (1975). Mushrooms and the Yoruba people of Nigeria. *Mycologia* 67: 271-279.

Oso, B.A. (1977). Mushrooms in Yoruba mythology and medicinal practices. *Economic Botany* 31: 367-371.

Parent, G. and D. Thoen (1977). Food value of edible mushrooms from Upper Shaba region. *Economic Botany* 31: 436-445.

Piearce, G.D. (1985). Livingstone and fungi in tropical Africa. *Bulletin of the British Mycological Society* 19: 39-50.

Samorini, G. (1992). The oldest representations of hallucinogenic mushrooms in the world (Sahara Desert, 9,000-7,000 BP). *Integration* 2/3: 69-78.

Samorini, G. (1995). Traditional use of psychoactive mushrooms in Ivory Coast? *Eleusis* 1: 22-27.

Van den Berg, J. and K. Biesbrouck (2000). The social dimension of rain forest management in Cameroon: Issues for co-management. *Tropenbos Cameroon Series* 4: 1-99.

Van Dijk, J.F.W. (1999). Non-timber forest products in the Bipindi-Akom II Region, Cameroon. A socio-economic and ecological assessment. *Tropenbos Cameroon Series* 1: 1-197.

Van Dijk, J.F.W., N.A. Onguene, and T.W. Kuyper (2003). Knowledge and utilization of edible mushrooms by local populations of the rain forest of south Cameroon. *Ambio* 32: 19-23.

Wasson, R.G. (1968). *Soma: Divine mushroom of immortality*. New York: Harcourt Brace Jovanovich.

Chapter 16

Aspects of Food Medicine and Ethnopharmacology in Morocco

Mohamed Eddouks

INTRODUCTION

The late King Hassan II of Morocco likened his country to a desert palm "rooted in Africa, watered by Islam and rustled by the winds of Europe." Morocco's location and resources have shaped its history.

The foods of Morocco take great advantage of the natural bounty of a country in which eating is a practical and social ritual. The strong Arab influence contributed greatly to Moroccan cuisine, as did the Andalusian sensitivities of the city of Tétouan and the Jewish traditions of the coastal city of Essaouira. The influence of these various cultures can be experienced in the best-loved Moroccan dishes: couscous (plump semolina grains), *bisteeya, mechoui,* and *djej emsherml* (Kadiri and Raiss, 1997). The cooks in the kitchens of the four royal cities (Fez, Meknes, Marrakesh, and Rabat) helped to define Moroccan cuisine, seasoned with spices and focused on fresh ingredients, and created the basis for what is known today as Moroccan cuisine. Moroccans are quick to point out that the best meals are not found in the restaurants but in the homes. Women do virtually all the cooking in this very traditional country. The meal usually begins with a series of hot and cold salads that are followed by a *tagine,* or stew (Kadiri and Raiss, 1997). The midday meal is the main meal, except during the holy month of Ramadan, and abundant servings are the norm. A soothing cup of sweet mint tea is the grace note to this repast.

Whereas spices have been imported to Morocco for thousands of years, many commonly used raw ingredients are home-grown. Moroccan cuisine is rich in spices that are used to enhance, not mask, the flavor of food (Kadiri and Raiss, 1997). The key spices in Moroccan cuisine are cinnamon, cumin, turmeric, ginger, cayenne, paprika, anise seed, sesame seed, black pepper, caraway, cloves, coriander seeds, and *Ras el hanout* (a mixture of twenty to thirty spices). The chief herbs are parsley, green coriander, marjoram, gray verbena, mint, and basil; also used to add flavor are fragrant waters, onions, garlic, and lemons (Kadiri and Raiss, 1997). Moroccan favorites are salads, *bisteeya,* couscous, fish, poultry, meat, desserts, and tea that has been steeped and then laced with sugar and fresh spearmint (Kadiri and Raiss, 1997).

Food retailing in Morocco can be broken down as follows:

1. *Wet markets:* These open-air markets are very common in urban and rural areas. In the cities, they typically sell fresh fruit and vegetables and are open daily, but in rural areas they sell all kinds of cheap local food and nonfood products and are held weekly. In most cities, wet-market retailers buy directly from the central city wholesale market. In the rural area, they often buy directly from farmers.
2. *Central markets:* Every major city in Morocco has at least one central market that contains a plethora of small shops.
3. *Traditional outlets:* These outlets are where food products are typically sold in Morocco. They offer several advantages to the Moroccan consumers, including credit and proximity.
4. *Supermarkets:* These are proliferating, particularly in major metropolitan areas (Casablanca, Rabat, Fez, Marrakech, Oujda, Mohammedia, El Jadia, and Agadir). They handle a significantly larger share of imported and more expensive products than any other type of outlet.

FOOD MEDICINE

It was Hippocrates who said, "Let food be your medicine, and medicine your food." Food medicine, the science and art of using food as an essential part of medicine, has been established for over 4,000 years. This medical resource is a major determinant of health that is directly under our control. Food is crucial to human existence, and because it is utilized many times each day, it has a major effect on the body. The twenty-first century is a turning point; the focus of medicine is returning to natural medicine because prescribed drug medications kill many thousands of people a year due to adverse effects and medical negligence.

The administration of foods to heal the body requires a mastery of natural medicine and food medicine coupled with knowledge of the physics, biology, and chemistry of individual foods. Food offers valuable insights into societies past and present and is perhaps the most distinctive expression of a culture, nation, or historical period.

One of the most respected conceptions by Moroccan people about natural medicine is "holistic" medicine. In the holy Qu'ran, food plants are often viewed as the gracious provision of God (Salman et al., 1999; Musselman, 1999). Islam also has extensive writings (extraqu'ranic literature or *hadith*) about food that are widely respected and used. Much more than providing food, fiber, and shelter, plants may also have religious significance. A good example is the use of trees as symbols of righteousness and stability. One of the scenes in Paradise in the Qur'an is a place where there are choice fruits and fowl to eat and the only greeting is "Peace! Peace." It is a place where the righteous will recline under the shade of thornless *sidr* (Ziziphus sp.) trees (Duwiejua et al., 1993).

The holy Qu'ran and Hadith include plants that have long been used for medicine. About twenty of the edible plants mentioned in the Qu'ran appear in the context of medicines. They include garlic *(Allium sativum)*, rock rose *(Cistus creticus)*, colocynth *(Citrullus colocynthis)*, tamarisk or tamarix *(Tamarix aphylla)*, myrrh (*Commiphora* spp.), mandrake *(Mandragora officinarum)*, black cummin *(Nigella sativa)*, and pomegranate *(Punica granatum)*. In the Qu'ran, the olive fruit is mentioned as a condiment (Danne et al., 1993). Ginger's present-day use is as a flavoring for drinks, which is also mentioned (Faraj, 1995).

Not all the plants mentioned in the Qu'ran are beneficial: *zaqqm* (arborescent *Euphorbia abyssinca*) is a terrible tree associated with hell (Baumann, 1996). It has fruits like devils' heads and a burning sap. This tree is the antithesis of the trees in the Garden of Paradise (Musselman, 1999). Like all species of *Euphorbia*, its milky latex is toxic and causes skin irritation in some people.

The domestic food sector supplies most of Morocco's needs for food products. Moroccans are conscious of the fact that what we ingest and how we treat our bodies on a daily basis have a very powerful effect on our health and quality of life. For many decades they have used food in the health care system, but until recently there had been no survey of the repertory of foods used as medicine. Drawing on the relevant published studies (Bellakhdar et al., 1991; Hmamouchi, 1999; Jouad, Haloui, et al., 2001; Eddouks et al., 2002), I propose to discuss the main plants used as food medicine in Morocco. Table 16.1 lists these plants, together with their scientific and vernacular names, the part of the plant used, and the medicinal use.

Most of the pharmacological effects related to food medicine in Morocco have not yet been studied. Those that have been reported, or have been demonstrated experimentally, are summarized below:

- Antidiabetic: *Brassica oleracea* (Roman-Ramos et al., 1995), *Eruca sativa* (El Missiry and El Gindy, 2000), *Opuntia ficus-indica* (Grover et al., 2002), *Artemisia herba-alba* (Marrif et al., 1995), *Sesanum indicum* (Takeuchi et al., 2001), *Olea europea* (Bennani-Kabchi et al., 2000), *Allium sativum* (Kasuga et al., 1999), *Allium cepa, Trigonella foenum graecum* (Grover et al., 2002), *Lupinus albus* (Sheweita et al., 2002), *Medicago sativa* (Gray and Flatt, 1997), *Lavendula dentata* (Gamez et al., 1988), *Citrullus collocynthis* (Abdel-Hassan et al., 2000), *Ammi visnaga* (Jouad et al., 2002a), *Lactuca sativa* (Roman-Ramos et al., 1995), and *Mangifera indica* (Aderibigbe et al., 1999)
- Cardiovascular disorders: *Daucus carota* (Gilani et al., 2000), *Lepidium sativum* (Vohora and Kahn, 1977), *Vitis vinifera* (Facino et al., 1999), *Allium sativum* (Orekhov and Grunwald, 1997), *Apium graveolens* (Ko et al., 1991), and *Mangifera indica* (Martinez Sanchez et al., 2001)
- Anti-inflammatory: *Apium graveolens* (Atta and Alkofahi, 1998) and *Mangifera indica* (Garcia et al., 2002)
- Gastrointestinal: *Cuminum cyminum* (Vasudevan et al., 2000; Nalini et al., 1998), *Foeniculum vulgare* (Vasudevan et al., 2000), *Berberis vulgaris* (Shamsa et al., 1999), and *Carum carvi*
- Antioxidant: *Opuntia ficus-indica* (Lee et al., 2002), *Apium graveolens* (Momin and Nair, 2002), and *Mangifera indica* (Scartezzini and Speroni, 2000).
- Anthelmintic: *Trigonella foenum-graecum* (Zia et al., 2001) and *Juglans regia* (Guarrera, 1999)
- Antimicrobial: *Foeniculum vulgare* and *Coriandrum sativum*
- Gynecologic: *Cuminum cyminum* (Malini and Vanithakumari, 1987)

TABLE 16.1. Main foods used as medicine in Morocco (nonexhaustive list).

Name of plants	Vernacular name	Part of plant	Medicinal use in Morocco	References
Anacardiaceae				
Mangifera indica	Anbaj, Anbaa	FR	Antidiarrheal	5
Apiaceae				
Ammi visnaga Lam.	Bachnikha	FR	D, dental hygiene, against headache, against vertigo, for nephritic colic	1,2,4
Ammodaucus leucotrichus Coss. Et Dur.	Kamoun sooufi	FR	CD	2
Apium graveo- lens L.	Kraffess	FR	CT, RD	2
Carum carvi L.	Karwiya	FR	RD	1, 2
Coriandrum sativum L.	Qezbour	FR	RD, magic, against scurvy, tonic, sto- machic, aphrodisiac, anti-inflammatory	1, 2, 3
Cuminum cymi- num L.	Kamoun	FR	CD	2
Daucus carota L.	Khizzou	FR	RD, antidiarrheal	1, 2, 5
Foeniculum dulce Mill.	Bessbass	FR	H, CD	1
Foeniculum vulgare Gaertn.	Nafaâ	FR	D, RD	1, 2
Petroselinum sativum Hoffm.	Maâdanous	AP	H, RD, diuretic, tonic	1, 2, 5
Berberidaceae				
Berberis vulgaris	Hamida	SD, FR, LE	H, CD	1
Cruciferae				
Brassica oleracea L.	Kroumb	AP	CD, D	2
Brassica nigra (L.) Koch	Khardal lakhal	SD	magic, calefacient	3
Eruca sativa Mill.	Fjel		D	1, 2
Lepidium sativum L.	Hebb rchad	SD	D, H, RD	1, 2

TABLE 16.1. *(continued)*

Name of plants	Vernacular name	Part of plant	Medicinal use in Morocco	References
Cactaceae				
Opuntia ficus indica Mill.	Hendiya, Kermous	FL	D, antidiarrheal, antispasmodic, diuretic	2, 5
Capparaceae				
Capparis spinosa L.	Kebbar	FR	D, appetite stimulant, diuretic, against painful menstruation	1, 2, 5
Compositae				
Artemisia absinthium L.	Chiba	AP	D, antiseptic, emmenagogue, vermifuge, febrifuge, digestive	1, 2, 5
Artemisia herba alba Asso.	Chih	AP	D, antimicrobial, anthelmintic, poison antidote	1, 2, 4
Artemisia vulgaris L.	Chih	–	–	–
Artemisia mesatlantica Maire	Chih	–	–	–
Carthamus tinctorium L.	Zaâfran	FL	RD, against skin infections	2, 5
Cerasus vulgaris Mill.	Hab lamlouk	FR	Depurgative, insecticide, hair care	5
Cynara cardunculus L.	Khorchouf	RT	D, CT, for digestive disorders	2, 3
Cynara scolymus L.	Khorchouf	LE, RT	Depurative, hypoglycemiant, diuretic	5
Helianthus annuus L.	Nouar Chems	SD	RD	1, 2
Lactuca sativa L.	Khouss	AP	D, CD	1, 2
Cucurbitaceae				
Citrullus vulgaris Schrad.	Dellah	FR	Antispasmodic, digestive, tonic	5
Cucurbita lagenaria Forsk	Slaoui	SD	Antiasthmatic, for bronchopulmonary infections	3
Cucurbita pepo L.	Gueraâ	SD	RD, antiasthmatic, for intestinal disorders	2, 3, 5

Name of plants	Vernacular name	Part of plant	Medicinal use in Morocco	References
Cucumis sativus L.	Khiyar	FR	D, RD	2
Cucumis sp.	Faqqous	FR	RD	2
Cucumis melo L.	Battikh	FR	RD	2
Cupuliferae				
Quercus lusitanica Lam.	El ballout	FR	Antidiarrheal	5
Fumariaceae				
Fumaria officinalis L.	El Bakoula	AP	H, CD	1
Graminae				
Hordeum vulgare L. and *H. distichon* L.	Chaâir	FR	Hypo	2
Zea mays L.	Dra	SM	RD	2
Triticum durum Desf.	Zraa	FR	Against digestive disorders	5
Iridaceae				
Crocus sativus L.	Zaâfran lhor	SM	RD, stimulant, cosmetic	2, 5
Juglandaceae				
Juglans regia L.	Guergaê	FR	D, tonic, astringent, depurative, cicatrizant, vermifuge, stomachic	2, 4
Lamiaceae				
Ajuga reptans L.	Chendgora	AP	D	2
Calamintha officinalis Moench.	Menta	AP	D	2
Lavandula dentata L.	Khzama	FL	D, H, carminative, sudorific, against bronchopulmonary infections	1, 2, 4
Medicago sativa L.	Fessae	AP	Antispasmodic	5
Mentha pulegium L.	Fliou	AP	D, against bronchopulmonary infections, antitussive, mouth hygiene, antispasmodic	1, 2, 4
Mentha viridis L.	Liqama, Naânaâ	LE	H, antispasmodic, analgesic, antiseptic, aphrodisiac, tonic, stimulant	1, 2, 5

TABLE 16.1. *(continued)*

Name of plants	Vernacular name	Part of plant	Medicinal use in Morocco	References
Ocimum basilicum L.	Lehbaq	FL	Stomachic, antispasmodic, against pulmonary diseases	5
Origanum najorana L.	Hbeq	AP	H	2
Rosmarinus officinalis L.	Merdedduch	LE	Against chill, antipyretic	3
Salvia officinalis L.	Salmia	LE	D, for throat diseases, refreshing, choleretic and stomachic, vulnerary, emmenagogue	1, 2, 4
Lauraceae				
Cinamomum cassia (L.) Presl.	L-Qrfa	AP	D, tonic, stimulant	1, 5
Laurus nobilis L.	Asat sidna mousa	LE	Dental hygiene, for liver disorders	3
Leguminosae				
Ceratonia siliqua L.	Kharoub	FR, GU	Antidiarrheal, antipyretic, laxative, against pulmonary infections	5
Cicer arietium L.	lhommss	FR	Tonic, reconstituant, aphrodisiac, cosmetic, dental hygiene	3, 5
Glycyrrhiza glabra L.	Arq souss	RT	RD, antispasmodic, aphrodisiac	2, 5
Glycine hispida Maxim. *soja sichet* Zucc.	Soja	FR	D	2
Lupinus albus L. (sensu Lato)	Foul mesri	SD	D	1, 2
Trigonella foenum-graecum L.	Halba	SD	D, H, antiasthmatic, anthelmintic, aphrodisiac, appetite stimulant, emollient, against aortic palpitations, blood cleansing	1, 2, 4, 5
Vicia faba L.	Foul	FR	Fortifying	5

Name of plants	Vernacular name	Part of plant	Medicinal use in Morocco	References
Vigna sinensis End.	Foul gnawa	SE	Hair care, pulmonary infections	3
Liliaceae				
Allium sativum L.	Touma	BU	D, H, CD, antispasmodic, cholagogue, against alopecia, urinary antiseptic	1, 2, 4
Allium cepa L.	Basla	BU	D, CD	1, 2
Linaceae				
Linum usitatissimum L.	Kattan	FR	Against pulmonary diseases, antidiabetic, laxative	1, 5
Malvaceae				
Hibiscus esculentus L.	Lmloukhiya	SE	Antiacid, calefacient	3
Malva sylvestris L.	Bakoula	RT	Laxative, emolient	3
Moraceae				
Ficus carica L.	Kermous	FR	D, antivitiligo, laxative, anti-inflammatory, antitussive, resolvent	2, 4, 5
Morus nigra L.	Tout	FR	Diuretic, hypoglycemiant, antidiarrheal	5
Myrtaceae				
Eugenia caryophyllata Thumb.	Qronfel	FL	D, H	1, 2
Oleaceae				
Olea europea L.	Zitoun, Zebbouj	LE, OI	D, H, CD, purgative, laxative	1, 2, 5
Palmae				
Phoenix dactylifera L.	Tmar	FR	Aphrodisiac, laxative	5
Pedaliaceae				
Sesamum indicum DC.	Jenjlan	SD	D	1, 2

TABLE 16.1. *(continued)*

Name of plants	Vernacular name	Part of plant	Medicinal use in Morocco	References
Punicaceae				
Punica granatum L.	Roumman	PE	RD, antiasthmatic, abortive	1, 2, 5
Ranunculaceae				
Malus communis Borkh.	Teffah	AP	H	1
Rhamnaceae				
Ziziphus lotus L.	Sedra, Nbeg	LE, FR	D, RD	2
Rosaceae				
Cydonia vulgaris Pers.	Sferjel	FR	D	2
Eriobotrya japonica Lindl.	Mzah	LE	Antidiarrheal for children, for digestive disorders, against hypertension	3, 5
Fragaria vesca L.	Fraiz berri	FR	D, RD, dental hygiene, antidiarrheal	2, 5
Pyrus communis L.	Bouaouied, Ngass	FR	RD	2
Prunus armeniaca L.	Alk Imchmach	GU	Aphrodisiac	3
Prunus carasus L.	Hob el molouk	FR	RD	2
Prunus amygdalus Stokes var. amara CD.	Louz Har	SD	D	2, 4
Prunus domestica L.	Berkouk	FR	Laxative, antidiarrheal	5
Prunus cerasus L.	Habelmlouk	FR	Antispasmodic	5
Rosa damascema Mill.	Lward	FL	Laxative, against headache, hair care, cosmetic	3
Rubus idaeus L.	Toute berri	FR	D, RD, cosmetic, tonic	2
Rubus fructicosis L.	Toute chaouki	LE	D, RD	2
Rubiaceae				
Ruta montana L.	Fijel	AP	D, RD	1, 2

Name of plants	Vernacular name	Part of plant	Medicinal use in Morocco	References
Rutaceae				
Citrus bigaradia Riss.	Ronge	FR, FL	D	1, 2
Citrus aurantium L.	Zhar limoun	FR	H, CD, against pulmonary infections, antispasmodic, sedative	1, 5
Citrus lemon (L.) Borm.	Laymoun lahlou	FR	Tonic, skin hygiene	5
Sapotaceae				
Argania spinosa (L.)	Argan	OI	Uterus diseases, cosmetic, stimulant	3
Solanaceae				
Atropa belladona L.	Zbib leydur	FR	D	2
Atropa baetica Willk.	Zbib leydur	FR	D	2
Capsicum annum L.	Felfla hamra	FR	Stimulant, aperitive	3, 5
Solanum tuberosus L.	Al-batates	FR	Antacid, antispasmodic	5
Ternstroemiaceae				
Thea sinensis Sims	Atay	FL	Diuretic, cardiotonic, astringent	5
Umbelliferae				
Cuminum cyminum L.	kamoun	FR	Against digestive disorders	5
Usneae				
Evernia prunastri Ach.	Lahyat shikh	AP	Cosmetic, liver complaints, making red blood corpuscles	3
Verbenaceae				
Lippia citriodora H.B.K.	Louiza	LE	H, diuretic, soporific, nervous diseases, against asthenia	1, 2, 4, 5
Viticeae				
Vitis vinifera L.	Inab	LE, FR	H, CD, diuretic, antiobesity	1, 5
Zingeberaceae				
Aframomum granum-paradisi K. Schum	Guza sahrawiya	SD	Stimulant, aphrodisiac	3

TABLE 16.1. *(continued)*

Name of plants	Vernacular name	Part of plant	Medicinal use in Morocco	References
Curcuma longa L.	Kharkoum	RH	Digestive stimulant, for blood diseases, against amnesia	3
Zingiber officinale	Skingebir	RH	Analgesic, D	2, 5
Not determined	Elwarguia	AP	D, against digestive diseases	1

1: Eddouks et al., 2002; 2: Jouad, Haloui, et al., 2001; 3: Bellakhdar et al., 1991; 4: Ziyyat et al., 1997; 5: Hmamouchi, 1999.

AP: aerial parts, EX: extract, FL: flowers, FR: fruits, GU: gum, LA: latex, LE: leaves, OI: oil, PE: pericarp, RH: rhizome, RT: roots, SD: seeds, SM: stigma, CD: cardiac disease, CT: cardiotonic, D: diabetes, H: hypertension, Hypo: hypotension, RD: renal disease.

Food safety is an essential public health priority throughout the world. The World Health Organization (WHO) estimates that up to one-third of the population in developing countries suffers from food-borne disease every year. Generally, though, the adverse effects of foods and of interactions between food and drugs are not taken seriously. Instead, researchers have paid attention to various food characteristics: biological (age, nature, shape and environmental requirements, physical values such as relationship of internal organs and organ systems, fluid mechanics, electrostatics, high energy physics, internal temperature, and vibrating bodies) chemical (water content, carbohydrates, fats, proteins, and vitamins and minerals), and trade elements.

PHYTOTHERAPY

In many developing countries the lack of resources has led the health system to depend heavily on traditional medicine and medicinal plants. In Africa, more than 80 percent of the population depends upon medicinal plants for health care. African medical systems vary between different cultural groups and regions.

The research on traditional medicines in Morocco dates from the colonial period. Studies have focused primarily on ethnobotanical and phytochemical aspects, but more recent research has examined how traditional health practices and herbal medicines can be integrated into modern medical systems. Although the flora and vegetation of Morocco are now well-known, only a few recent field studies have been done on traditional medicine (Eddouks et al., 2002; Jouad, Haloui, et al., 2001; Ziyyat et al., 1997; Bellakhdar et al., 1991; Bellakhdar, 1997). The diversity of biotopes has allowed a rich flora to develop, including 4,200 endemic species and about 1,500 introduced species (industrial, alimentary, ornamental, and so on). The strategic geographical location of Morocco, at the crossroads of Europe and Africa, has favored meetings between people and cultures. In Morocco there are three main medical traditions: classical Arab medicine, based largely on the humoral theories; local popular medicine, which is the standard throughout the country; and magico-religious practices, based on indigenous beliefs about the spiritual causes of diseases (Bellakhdar, 1997).

The art of healing is a part of the Muslim tradition of this country (Bellakhdar, 1997). Many authors have studied the traditional pharmacopoeia in different areas of Morocco: Bellakhdar and colleagues (1991), Claisse (1990), Sijelmassi (1993), Ziyyat and colleagues (1997), Jouad, Haloui, and colleagues (2001), and Eddouks and colleagues (2002). Numerous medicinal plants are described for treatment of many diseases.

All Moroccans keep stocks of some traditional home remedies (Weniger, 1991). The main ingredients of these remedies are plants. Even today, plant medicines are freely available to Moroccans, without prescription.

Research on the Medicinal Plants
Used in the Tafilalet and Fez Regions

The Tafilalet region in southeastern Morocco has played an important role historically, as it is crossed by the desert caravans travelling between the south and north of Africa. It is considered to be one of the regions of Morocco in which knowledge of phytotherapy is very developed. Its climate is arid, so many of the plant species have high concentrations of active substances.

In the Fez region (the northern part of central Morocco) traditional plant medicines have always held a strong position. Here, the Quarawiyine University in Fez is renowned for its medical research. Recent studies have described the medicinal plants used in treating diabetes (especially type 1 and type 2 diabetes mellitus), hypertension and cardiac diseases, and renal diseases in the Tafilalet and Fez regions of Morocco (Jouad, Haloui, et al., 2001; Eddouks et al., 2002). The findings are discussed following.

Ethnobotanic enquiries were performed in different areas of the Tafilalet (Eddouks et al., 2002) and Fez-Boulemane regions (Jouad, Haloui, et al., 2001). In the Tafilalet region 700 patients were questioned: 320 were diabetics and 380 had hypertension and/or cardiac disorders (Eddouks et al., 2002). In the Fez-Boulemane region, 1,527 patients were questioned: 1,095 (72 percent) of them were diabetics, 274 (18 percent) had renal diseases, and 158 (10 percent) had cardiac disorders (Jouad, Haloui, et al., 2001). The reported use of phytotherapy was 80 percent in Tafilalet and 76 percent in Fez-Boulemane. These percentages, which are high compared with other regions of Morocco (Jouad, Haloui, et al., 2001), show clearly that phytotherapy has always been practiced in these areas.

In previous studies in Morocco, many authors found that the percentage of the population using phytotherapy ranged from 55 percent to 90 percent, depending on the region (Bellakhdar, 1997; El Beghdadi, 1991; Jaouad, 1992; Magoua, 1991; Nabih, 1992; Sekkat, 1987; Ziyyat et al., 1997). The long-standing use of medicinal plants testifies to their medicinal efficacy and safety. In many regions of Morocco (and also in other countries), as well as in Tafilalet and Fez-Boulemane, medicinal plants are freely available to the public without prescription: 65 percent of the informants reported having obtained such remedies. Nearly half (49 percent) of the informants consulted a traditional herbal healer; only 1 percent consulted a pharmacist (Eddouks et al., 2002).

Both regions showed a clear gender difference, with women using medicinal plants more: the percentages were 63 and 69 percent of the female informants in Tafilalet and Fez-Boulemane, respectively, and the comparable figures for male informants were 37 and 31 percent (Eddouks et al., 2002; Jouad, Haloui, et al., 2001). Some previous studies have also shown this trend in other Moroccan populations, with percentages ranging from 61 to 65 percent for females and 35 to 39 percent for males (El Beghdadi, 1991; Jaouad, 1992; Nabih, 1992; Ziyyat et al., 1997). Reasons for the high percentage of women users include the high illiteracy rate among women in this society, the ease of transmission of information between women, and the great store attached by women to traditional knowledge (Jaouad, 1992; Nabih, 1992). Also, women were most often at home during the hours of the survey (Jouad, Lacaille-Dubois, and Eddouks, 2001).

The studies (Eddouks et al., 2002; Jouad, Haloui, et al., 2001) reported that the interviewed patients used medicinal plants to treat diabetes mellitus and hypertension and cardiac diseases because phytotherapy is cheaper (53 to 58 percent), more efficient (40 percent), and better (65 percent) than modern medicine. About 72 percent of all informants said they were satisfied with the treatment and the use of phytotherapy and preferred using medicinal plants rather than synthetic drugs. The patients included in the studies were generally illiterate (63 percent) and professionally inactive (52 percent). In all groups, the number of plant users was very important and did not depend on sex, age, or sociocultural level (Eddouks et al., 2002; Jouad, Haloui, et al., 2001).

Seventy percent of the patients respected neither the precision of doses when using medicinal plants nor the duration of the treatment. Furthermore, the patients did not take into account that the prolonged use of plants could lead to some constituents accumulating in the body, which could provoke severe side effects and could also aggravate the disorder. These findings might explain why there are accidental poisonings by medicinal plants (Eddouks et al., 2002).

In almost all the studies that have inventoried medicinal plants, the authors have reported only the therapeutic plants, not the toxic plants known by the traditional herbal healers. Yet the recording of the latter plants can provide useful information and should be taken into consideration by researchers. In our study we found that 12 to 25 percent of the total users of medicinal plants have a little information about toxic plants (Jouad, Haloui, et al., 2001; Eddouks et al., 2002). Fourteen plants were known to be toxic: *Atractylis gummifera, Nerium oleander, Citrullus colocynthis, Cannabis sativa, Peganum harmala, Colchicum autumnale, Lycium vulgare, Datura stramonium, Atropa belladona, Ferula assa-foetida, Papaver somniferum, Mandragora autumnalis, Zygophyllum geatulum,* and *Ricinus communis.*

In general, indigenous tribal plant medicines that are not prescription medicines are mostly used for automedication and are frequently dispensed by ignorant people (Keller, 1991). When this is the case, it is necessary to inform the public and raise awareness about toxic plants, in order to prevent at least some cases of accidental poisoning caused by ignorance. In our study we found that medical knowledge was passed on orally; this had led to some impoverishment of traditional knowledge (Jouad, Haloui, et al., 2001). At present, the transmission of traditional medical knowledge from generation to generation is currently in danger, because transmission between old people and the younger generation is not always assured (Weniger, 1991): the traditional practitioners of today are less instructed and organized than their predecessors.

As regards diabetes pathology, the majority (75 percent) of the interviewees with diabetes mellitus suffered from type 2 (Eddouks et al., 2002). Of these, 25 percent relied solely on medicinal plants and 75 percent used phytotherapy in conjunction with modern drugs. By comparison, only 10 percent of the type 1 diabetic patients frequently used medicinal plants, in addition to insulin treatment (Eddouks et al., 2002). Generally, it is very dangerous to use hypoglycemic plants to treat diabetes mellitus, especially type 1 diabetes mellitus. It seems that some of the medicinal plants had induced hypoglycemic accidents in type 1 diabetic patients and also in poorly controlled type 2 diabetic patients (Eddouks et al., 2002).

Our inventory of medicinal plants included over 150 that were used to treat diabetes mellitus, hypertension, renal disease, and cardiac disease (Eddouks et al., 2002; Jouad, Haloui, et al., 2001).

Ninety plants were used to treat diabetes mellitus. Those most frequently mentioned were *Ammi visnaga, Artemisia herba-alba, Trigonella foeniculum-granum, Marrubium vulgare, Nigella sativa, Globularia alypum, Allium sativum, Olea europaea, Citrullus colocynthis, Aloe succotrina, Artimisia absinthium, Rosmarinus officinalis, Thymus vulgaris, Eucalyptus globulus, Mentha pulegium, Myrtus communis, Linum usitatissimum, Carum carvi* (El warguia), *Zygophyllum gaetulum, Centaurium erythraea, Allium cepa, Spergularia purpurea, Urtica dioica, Cynara cardunculus, Opuntia ficus-indica,* and *Rubus fructicosus* (Jouad, Haloui, et al., 2001; Eddouks et al., 2002). Some of these plants have been experimentally studied and their hypoglycemic activity demonstrated; they include *Allium sativum* (Chang and Johnson, 1980), *Allium cepa* (Alaoui et al., 1992), *Artemisia herba-alba* (Khazraji et al., 1993), *Ammi visnaga* (Jouad et al, 2004), *Centaurium erythraea* (Alaoui et al., 1992), *Nigella sativa*

(Labhal et al., 1999), *Trigonella foenum- graecum* (Raghuram et al., 1994), *Zygophyllum gaetulum* (Jaouhari et al., 1999), *Rosmarinus officinalis* (Erenmemisoglu et al., 1997), *Eucalyptus globulus* (Jouad et al., 2004), *Crataegus oxyacantha* (Jouad et al., 2002a), *Globularia alypum* (Jouad et al., 2002b), *Rubus fructicosus* (Jouad et al., 2002b), *Opuntia ficus-indica,* and *Spergularia purpurea* (Jouad et al., 2000; Eddouks et al., 2003).

One hundred plants were reported for treating hypertension and cardiac diseases (Eddouks et al., 2002; Jouad, Haloui, et al., 2001). Those most often used were *Allium sativum, Olea europaea, Pimpinella anusum, Artemisia herba-alba, Globularia alypum, Artemisia absinthium, Citrullus colocynthis, Fumaria officinalis, Marrubium vulgare, Mentha pulegium, Thymus serphyllum, Satureia montana, Glycyrrhiza glabra, Nigella sativa, Origanum vulgare, Rosmarinus officinalis, Carum carvi, Lippia citriodora, Foeniculum dulce, Myrtus communis, Rubia tinctorum, Peganum harmala, Urtica dioica, Petroselinum sativum, Trigonella foenum-graecum, Lippia citriodora, Herniaria glabra,* and *Spergularia purpurea* (Jouad, Haloui, et al., 2001; Eddouks et al., 2002).The antihypertensive activity of some of these plants has previously been demonstrated: *Peganum harmala* (Aarons et al., 1977), *Allium sativum* (Pantoja et al., 1991), *Olea europaea* (Circosta et al., 1986), *Rosmarinus officinalis* (Aqel, 1991), *Herniaria glabra* (Rhiouani et al., 1999), *Nigella sativa* (Labhal et al., 1994), *Spergularia purpurea* (Jouad, Lacaille-Dubois, Lyoussi, et al., 2001; Jouad, Lacaille-Dubois, and Eddouks, 2001), and *Arbutus unedo* (Abdalla et al., 1994).

Thirty-three plants were mentioned for treating renal disease (Jouad, Haloui, et al., 2001). Those most used were *Herniaria glabra, Coriandrum sativum, Carum carvi, Daucus carota, Pimpinella anisum, Lepidium sativum, Silene* sp., *Cucurbita pepo, Cucumis melo, Zea mays, Crocus sativus, Ziziphus lotus, Petroselinum sativum, Punica granatum, Foeniculum vulgare, Glycyrrhiza glabra, Linum usitatissinum, Pyrus communis, Prunus carasus, Rubia tinctorium, Ruta montana,* and *Spergularia purpurea.* Scientific studies have demonstrated the renal effect of some of these plants, such as *Herniaria glabra* (Rhiouani et al., 1999), *Foeniculum vulgare* (Tanira et al., 1996), *Zea mays* (Dat et al., 1992), *Centaurium erythraea, Rosmarinus officinalis,* and *Spergularia purpurea* (Jouad, Lacaille-Dubois, and Eddouks, 2001).

Eleven plants were mentioned for treating cardiac diseases (Jouad, Haloui, et al., 2001). The most used were *Arbutus unedo, Ammodaucus leucotrichus, Apium graveolens, Cuminum cyminum, Brassica oleracea, Cynara cardunculus, Lactuca sativa,* and *Thymus vulgaris.* The only one to have been scientifically studied is *Arbutus unedo* (Ziyyat and Boussairi, 1998).

The mechanism of action of the pharmacological activity of the plants mentioned in the preceding paragraphs remains to be identified. Though the therapeutic properties of the other plants mentioned in Table 16.1 have not been scientifically investigated, they are well-known in traditional folk medicine in the Tafilalet and Fez-Boulemane regions.

Sixteen of the 19 species used to relieve hypertension were also used to treat diabetes (Jouad, Haloui, et al., 2001). These were *Petroselinum sativum, Herniaria glabra, Spergularia purpurea, Juniperus communis, Lepidium sativum, Arbutus unedo, Lavandula dentata, Origanum compactum, Rosmarinus officinalis, Trigonella foenum-graecum, Allium sativum, Eucalyptus globulus, Eugenia caryophyllata, Olea europaea, Urtica dioica,* and *Peganum harmala.*

Six of the 11 plants used for cardiac diseases were used for diabetes treatment (Jouad, Haloui, et al., 2001). These were: *Brassica oleracea, Cynara cardunculus, Lactuca sativa, Allium sativum, Allium cepa,* and *Olea europaea.*

Another remarkable feature in the ethnopharmacopoeia of many African populations is the use of food substances as medicinal agents. Our survey revealed 20 such edible plants, such as *Daucus carota, Brassica oleracea, Eruca sativa, Opuntia ficus-indica, Cynara cardunculus, Lactuca sativa, Cucumis sativus, Cucumis melo, Arbutus unedo, Zea mays, Cucurbita pepo, Lupinus albus, Allium sativum, Allium cepa, Ficus carica, Olea europaea, Punica granatum, Cydonia vulgaris, Pyrus communis,* and *Prunus cerasus.* Many patients used more than one plant in order to treat the same disease.

Further systematic investigations into the chemical constituents, pharmacological actions, and toxicity of the plant materials will be needed to prove their medicinal worth. In addition, the cellular and molecular mechanisms of the recorded plants still need to be determined in animal models, and detailed information on their usage, duration, and dosage must be investigated before they can be prescribed in human health care.

The comparative analysis of the ethnobotanical surveys in Tafilalet and Fez-Boulemane regions (Eddouks et al., 2002; Jouad, Haloui, et al., 2001) shows that the plants most frequently used to treat diabetes mellitus and cardiac disorders are similar. However, over 45 medicinal plants used in the Tafilalet region were not used in the Fez region (Eddouks et al., 2002). This indicates that despite the fact that some plants are widely used for the treatment of some pathologies across Morocco, each region also has very specific knowledge of phytotherapy. This can be explained by such factors as local climate, culture, and ethnology.

Our study confirms that in the Tafilalet and Fez-Boulemane regions phytotherapy is highly developed. It represents a part of the local heritage (Eddouks et al., 2002). We can thus confirm that in Morocco phytotherapy is an integral part of the human health care system. One of many reasons for the development of phytotherapy is the low socioeconomic level of some regions. Furthermore, many of the plant species used are region-specific. Empirical and clinical tests will show whether the medicinal plants identified have therapeutic value. Meanwhile, serious efforts must be made to alert the local population to the dangers of anarchic usage of phytotherapy, especially the use of toxic plants and hypoglycemic medicinal herbs in the treatment of type 1 and poorly controlled type 2 diabetes mellitus.

Other Research on Medicinal Plants in Morocco

When traditional healers in the six main provinces of Morocco were surveyed (Bellakhdar et al., 1991) in order to obtain the repertory of the main phytotherapeutic plants, 231 medicinal plants were identified. Of these, 27 percent were cultivated species, 15.5 percent were imported species and 6.5 percent were endemic species from the Maghreb or Sahara. Most (51 percent) were wild species from the Mediterranean flora (Bellakhdar et al., 1991). The study reported that the major diseases cured by Moroccan traditional medicine relate to digestive pathology (mainly intestinal, antiseptic, and anthelmintic): 62 plants. Other disorders treated had to do with the skin (54 plants); hair (30 plants); bronchopulmonary system (28 plants); urinary system (27 plants); and liver (28 plants). Twenty-six plants were used in emmenagogic and other gynaecologic cures (Bellakhdar et al., 1991).

In addition, laxative (23 plants), depurative (5 plants), analgesic, and anti-inflammatory (30 species) uses were also reported.

Another enquiry across Morocco reported that more than 800 spontaneous, cultivated, or imported species (Hmamouchi, 1999) were used for the treatment of 27 diseases. The main disorders were digestive, pulmonary, cardio-vascular, and skin diseases (Hmamouchi, 1999).

An earlier survey in different areas of oriental Morocco (Ziyyat et al., 1997) aimed to determine the main medicinal plants used in folk medicine to treat arterial hypertension and/or diabetes. The patients (370 women and 256 men) were divided into three groups: diabetics (61 percent), hypertensive (23 percent), and hypertensive diabetic persons (16 percent). On average, 67 percent of the patients regularly used medicinal plants. The proportion was the same in all groups and did not depend on sex, age, or sociocultural level. This result shows how widespread phytotherapy is in northeastern Morocco. Eighteen species were reported as being used in hypertension therapy, compared with 38 species being used to treat diabetes. The problems of phytotherapy in oriental Morocco reported by the authors included medical diagnosis by the herbal healers, the bad packaging of the plants on the herbalists' stalls, and damage to the plants caused by permanent exposure to the sun. The authors concluded that phytotherapy continues to be the means of primary health care in this region due to the high cost of medicaments and the fact that the efficacy of folk pharmacopoeia is well proven (Ziyyat et al., 1997).

CONCLUSIONS

Food medicine represents an integral part of the health care system in Morocco. Many pathologies have been treated naturally, for a long time, using foods. However, much remains to be done in order to educate the local population about the rational scientific use of this valuable resource. If we are to conserve these resources, decision makers must rationalize their efforts and promote the exchange of information between the many actors such as research institutions, the pharmaceutical industry, NGOs, small businesses, and governments.

Thanks to the diversity of the environment and flora of Morocco, the traditional pharmacopoeia comprises a wide arsenal of plant remedies. In all the regions surveyed, most of the interviewees had few resources and could not afford modern health care. Phytotherapy should not be the medicine of the poor; it should be a real tool for all. We should study these drugs in order to identify the real therapeutic uses and to prevent charlatanism, which could affect public confidence (Eddouks et al., 2002). Increased awareness of the need for biodiversity conservation, of intellectual property rights issues, and of the value of indigenous knowledge have also contributed to the development of new research activities.

The safety, effectiveness, and accessibility of natural medicine to local populations must be guaranteed, and the equitable and sustainable use of these plants must be enhanced. We must develop programs supporting strategic research; foster partnerships between the key stakeholders, including donors; and encourage regional and international networking.

REFERENCES

Aarons, D.H., G.V. Rossi, and R.F. Orzechowski (1977). Cardiovascular actions of three harmala alcaloids: harmine, harmaline and harmalol. *Journal of Pharmaceutical Sciences* 66: 1244-1248.

Abdalla, S., M. Abu-Zarga, and M. Sabri (1994). Effects of the flavone luteolin, isolated from *Colchicum richii* on guinea-pig isolated smooth muscle and heart and on blood pressure and blood flow. *Phytotherapy Research* 8: 265-270.

Abdel-Hassan, I.A., J.A. Abdel-Barry, and S. Tariq Mohammeda (2000). The hypoglycaemic and antihyperglycaemic effects of *Citrullus colocynthis* fruit aqueous extract in normal and alloxan diabetic rabbits. *Journal of Ethnopharmacology* 71 (1-2): 325-330.

Aderibigbe, A.O., T.S. Emudianughe, and B.A. Lawal (1999). Antihyperglycaemic effect of *Mangifera indica* in rat. *Phytotherapy Research* 13 (6): 504-507.

Alaoui, T., I. Benabdelkrim, and A. Zaid (1992). Etude de l'effet hypoglycémiant sur des rats d'une association d'*Ammi visnaga, Erythraea centaurium* et *Thymus ciliatus* utilisées en médecine traditionnelle marocaine. *Al Biruniya* 8: 37-44.

Al Faraj, S. (1995). Haemorrhagic colitis induced by *Citrullus colocynthis. Annals of Tropical Medicine and Parasitology* 89 (6): 695-696.

Al Khazraji, S.M., L.A. Al Shamaony, and H.A. Twaij (1993). Hypoglycaemic effect of *Artemesia herba alba*. Effect of different parts and influence of the solvent on hypoglycaemic activity. *Journal of Ethnopharmacology* 40: 163-166.

Aqel, M.B. (1991). Relaxant effect of the volatile oil of *Rosmarinus officinalis* on tracheal smooth muscle. *Journal of Ethnopharmacology* 33: 57-62.

Atta, A.H. and A. Alkofahi (1998). Anti-nociceptive and anti-inflammatory effects of some Jordanian medicinal plant extracts. *Journal of Ethnopharmacology* 60 (2): 117-124.

Baumann, H. (1996). *The Greek plant world in myth, art and literature*. Portland: Timber Press.

Bellakhdar, J. (1997). *La pharmacopée Marocaine traditionnelle. Médecine Arabe ancienne et savoirs populaires*. Casablanca: Edition le Fennec et Ibis Press.

Bellakhdar, J., R. Claisse, J. Fleurentin, and C. Younos (1991). Repertory of standard herbal drugs in the Moroccan pharmacopoeia. *Journal of Ethnopharmacology* 35: 123-143.

Bennani-Kabchi, N., H. Fdhil, Y. Cherrah, F. El Bouayadia, L. Kehel, and G. Marquie (2000). Therapeutic effect of *Olea europea* var. oleaster leaves on carbohydrate and lipid metabolism in obese and prediabetic sand rats *(Psammomys obesus)*. *Annales Pharmaceutiques Francaises* 58 (4): 271-277.

Chang, M. and M. Johnson (1980). Effect of garlic on carbohydrate metabolism and lipid synthesis in rats. *Journal of Nutrition* 110: 931-936.

Circosta, C., F. Occhiuto, S. Toigo, A. Gregorio (1986). Studio comparativo dell'attivitá cardiovasculare di germogli e di foglie di *Olea europaea*. I. Attivitá elettrica e sulla pressione arteriosa. *Pharmacia Mediterranea* 16: 157-166.

Claisse, R. (1990). Pharmacopée traditionnelle au Maroc: Marché populaire de Yacoub El Mansour. *Actes du 1er Colloque Européen d'Ethnopharmacologie*, pp. 448-449. Paris: ORSTOM.

Danne, A., F. Peterett, and A. Nahrstedt (1993). Proanthocyanidins from *Cistus incanus*. *Phytochemistry* 34 (4): 1129-1133.

Dat, D.D., N.N. Ham, D.H. Khac, N.T. Lam, P.T. Son, N.V. Dau, M. Grabe, R. Johansson, G. Lindgren, N.E. Stjernströn (1992). Studies on the individual and combined diuretic effects of four Vietnamese traditional herbal remedies *(Zea mays, Imperata cylindrica, Plantago major,* and *Orthosiphon stamineus)*. *Journal of Ethnopharmacology* 36: 225-231.

Duwiejua M., I.J. Zeitlin, P.G. Waterman, J. Chapman, G.J. Mhango, and G.J. Provan (1993). Anti-inflammatory activity of resins from some species of the plant family Burseraceae. *Planta Medica* 59 (1): 12-16.

Eddouks, M., H. Jouad, M. Maghrani, A. Lemhadri, R. Burcelin (2003). Inhibition of endogenous glucose production accounts for hypoglycaemic effect of *Spergularia purpurea* in streptozotocin mice. *Phytomedicine* 10 (6-7): 594-599.

Eddouks, M., M. Maghrani, A. Lemhadri, M.L. Ouahidi, and H. Jouad (2002). Ethnopharmacological survey of medicinal plants used for the treatment of diabetes mellitus, hypertension and cardiac diseases in the south-east region of Morocco (Tafilalet). *Journal of Ethnopharmacology* 82: 97-103.

El Beghdadi, M. (1991). Pharmacopée traditionnelle du Maroc. Les plantes médicinales et les affections du système cardio-vasculaire. PharmD thesis. University of Mohamed IV, Rabat, Morocco.

El Missry, M.A. and A.M. El Gindy (2000). Amelioration of alloxan-induced diabetes mellitus and oxidative stress in rats by oil of *Eruca sativa* seeds. *Annals of Nutrition & Metabolism* 44 (3): 97-100.

Erenmemisoglu, A., R. Saraymen, and H. Ustun (1997). Effect of *Rosmarinus officinalis* leaf extract on plasma glucose levels in normoglycaemic and diabetic mice. *Pharmazie* 52 (8): 645-646.

Facino, R.M., M. Carini, G. Aldini, F. Berti, G. Rossoni, E. Bombardelli, and P. Morazzoni (1999). Diet enriched with procyanidins enhances antioxidant activity and reduces myocardial post-ischaemic damage in rats. *Life Sciences* 64 (8): 627-642.

Gamez, M.J., A. Zazuelo, S. Risco, P. Utrilla, and J. Jimenez (1988). Hypoglycemic activity in various spices of the genus *Lavandula*. Part 2: *Lavandula dentala* and *Lavandula latifolia*. *Pharmazie* 43 (6): 441-442.

Garcia, D., R. Delgado, F.M. Ubeira, and J. Leiro (2002). Modulation of rat macrophage function by the *Mangifera indica* L. extracts vimang and mangiferin. *International Immunopharmacology* 2 (6): 797-806.

Gilani, A.H., E. Shaheen, S.A. Saeed, S. Bibi, M. Sadiq, and S. Faizi (2000). Hypotensive action of coumarin glycosides from *Daucus carota*. *Phytomedicine* 7 (5): 423-642.

Gray, A.M. and P.R. Flatt (1997). Pancreatic and extra-pancreatic effects of the traditional and anti-diabetic plants, *Medicago sativa* (lucerne). *The British Journal of Nutrition* 78 (2): 325-334.

Grover, J.K., S. Yadav, V. Vats (2002). Medicinal plants of India with anti-diabetic potential. *Journal of Ethnopharmacology* 81 (1): 81-100.

Guarrera, P.M. (1999). Traditional anthelmintic, antiparasitic and repellent uses of plants in Central Italy. *Journal of Ethnopharmacology* 68: 183-192.

Hmamouchi, M. (1999). *Les plantes médicinales et aromatiques Marocaines. Utilisations, Biologie, Écologie, Chimie, Pharmacologie, Toxicologie et Lexiques*. Rabat, Fédala: Rabat-Institutes.

Jaouad, L. (1992). Enquête ethnobotanique: La part de la médecine traditionnelle dans les différentes couches socio-économiques de la population de Casablanca. PharmD thesis. University of Mohamed IV, Rabat, Morocco.

Jaouhari, J.T., H.B. Lazrek, A. Seddik, and M. Jana (1999). Hypoglycaemic response to *Zygophyllum gaetulum* extracts in patients with non-insulin-dependent diabetes mellitus. *Journal of Ethnopharmacology* 64: 211-217.

Jouad, H., M. Eddouks, M.A. Lacaille-Dubois, and B. Lyoussi (2000). Hypoglycaemic effect of *Spergularia purpurea* in normal and streptozotocin-induced diabetic rats. *Journal of Ethnopharmacology* 71: 169-177.

Jouad, H., M. Haloui, H. Rhiouani, J. El Hilaly, and M. Eddouks (2001). Ethnobotanical survey of medicinal plants used for the treatment of diabetes, cardiac and renal diseases in the North center region of Morocco (Fez-Boulemane). *Journal of Ethnopharmacology* 77: 175-182.

Jouad, H., M.A. Lacaille-Dubois, and M. Eddouks (2001). Chronic diuretic effect of the water extract of *Spergularia purpurea* in normal rats. *Journal of Ethnopharmacology* 75: 219-223.

Jouad, H., M.A. Lacaille-Dubois, B. Lyoussi, and M. Eddouks (2001). Effects of the flavonoids extracted from *Spergularia purpurea* Pers. on arterial blood pressure and renal function in normal and hypertensive rats. *Journal of Ethnopharmacology* 76: 159-163.

Jouad, H., M. Maghrani, R. Ameziane El Hassani, and M. Eddouks (2004). Hypoglycemic activity of aqueous extract of *Eucalyptus globulus* in normal and streptozotocin-induced diabetic rats. *Journal of Herbs Spices & Medicinal Plants* 10 (4): 19-28.

Jouad, H., M. Maghrani, and M. Eddouks (2002a). Hypoglycemic effect of aqueous extract of *Ammi visnaga* in normal and streptozotocin-induced diabetic rats. *Journal of Herbal Pharmacotherapy* 2 (4): 19-30.

Jouad, H., M. Maghrani, and M. Eddouks (2002b). Hypoglycaemic effect of *Rubus fructicosis* and *Globularia alypum* L. in normal and streptozotocin-induced diabetic rats. *Journal of Ethnopharmacology* 81: 351-356.

Kadiri, A. and S. Raiss (1997). *Moroccan cuisine: Modern and traditional. Addar al Alamia lil Kitab.* Casablanca.

Kasuga, S., M. Ushijima, N. Morihara, Y. Itakura, and Y. Nakata (1999). Effect of aged garlic extract (AGE) on hyperglycemia induced by immobilization stress in mice. *Nippon Yakurigaku Zasshi* 114 (3):191-197.

Keller, K. (1991). Legal requirements for the use of phytopharmaceutical drugs in the Federal Republic of Germany. *Journal of Ethnopharmacology* 32: 225-229.

Ko, F.N., T.F. Huang, and C.M. Teng (1991). Vasodilatory action mechanisms of apigenin isolated from *Apium graveolens* in rat thoracic aorta. *Biochimica et Biophysica Acta* 1115 (1): 69-74.

Labhal, A., A. Settaf, Y. Cherrah, A. Ettaib, S. El Kabbaj, A. Amrani, R. El Fassi, M. Hassar, M. Seqat, and A. Slaoui (1994). Action antihypertensive de *Nigella sativa* chez le rat spontanément hypertendu (SHR). *Actes du Ivème Congrès National d'Endocrinologie Comparée, Marrakech*, p. 106 (Abstracts). Morocco.

Labhal, A., A. Settaf, F. Zalagh, Y. Cherrah, M. Hassar, and A. Slaoui (1999). Propriétés antidiabétiques des graines de *Nigella sativa* chez le Merione Shawi obèse et diabétique. *Espérance Médicale* 47: 72-74.

Lee, J.C., H.R. Kim, J. Kim, and Y.S. Jang (2002). Antioxidant property of an ethanol extract of the stem of *Opuntia ficua-indica* var. Saboten. *Journal of Agricultural and Food Chemistry* 50 (22): 6490-6496.

Magoua, N. (1991). Les recettes familiales à base de plantes médicinales dans la Province de Salé. PharmD thesis. University of Mohamed IV, Rabat, Morocco.

Malini, T. and G. Vanithakumari (1987). Estrogenic activity of *Cuminum cyminum* in rats. *Indian Journal of Experimental Biology* 22: 442-444.

Marrif, H.I., B.H. Ali, and K.M. Hassan (1995). Some pharmacological studies on *Artemisia herba-alba* (Asso.) in rabbits and mice. *Journal of Ethnopharmacology* 49 (1): 51-55.

Martinez Sanchez, G., E. Candelario-Jalil, A. Giuliani, O.S. Leon, S. Sam, R. Delgado, and A.J. Nunez Selles (2001). *Mangifera indica* L. extract (QF808) reduces ischaemia-induced neuronal loss and oxidative damage in the gerbil brain. *Free Radical Research* 35 (5): 465-473.

Momin, R.A. and M.G. Nair (2002). Antioxidant, cyclooxygenase and topoisomerase inhibitory compounds from *Apium graveolens* Linn. Seeds. *Phytomedicine* 9 (4): 312-318.

Musselman, L.J. (1999). A Biblical view of creation. *Al Reem, Journal of the Royal Society for the Conservation of Nature (Jordan)* 65: 8-9.

Nabih, M. (1992). Secrets et vertus thérapeutiques des plantes médicinales utilisées en médecine traditionnelle dans la Province de Settat. PharmD thesis. University of Mohamed IV, Rabat, Morocco.

Nalini, N., K. Sabitha, P. Viswanathan, and V.P. Menon (1998). Influence of spices on the bacterial (enzyme) activity in experimental colon cancer. *Journal of Ethnopharmacology* 62 (1): 15-24.

Orekhov, A.N. and J. Grunwald (1997). Effects of garlic on atherosclerosis. *Nutrition* 13 (7-8): 656-663.

Pantoja, C.V., C.H. Chiang, B.C. Norris, and J.B. Concha (1991). Diuretic, natriuretic and hypotensive effects produced by *Allium sativum* (Garlic) in anaesthetized dogs. *Journal of Ethnopharmacology* 31: 325-331.

Raghuram, T.C., R.D. Sharma, B. Sivakumar, and B.K. Sahay (1994). Effect of fenugreek seeds on intravenous glucose disposition in non-insulin-dependent diabetic patients. *Phytotherapy Research* 8: 83-86.

Rhiouani, H., A. Settaf, B. Lyoussi, Y. Cherrah, and M. Hassar (1999). Action diurétique des saponines de *Herniaria glabra* chez le rat spontanément hypertendu. *Espérance Médicale* 47: 68-71.

Roman-Ramos, R., J.L. Flores-Saenz, F.J. Alarcon-Aguilar (1995). Anti-hyperglycemic effect of some edible plants. *Journal of Ethnopharmacology* 48 (1): 25-32.

Salman, H., M. Bergman, H. Bessler, I. Punksy, and M. Djaldetti (1999). Effect of a garlic derivative (alliin) on peripheral blood cell immune responses. *International Journal of Immunopharmacology* 21 (9): 589-597.

Scartezzini, P. and E. Speroni (2000). Review on some plants of Indian medicine with antioxidant activity. *Journal of Ethnopharmacology* 71: 23-43.

Sekkat, C. (1987). Le diabète et la phytothérapie. Enquête auprès de 100 D.I.D. et 100 D.N.I.D. PharmD thesis. University of Mohamed VI, Rabat, Morocco.

Shamsa, F., A. Ahmadiani, and R. Khosrokhavar (1999). Antihistaminic and anticholinergic activity of barberry fruit *(Berberis vulgaris)* in the guinea-pig ileum. *Journal of Ethnopharmacology* 64 (2): 161-166.

Sheweita, S.A., A.A. Newairy, H.A. Mansour, and M.I. Yousef (2002). Effect of some hypoglycemic herbs on the activity of phase I and II drug-metabolizing enzymes in alloxan-induced diabetic rats. *Toxicology* 174 (2): 131-139.

Sijelmassi, A. (1993). *Les plantes médicinales du Maroc.* Casablanca: Le Fennec.

Takeuchi, H., L.Y. Mooi, Y. Inagaki, and P. He (2001). Hypoglycemic effect of a hot-water extract from defatted sesame (*Sesamum indicum* L.) seed on the blood glucose level in genetically diabetic KK-Ay mice. *Bioscience, Biotechnology, and Biochemistry* 65 (10): 2318-2321.

Tanira, M.O., A.H. Shah, A. Mohsin, A.M. Ageel, and S. Qureshi (1996). Pharmacological and toxicological investigations on *Foeniculum vulgare* dried fruit extract in experimental animals. *Phytotherapy Research* 10: 33-36.

Vasudevan, K., S. Vembar, K. Veeraraghavan, and P.S. Haranath (2000). Influence of intragastric perfusion of aqueous spice extracts on acid secretion in anesthetized albino rats. *Indian Journal of Gastroenterology* 19 (2): 53-56.

Vohora, S.B. and M.S. Khan (1977). Pharmacological studies on *Lepidium sativum*, linn. *Indian Journal of Physiology and Pharmacology* 21 (2): 118-120.

Weniger, B. (1991). Interest and limitation of a global ethnopharmacological survey. *Journal of Ethnopharmacology* 32: 37-41.

Zia, T., I.A. Siddiqui, and A. Nazrul-Hasnain (2001). Nematicidal activity of *Trigonella foenum-graecum* L. *Phytotherapy Research* 15: 538-540.

Ziyyat, A. and E.H. Boussairi (1998). Cardiovascular effects of *Arbutus unedo* L. in spontaneously hypertensive rats. *Phytotherapy Research* 12: 110-113.

Ziyyat, A., A. Legssyer, H. Mekhfi, A. Dassouli, M. Serrhouchni, and W. Benjelloun (1997). Phytotherapy of hypertension and diabetes in oriental Morocco. *Journal of Ethnopharmacology* 58: 45-54.

Index

Page numbers followed by the letter "f" indicate figures; those followed by the letter "t" indicate tables.

Order a copy of this book with this form or online at:
http://www.haworthpress.com/store/product.asp?sku=5254

EATING AND HEALING
Traditional Food As Medicine

_____ in hardbound at $59.95 (ISBN-13: 978-1-56022-982-7; ISBN-10: 1-56022-982-9)

_____ in softbound at $39.95 (ISBN-13: 978-1-56022-983-4; ISBN-10: 1-56022-983-7)

Or order online and use special offer code HEC25 in the shopping cart.

COST OF BOOKS_____	☐ **BILL ME LATER:** (Bill-me option is good on US/Canada/Mexico orders only; not good to jobbers, wholesalers, or subscription agencies.)
	☐ Check here if billing address is different from
POSTAGE & HANDLING_____	shipping address and attach purchase order and
(US: $4.00 for first book & $1.50	billing address information.
for each additional book)	
(Outside US: $5.00 for first book	Signature_____
& $2.00 for each additional book)	
SUBTOTAL_____	☐ **PAYMENT ENCLOSED: $_____**
IN CANADA: ADD 7% GST_____	☐ **PLEASE CHARGE TO MY CREDIT CARD.**
STATE TAX_____	☐ Visa ☐ MasterCard ☐ AmEx ☐ Discover
(NJ, NY, OH, MN, CA, IL, IN, PA, & SD	☐ Diner's Club ☐ Eurocard ☐ JCB
residents, add appropriate local sales tax)	Account #_____
FINAL TOTAL_____	
(If paying in Canadian funds,	Exp. Date_____
convert using the current	
exchange rate, UNESCO	Signature_____
coupons welcome)	

Prices in US dollars and subject to change without notice.

NAME_____

INSTITUTION_____

ADDRESS_____

CITY_____

STATE/ZIP_____

COUNTRY_____ COUNTY (NY residents only)_____

TEL_____ FAX_____

E-MAIL_____

May we use your e-mail address for confirmations and other types of information? ☐ Yes ☐ No
We appreciate receiving your e-mail address and fax number. Haworth would like to e-mail or fax special
discount offers to you, as a preferred customer. **We will never share, rent, or exchange your e-mail address
or fax number.** We regard such actions as an invasion of your privacy.

Order From Your Local Bookstore or Directly From
The Haworth Press, Inc.
10 Alice Street, Binghamton, New York 13904-1580 • USA
TELEPHONE: 1-800-HAWORTH (1-800-429-6784) / Outside US/Canada: (607) 722-5857
FAX: 1-800-895-0582 / Outside US/Canada: (607) 771-0012
E-mail to: orders@haworthpress.com

For orders outside US and Canada, you may wish to order through your local
sales representative, distributor, or bookseller.
For information, see http://haworthpress.com/distributors

(Discounts are available for individual orders in US and Canada only, not booksellers/distributors.)

PLEASE PHOTOCOPY THIS FORM FOR YOUR PERSONAL USE.
http://www.HaworthPress.com   BOF06

PGIL2020USA